Dysphagia

Dysphagia: Diagnosis and Management

Third Edition

Michael E. Groher, Ph.D.
Chief of Audiology, Speech Pathology Service, James A. Haley Veterans Administration Hospital, Tampa, Florida

Butterworth–Heinemann

Boston Oxford Johannesburg Melbourne New Delhi Singapore

Every effort has been made to ensure that the drug dosage schedules within this text are accurate and conform to standards accepted at time of publication. However, as treatment recommendations vary in the light of continuing research and clinical experience, the reader is advised to verify drug dosage schedules herein with information found on product information sheets. This is especially true in cases of new or infrequently used drugs.

Recognizing the importance of preserving what has been written, Butterworth–Heinemann prints its books on acid-free paper whenever possible.

Library of Congress Cataloging-in-Publication Data
Dysphagia : diagnosis and management / [edited by] Michael E. Groher.
— 3rd ed.
p. cm.
Includes bibliographical references and index.
ISBN 0-7506-9730-X
1. Deglutition disorders. I. Groher, Michael E.
[DNLM: 1. Deglutition Disorders—diagnosis. 2. Deglutition Disorders—therapy. WI 250 D998 1997]
RC815.2.D87 1997
616.3'1—dc21
DNLM/DLC
for Library of Congress 96-47477
CIP

British Library Cataloguing-in-Publication Data
A catalogue record for this book is available from the British Library.

The publisher offers special discounts on bulk orders of this book.

For information, please contact:
Manager of Special Sales
Butterworth–Heinemann
313 Washington Street
Newton, MA 02158–1626
Tel: 617-928-2500
Fax: 617-928-2620

For information on all B–H medical publications available, contact our World Wide Web home page at: http://www.bh.com/med

10 9 8 7 6 5 4 3 2 1

Printed in the United States of America

Contents

Contributing Authors

Wendy Avery-Smith, M.S., O.T.R.
Occupational Therapist, Optimum Rehabilitation, Boston; Professional Associate, Department of Rehabilitation Medicine, The New York Hospital, New York

Norman H. Bass, M.D.
Professor of Neurology and Pediatrics, Boston University School of Medicine and Boston University Medical Center, Boston

James F. Bosma, M.D.
Research Professor, Department of Pediatrics, University of Maryland School of Medicine, Baltimore

David W. Buchholz, M.D.
Associate Professor of Neurology, The Johns Hopkins University School of Medicine, Baltimore; Director, Neurological Consultation Center, The Johns Hopkins Medical Institutions, Baltimore

Jean E. Curran, M.S., R.D., C.D.N.
Dietitian and Geriatric Neuro-Dysphagia Specialist, Nutrition and Food Service, Veterans Affairs Medical Center, Bronx, New York

Olle Ekberg, M.D., Ph.D.
Professor and Head of Gastrointestinal Section, Department of Radiology, University Hospital, Malmö, Sweden

Susan M. Fleming, Ph.D.
Lecturer in Audiology and Speech-Language Pathology and Adjunct Assistant Professor of Medicine and Surgery, Wayne State University School of Medicine, Detroit; Adjunct Assistant Professor of Audiology and Speech Sciences, Michigan State University College of Human Medicine, East Lansing; Consultant, Lakeshore Communication Disorders Center, St. Clair Shores, Michigan

Barbara A. Griggs, R.N., M.A.
CORTAK MedSystems, Wheeling, Illinois

Michael E. Groher, Ph.D.
Chief of Audiology, Speech Pathology Service, James A. Haley Veterans Administration Hospital, Tampa, Florida

Gregory Hulka
Assistant Professor of Otolaryngology, Duke University Medical Center, Durham, North Carolina

Robert M. Miller, Ph.D.
Clinical Associate Professor of Speech and Hearing Sciences, Rehabilitation Medicine and Otolaryngology, University of Washington, Seattle; Chief, Audiology and Speech Pathology Service, Veterans Administration Puget Sound Health Care System, Seattle and Tacoma

Harold C. Pillsbury III, M.D.
Thomas J. Dark Distinguished Professor and Chief, Division of Otolaryngology/Head and Neck Surgery, University of North Carolina at Chapel Hill School of Medicine; Attending Physician and Surgeon, University of North Carolina Hospitals, Chapel Hill

William J. Ravich, M.D.
Associate Professor of Gastroenterology and Clinical Director, The Johns Hopkins Swallowing Center, Department of Medicine, Division of Gastroenterology, Johns Hopkins University School of Medicine, Baltimore; Active Attending Physician, The Johns Hopkins Hospital, Baltimore

Jonathan R. Workman
Senior Resident in Otolaryngology, Division of Otolaryngology/Head and Neck Surgery, University of North Carolina at Chapel Hill School of Medicine, Chapel Hill

Preface

Health care providers agree that good nutrition is a prerequisite for maintaining and improving health and that receiving this nutrition orally is most expedient and psychologically pleasurable. It is surprising, then, that only in the past decade have we begun in earnest to systematically evaluate and treat patients with swallowing disorders in an effort to provide quality nutritional care. Documentation of these efforts resulted in the first edition of *Dysphagia: Diagnosis and Management*. Since its publication, dysphagia diagnosis and management has become a recognized subspecialty of care, both in the United States and abroad. Dysphagia team formation in the Department of Veterans Affairs has increased from 59 in 1988 to over 100 in 1995. In Japan, the Japanese Society of Dysphagia Rehabilitation holds annual meetings of representatives from diverse disciplines. In southern Sweden, a multidisciplinary study group devoted to a better understanding of how to manage the dysphagic patient meets monthly. In the United States, the Dysphagia Research Society holds annual meetings. This third edition provides the clinician with an update and review of the explosion of information that has improved the management of patients with dysphagia in the past decade.

Before the early 1970s, patients incapable of swallowing were managed by feeding gastrostomy or by nasogastric tube feedings. Return to oral feeding was a primary goal, but attempts to move in this direction were half-hearted, partly from ignorance, partly from lack of time. To complicate matters, no one person had direct responsibility for monitoring patients' feeding and swallowing.

Health care professionals have discovered that active intervention with dysphagic patients, including carefully planned diagnostic evaluations and subsequent management and rehabilitative techniques, often assists a patient's return to normal feeding and swallowing, a result that speeds recovery and enhances the quality of life. Demonstrations of this improvement in care are now documented in the literature.

It is apparent to me that our efforts to provide this care require the close cooperation of a professional, multidisciplinary staff, wherein each member possesses particular expertise. It is the combined expertise that links diagnosis and treatment. A diagnosis is established through cooperation between the physician, with primary care responsibility and consultants in neurology, radiology, gastroenterology, surgery, and psychiatry. Further evaluation by the nurse and speech-language pathologist is critical to measure the level of function and to follow the rate of improvement during treatment sessions. The dietitian and therapist must join forces to ensure adherence to dietary requirements and appropriateness of food formula and consistency. The speech-language pathologist, physical therapist, and occupational therapist must design and implement a program of rehabilitation tailored to each individual, always in cooperation with the nursing staff, who are responsible for daily management of the patient.

Because dysphagia management involves multiple disciplines, our basic core of knowledge is dispersed among many different journals, making it difficult for the beginning clinician to read about and understand the current state of the art. Since the publication of the first edition of this volume, the emergence of the journal *Dysphagia* has helped to provide both multidisciplinary and international contributions, bridging the gap that previously existed among disciplines concerned with the dysphagic patient. This third edition is an extension of the development of the subspeciality of dysphagia, combining each discipline's perspective toward a common goal and allowing an understanding of how each affects the care of dysphagic patients.

We know that disorders of the swallowing mechanism can result from a broad spectrum of disabilities and that each stage of swallow has potential interactions with another, as facilitators in the normal process and as contributors to disability. These disorders range from minimal difficulty swallowing foods and liquids to inability to swallow without a high risk of aspiration in a patient who may require gastrostoma or a feeding tube for nutritional maintenance. At one extreme the disability is severe, the cause usually clear, and the therapy urgent. At the other are patients with mild-to-moderate dysphagia, no clear diagnosis, but a significant disability that may become life-threatening. This book is written with both groups of patients in mind.

While the focus is the adult population, a chapter on pediatric issues has been included in an effort to detail disorders specific to the first years of life. Those working with this population also will benefit from the chapters on diagnosis, evaluation, and program development. Some discussions of management and rehabilitative techniques will not directly apply to newborns and infants, but certain conceptual frameworks will—for example, the importance of a thorough physical and laboratory evaluation, and the use of diet modifications to circumvent disability.

Throughout the text, the distinction between neurologic and mechanical disorders of the swallowing mechanism is maintained. This is done for several reasons. Diagnostically, the two categories often are mutually exclusive, and attempts to classify the more subtle disorders should be made with this separation in mind. The distinction is also valid in therapy, since some of the techniques and the level of patient cooperation may differ between those with mechanical disorders and those with neurologic mechanisms of impairment. From the outset, the careful clinician must have the differential diagnosis of dysphagia clearly in mind and must not stop after the first few common disorders have been ruled out. To leave the patient with no diagnosis or to conclude that the origin is psychiatric when persistent investigation would uncover a treatable cause is the pitfall that we hope this resource will help clinicians avoid.

It is my firm conviction that resorting immediately to tube or gastrostomy feedings in patients with dysphagia is a mistake, particularly if the condition has not been adequately diagnosed and other therapeutic measures have not been tried. The limitations and the compromise of quality of life to the patient are unacceptable.

Not all patients will respond to our rehabilitative efforts; however, improved management of their swallowing dysfunction short of total rehabilitation should not be underestimated. The importance of delivering adequate nutrition to hospitalized patients, particularly those who cannot receive nourishment by mouth, should be clear to all who invest their time with this patient group. More rapid wound healing, a briefer hospital stay, less morbidity and mortality, and an improved psychological outlook for the patient are important dividends.

Techniques used in establishing a clear diagnosis followed by the development of creative and realistic treatment protocols require in-depth didactic preparation and clinical exposure. They require a well-trained staff for implementation, cooperation on the part of the patient and family, considerable time and patience, and, most important, a team approach.

Michael E. Groher

1

Nature of the Problem

Michael E. Groher

DEFINITION

Dysphagia is characterized by abnormality in the transfer of a bolus from the mouth to the stomach. Abnormalities may involve the oral, pharyngeal, or esophageal stage of the swallowing sequence. Impairment ranges from delay in transfer to absence of transfer and includes misdirections of transference, as in airway penetration. A more functional definition is that dysphagia is a condition resulting from an interruption in either eating pleasure or the maintenance of nutrition and hydration (Buchholz 1996).

DYSPHAGIA AS A SYMPTOM

Dysphagia is commonly a symptom of underlying disease, usually disease of neurogenic or mechanical (obstructive) origin. It may be secondary to psychiatric disease (Bazemore et al. 1991) or to iatrogenic factors such as tracheostomy or medications (Kikendall et al. 1983; Stoschus and Allescher 1993; Buchholz 1994). Dysphagic symptoms may be occult or overt. Occult dysphagia might be defined as an unrecognized problem in which the patient offers no complaint, or a problem that patients compensate well for. For instance, Hagen (1963) found that 20–30% of those who suffered café coronary did not complain of previous swallowing difficulty. Ekberg and Feinberg (1991) found a significant number of radiographic swallowing abnormalities in a group of 56 healthy elderly patients, none of whom complained of dysphagia. Similar results (i.e., dysphagia without complaint) in a group of patients aged 87 or older were reported from a community in the Netherlands (Bloem et al. 1990). Overt dysphagic symptoms include difficulty in chewing or bolus preparation, excessive drooling, choking or regurgitation, food sticking at any level of the alimentary tract, and painful swallow. These overt symptoms are most significant when associated with aspiration pneumonia, weight loss, compromised nutritional status, or any combination of these.

PREVALENCE AND INCIDENCE

Groher and Bukatman (1986) studied the prevalence of dysphagia in patients at two large teaching centers. They collected their data from the medical records and nursing reports. At the time of the study, nearly one-third of those hospitalized were dysphagic, either from disorders of suspected oropharyngeal or esophageal origin, or because their illness precluded oral alimentation. The largest percentage of patients with dysphagia were in intensive care units. Reporting on 937 patients admitted to the Rehabilitation Institute of Chicago, Cherney (1994) found a 32% incidence of dysphagia. Most of these were secondary to bilateral strokes.

DYSPHAGIA AND STROKE

In 452 consecutive patients admitted for stroke who could cooperate with formalized testing, 45% evidenced some swallowing abnormality (Wade and Hewer 1987). Of these patients, 14% had choking episodes, 6% had abnormal swallowing patterns, and 23% had swallow delay. In a series of 38 post-stroke patients, swallowing disorders were present in one-third of the group (Veis and Logemann 1985). The most common radiographic finding in this group was delay in swallow initiation. Of the 70 post-stroke patients with bilateral disease who were referred for suspected dysphagia and videofluoroscopic studies, 49% aspirated (Horner et al. 1990). Those that aspirated were more likely to have had strokes involving the posterior circulatory system with physical findings of abnormal cough, gag, and dysphonia. In 91 consecutive admissions for acute stroke, Gordon and colleagues (1987) reported that 45% were dysphagic, and that after 14 days, 90% of this group did not show dysphagia when tested by their response to drinking water. The majority of these patients evidenced single, hemispheric brain lesions.

LESION SITE

Because of the bilateral innervation of the volitional muscles of deglutition, traditional wisdom dictates that oropharyngeal dysphagia only results from brain lesions that are bilateral. However, there are numerous studies that demonstrate that unilateral stroke may precipitate dysphagic symptomatology. Further interest in this issue is warranted, because studying the effects of unilateral brain lesions on swallow may provide insight into the neurologic organization of the swallow response. In a study that took special care to document lesion site, Robbins and Levine (1988) found differences in the swallow response between dysphagic patients with right hemisphere brain lesions and those with left hemisphere brain lesions. In three of the eight patients with right hemisphere involvement, aspiration was apparent, but it was not a finding in any of those with left hemisphere impairment. Patients with right hemisphere lesions had more impairment in pharyngeal function; those with left hemisphere lesions had more oral stage involvement. In contrast to these findings, Chen and associates (1990) did not find any differences between dysphagic patients with right and left brain lesions in videoradiographic swallowing studies. Teasell and colleagues (1994) found that of the 54 post-stroke patients who aspirated on videoradiographic studies, 9.9% had right unilateral lesions, 24% had bilateral lesions, and 40% had lesions in the brain stem. A high incidence of silent aspiration is associated with brain stem lesions (Linden and Siebens 1983) and lesions involving the cortex and brain stem (Horner et al. 1988). The majority of studies that tested the relationship between rehabilitation and medical outcomes in those with and without dysphagia following stroke have found that those with dysphagia had increased mortality and morbidity, and rehabilitation was delayed because of their dysphagia (Gordon et al. 1987; Barer 1989; Young and Durant-Jones 1990).

Dysphagia and Traumatic Brain Injury

The incidence of acute dysphagic complications in a large series of patients following traumatic brain injury has not been reported. One would expect that the incidence of dysphagia would be high in severe injury, secondary to the primary neurologic complications of the injury and frequent need for placement of tracheostomy tubes with ventilator support. Prevalence data exist for patients who survive their injury and proceed to rehabilitation. In general, one can expect that almost one-third of those with head injury who are entering rehabilitation will have oropharyngeal dysphagia (Winstein 1983; Lazarus and Logemann 1987; Field and Weiss 1989). Winstein found that of patients with dysphagia at admission, 94% were feeding orally at 5 months post-injury following treatment (Winstein 1983).

Dysphagia and Parkinson's Disease

Dysphagia in those with Parkinson's disease appears to be common, although precise estimates of incidence are restricted by definitions of disease stage, mental status, and methods of dysphagia documentation. Prevalence of dysphagia, usually characterized by involvement of both oral and pharyngeal swallow stages, has been reported to be over 50% (Lieberman et al. 1980) and is often associated with aspiration pneumonia (Bine et al. 1995). In those with suspected swallowing disorders, 95% will evidence abnormality on videoradiographic studies (Robbins et al. 1986).

DYSPHAGIA AND AGING

The higher incidence of dysphagia in older populations is due in part to changes in the swallow mechanism secondary to the aging process and to the increased incidence of disease such as stroke and other neurologic sequelae in individuals over 65. In the elderly without dysphagia who are in good health, the changes in swallow physiology associated with aging rarely precipitate dysphagic symptoms (Sonies et al. 1984; Borgstrom and Ekberg 1988; Robbins et al. 1992).

In a survey of 556 men and women aged 50–79, Lindgren and Janzon (1991) found that 35% complained of dysphagia, which was usually associated with complaints of the globus sensation and gastroesophageal reflux. Reports of elderly patients hospitalized with chronic disease reveal a high incidence of dysphagia. In a 240-bed nursing home, Siebens et al. (1986) found that 59% of the residents were unable to feed or swallow normally. Dysphagia was found most often in patients who were unable to feed themselves. Using a detailed index for dysphagia detection in a 668-bed neuropsychiatric facility, Layne and coworkers (1989) found a 66% incidence of dysphagia.

CONCLUSION

Dysphagia is a symptom of underlying disease that is most prevalent in elderly patients with neurologic disease and commonly the result of medical complications related to that disease. Dysphagic symptoms may be occult or obvious. Patients may not have swallowing complaints, yet laboratory studies reveal abnormalities. Other patients may have complaints that diagnostic testing is unable to explain. The incidence of dysphagia with its attendant morbidity and mortality in hospitals and long-term care centers is sufficiently high to warrant medical attention.

REFERENCES

Barer DH. The natural history and functional consequences of dysphagia after hemisphere stroke. J Neurol Neurosurg Psychiatry 1989;52:236.

Bazemore PH, Tonkonogy J, Ananth R. Dysphagia in psychiatric patients: clinical and fluoroscopy study. Dysphagia 1991;6:2.

Bine JE, Frank EM, McDade HL. Dysphagia and dementia in subjects with Parkinson's disease. Dysphagia 1995;10:160.

Bloem BR, Lagaay AM, vanBeck W, et al. Prevalence of subjective dysphagia in community residents aged over 87. Br Med J 1990;300:721.

Borgstrom PS, Ekberg O. Speed of peristalsis in pharyngeal constrictor musculature: correlation to age. Dysphagia 1988;2:140.

Buchholz DW. Neurogenic dysphagia: what is the cause when the cause is not obvious? Dysphagia 1994;9:245.

Buchholz D. Editorial: what is dysphagia? Dysphagia 1996;11:23.

Chen MYN, Ott DJ, Peele VN, Gelfand DW. Oropharynx in patients with cerebrovascular disease: evaluation with videofluoroscopy. Radiology 1990;176:641.

Cherney LR. Dysphagia in Adults with Neurologic Disorders: An Overview. In LR Cherney (ed), Clinical Management of Dysphagia in Adults and Children. Gaithersburg, MD: Aspen, 1994.

Ekberg O, Feinberg M. Altered swallowing function in elderly patients without dysphagia: radiologic findings in 56 cases. AJR Am J Roentgenol 1991;156:1181.

Field LH, Weiss CJ. Dysphagia with head injury. Brain Inj 1989;3:19.

Gordon C, Hewer RL, Wade DT. Dysphagia in acute stroke. Br Med J 1987;295:411.

Groher M, Bukatman R. Prevalence of dysphagia in two teaching hospitals. Dysphagia 1986;1:3.

Hagen RK. The café coronary: sudden deaths in restaurants. JAMA 1963;186:142.

Horner J, Massey EW, Brazier SR. Aspiration in bilateral stroke patients. Neurology 1990;40:1686.

Horner J, Massey EW, Riski JE, et al. Aspiration following stroke: clinical correlates and outcome. Neurology 1988;38:1359.

Kikendall JW, Friedman AC, Oyewole MA, Fleisher D, Johnson LS. Pill-induced esophageal injury: case reports and review of the medical literature. Dig Dis 1983;28:174.

Layne KA, Losinski DS, Zenner PM, Ament JA. Using the Fleming Index of Dysphagia to establish prevalence. Dysphagia 1989;4:39.

Lazarus C, Logemann, JA. Swallowing disorders in closed head trauma patients. Arch Phys Med Rehabil 1987;68:79.

Lieberman AN, Horowitz L, Redmond P, et al. Dysphagia in Parkinson's disease. Ann Neurol 1980;74:157.

Linden P, Siebens AA. Dysphagia: predicting laryngeal penetration. Arch Phys Med Rehabil 1983;64:281.

Lingren S, Janzon L. Prevalence of swallowing complaints and clinical findings among 50–79 year old men and women in an urban population. Dysphagia 1991;6:187.

Robbins JA, Hamilton J, Lof G, Kemster G. Oropharyngeal swallowing in normal adults of different ages. Gastroenterology 1992;103:823.

Robbins JA, Levine RL. Swallowing after unilateral stroke of the cerebral cortex: preliminary experience. Dysphagia 1988;3:11.

Robbins JA, Logemann JA, Kirshner HS. Swallowing and speech production in Parkinson's disease. Ann Neurol 1986;19:283.

Siebens H, Trupe E, Siebens AA, et. al. Correlates and consequences of eating dependency in institutionalized elderly. J Am Geriatr Soc 1986;34:192.

Sonies BC, Stone M, Shawker T. Speech and swallowing in the elderly. Gerontology 1984;3:115.

Stoschus B, Allescher HD. Drug-induced dysphagia. Dysphagia 1993;8:154.

Teasell RW, Bach D, McRae M. Prevalence and recovery of aspiration post-stroke: a retrospective analysis. Dysphagia 1994;9:35.

Veis SL, Logemann JA. Swallowing disorders in persons with cerebrovascular accident. Arch Phys Med Rehabil 1985;66:372.

Wade DT, Hewer RL. Motor loss and swallowing difficulty after stroke: frequency, recovery, and prognosis. Acta Neurol Scand 1987;76:50.

Winstein CJ. Neurogenic dysphagia: frequency, progression, and outcome in adults following head injury. Phys Ther 1983;63:1992.

Young EC, Durant-Jones L. Developing a dysphagia program in an acute care hospital: a needs assessment. Dysphagia 1990;5:159.

2

The Neurology of Swallowing

Norman H. Bass

Normal swallowing includes an integrated interdependent group of complex feeding behaviors emerging from interacting cranial nerves of the brain stem and governed by neural regulatory mechanisms in the medulla, as well as in sensorimotor and limbic cortical systems. Such sensory-guided discriminatory feeding and sensory-cued, stereotyped swallowing behaviors may be, for purposes of simplification, divided into three stages: (1) the oral stage is the transfer of material from the mouth to the oropharynx; (2) the pharyngeal stage is the highly coordinated transport of material away from the oropharynx, around an occluded laryngeal vestibule, and through a relaxed cricopharyngeus muscle into the upper esophagus; and (3) the esophageal stage is the transport of material along the esophagus into the gastric cardia (Figure 2.1). It is important to remember that the anatomic arrangement mediating the pharyngeal stage of swallowing involves complex behavioral interactions of the hypopharynx and larynx, where neurologic dysfunction can result in life-threatening aspiration (Ardran and Kemp 1951, 1952). Hence, the anatomic and physiologic aspects of this interdependent group of voluntary and involuntary behaviors requires detailed understanding if we are to rehabilitate persons with dysphagia caused by a wide array of neurologic impairments that result from injury or disease affecting the central nervous system, cranial nerves, and muscles.

The oral cavity extends from the lips anteriorly to the nasopharynx posteriorly and contains the tongue, gums, and teeth (Figure 2.2). The oral cavity is separated from the nasal cavity by the bony palate and muscular palate. It is composed of a highly mobile lower jaw, or mandible, consisting of a U-shaped body containing important ridges for muscle attachments. The upper jaw, or maxilla, meets the zygomatic or cheek bone and is adjoined by the L-shaped palatine bones, lying posterior to the nasal cavity. The perpendicular part of the palatines forms the back of the nasal cavity, whereas the horizontal part forms the back of the bony palate. The muscular palate and posterior nasopharyngeal wall work to seal and open communication between the nasal and oral cavities during swallowing and respiratory behaviors, respectively. The nasopharynx lies above the muscular palate, and the oropharynx lies posterior to the mouth. The pharynx extends below to the esophagus; its inferior portion is called the hypopharynx and is separated from the esophagus by the cricopharyngeal muscle. The cartilaginous larynx lies anterior to the hypopharynx at the upper end of the trachea, suspended by muscles attached to the hyoid bone (Hamilton and

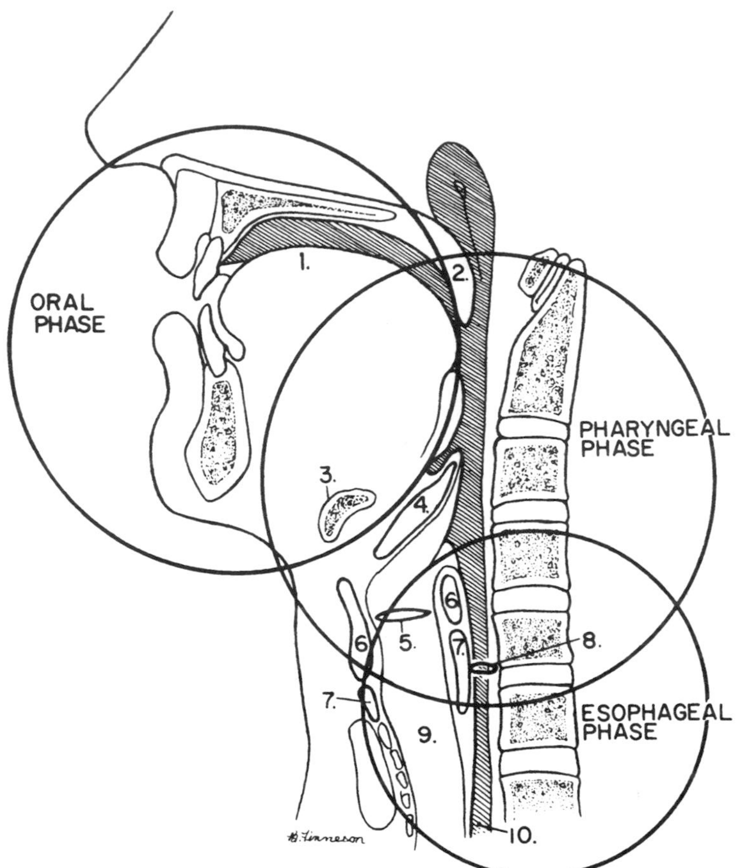

Figure 2.1 The normal swallow involves three separate stages that are interdependent and highly coordinated: (1) tongue, (2) soft palate, (3) hyoid bone, (4) epiglottis, (5) vocal folds, (6) thyroid cartilage, (7) cricoid cartilage, (8) pharyngoesophageal sphincter, (9) trachea, and (10) esophagus. (Reprinted with permission from A Schultz, P Niemtzow, S Jacobs, F Naso. Dysphagia associated with cricopharyngeal dysfunction. Arch Phys Med Rehabil 1979;60:381.)

Harrison 1971). The cricoid cartilage lies above the trachea, with the thyroid cartilage above it. Both are suspended from muscles attached to the hyoid bone, which in itself is suspended between the jaw, tongue, and sternum by suprahyoid and infrahyoid musculature.

The respiratory system is protected during pharyngeal swallow by occlusive muscular constriction of the vestibule and downward displacement of the epiglottis. The true vocal cords are at the inferior margin of the laryngeal ventricle and are attached anteriorly at the thyroid cartilage and posteriorly at the ary-

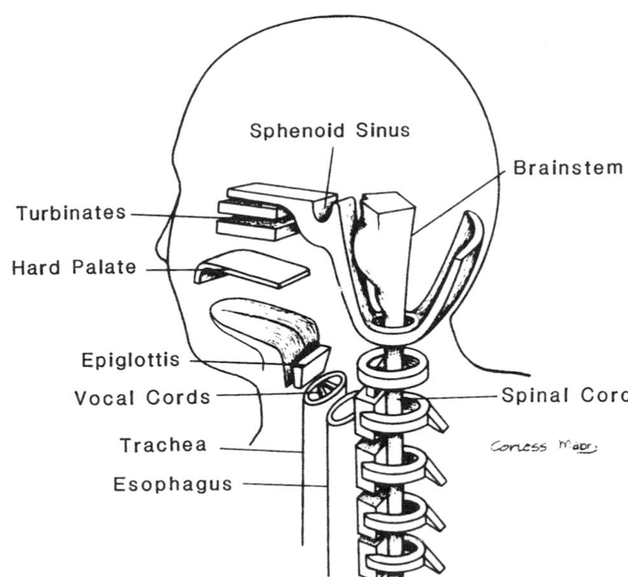

Figure 2.2 Relationship between bony and muscular structures associated with normal swallowing.

tenoid cartilages. The false vocal folds separate the ventricle and the vestibule. The epiglottis extends from the base of the tongue into the pharyngeal cavity.

The valleculae are lateral recesses at the base of the tongue on each side of the epiglottis (Figure 2.3). The piriform sinuses are lateral recesses between the larynx and the anterior hypopharyngeal wall. These recesses serve as important anatomic landmarks in videoradiographic assessment of pharyngeal swallow.

MUSCULOSKELETAL ACTIONS

Oral Stage

The mandibular branch of the trigeminal nerve (cranial nerve V) innervates the principal muscles for chewing behaviors. The primary muscles of chewing are the masseter, temporalis, and pterygoid muscles, which attach to the sphenoid wing of the temporal bone (Table 2.1). The masseter closes the jaw while the temporalis moves it up, forward, or backward. The medial pterygoid muscles work bilaterally to elevate the mandible while they shift the jaw to the opposite side unilaterally. The lateral pterygoid muscles work together, pulling down or forward while moving the jaw or chin to the opposite side unilaterally. Both sets of pterygoid muscles cooperate to grind in mastication.

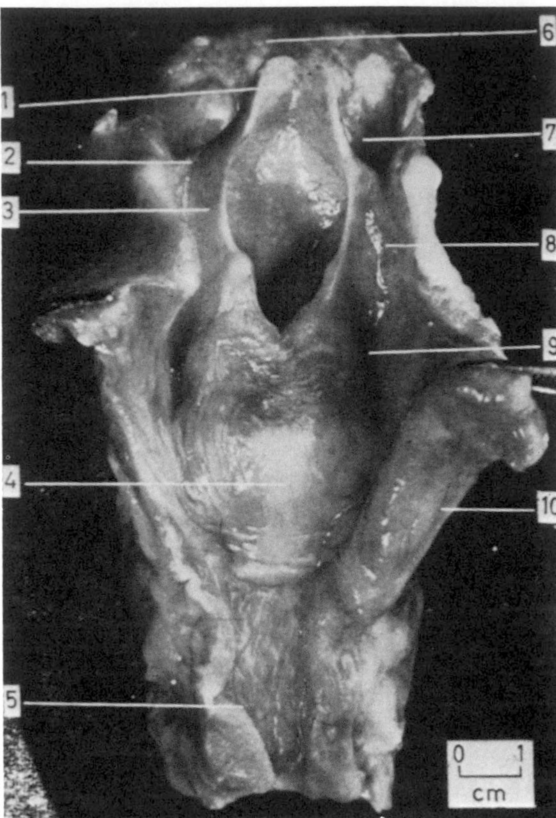

Figure 2.3 The vallecular (7) and piriform spaces (8, 9) are potential sites for abnormal retention of food and liquid. Note their relationship to other laryngeal structures: (1) epiglottis; (2) pharyngoepiglottic fold; (3) aryepiglottic fold; (4) postcricoid region; (5) cervical esophagus; (6) base of tongue; and (10) posterolateral pharyngeal wall. (Reprinted with permission from J Ballantyne, J Groves (eds). Disease of the Ear, Nose, and Throat. London: Butterworth, 1971.)

The facial nerve (cranial nerve VII) innervates lower facial muscles attached to the maxillae and mandible of the skull (Table 2.2). These include the buccinator muscles, which compress the lips and flatten the cheeks in the movement of food across the teeth. The buccinator fibers blend with those of the orbicularis oris—the sphincter of the lips.

The hypoglossal nerve (cranial nerve XII) innervates the tongue, which contains four separate intrinsic muscle masses that have different effects on the shape, contour, and function of the tongue.

Pharyngeal Stage

The pharyngeal cavity of the neck, which is suspended from the base of the skull and anchored to the top of the sternum, is formed by 26 pairs of striated muscles innervated by six cranial and four cervical nerves. The horseshoe-shaped hyoid bone in the neck serves as a fulcrum that provides a mechanical advantage for pharyngeal musculature associated with swallowing behaviors of the posterior tongue, pharynx, and larynx.

Table 2.1 Muscles of Mastication

Muscle	*Origin*	*Insertion*	*Nerve*	*Action*
Temporalis	Temporal fossa of skull	Ramus and coronoid process of mandible	Trigeminal	Elevates or closes mandible; retracts mandible
Masseter	Zygomatic arch	Ramus of mandible	Trigeminal	Elevates or closes mandible
Medial pterygoid	Palatine bone, lateral ptery-goid plate, tuberosity of maxilla	Ramus of mandible	Trigeminal	Elevates or closes mandible
Lateral pterygoid	Great wing of sphenoid and lateral ptery-goid plate	Neck of con-dyle of mandible	Trigeminal	Depressor or opener of mandible; pro-trudes mandible; permits side-to-side movement of mandible

In the nasopharynx, five muscles adjust the position of the muscular palate with respect to the food bolus (Table 2.3): the palatoglossal and levator veli palatini muscles (pharyngeal plexus and accessory nerve), which elevate the soft palate and seal the nasopharynx; the tensor veli palatini (mandibular branch of the trigeminal nerve), which tenses the palate and dilates the orifice of the eustachian tube; the palatopharyngeal muscle (pharyngeal plexus and spinal accessory nerve), which depresses the soft palate, approximates the palate or pharyngeal folds, and constricts the pharynx; and the muscularis uvula (spinal accessory nerve), which shortens the soft palate.

The hypoglossal (cranial nerve XII), trigeminal (V), and facial (VII) nerves innervate the suprahyoid group of muscles (Table 2.4). The hypoglossal nerve supplies the geniohyoid, which draws the hyoid bone up and forward, depressing the jaw, and the trigeminal nerve supplies the mylohyoid, which elevates the hyoid bone and tongue and depresses the jaw. The digastric muscles contain anterior and posterior bellies. The anterior belly is innervated by the mandibular branch of the trigeminal nerve and depresses the jaw or raises the hyoid, whereas the posterior portion is innervated by the facial nerve (VII) and elevates or retracts the hyoid. The facial nerve (VII) innervates the stylohyoid muscle, which elevates the hyoid bone during swallowing. In addition, the hyoglossus and the genioglossus serve as laryngeal elevators, as well as extrinsic tongue muscles, and are designed to depress the tongue or help to elevate the hyoid bone when the tongue is fixed. The accessory nerve (cranial nerve XI), in association with the

Table 2.2 Muscles of the Face

Muscle	*Origin*	*Insertion*	*Nerve*	*Action*
Orbicularis oris	Neighboring muscles, mostly buccinator; has many layers of tissue around the lips	Skin around lips and angles of the mouth	Facial	Closes, opens, protrudes, inverts, and twists lips
Zygomaticus minor	Zygomatic bone	Orbicularis oris in upper lip	Facial	Draws upper lip upward and outward
Levator labii superioris	Below infraorbital foramen in maxilla	Orbicularis oris in upper lip	Facial	Pulls up or elevates upper lip
Levator labii superioris alaeque nasi	Process of maxilla	Skin at mouth angle, orbicularis oris	Facial	Raises angle of the mouth
Zygomaticus major	Zygomatic bone	Fibers of the orbicularis oris, angle of the mouth	Facial	Draws upper lip upward; draws angle of mouth upward and backward; the smiling muscle
Levator anguli oris (caninus)	Canine fossa of maxilla	Lower lip near angle of the mouth	Facial	Pulls down corners of mouth
Depressor anguli oris	Outer surface and above lower border of mandible	Skin of cheek, corner of mouth, lower border of mandible	Facial	Draws lower lip down; draws angle of mouth down and inward
Depressor labii inferioris	Lower border of the mandible	Skin of lower lip, orbicularis oris	Facial	Depresses lower lip
Mentalis	Incisor fossa of mandible	Skin of chin	Facial	Pushes up lower lip; raises chin
Risorius	Platysma, fascia over the masseter skin	Angle of mouth, orbicularis oris	Facial	Draws corners or angle of mouth outward; causes dimples; gives expression of strain to face
Buccinator	Alveolar process of maxilla, buccinator ridge of mandible	Angle of mouth, orbicularis oris	Facial	Flattens cheek; holds food in contact with teeth; retracts angles of the mouth

Table 2.3 Muscles of the Palate

Muscle	*Origin*	*Insertion*	*Nerve*	*Action*
Levator veli palatini	Apex of temporal bone	Palatine aponeurosis of soft palate	Vagus and accessory	Raises soft palate
Tensor veli palatini	Fossa of sphenoid bone	Palatine aponeurosis of soft palate	Trigeminal	Stretches soft palate
Palatoglossus	Undersurface of soft palate	Side of tongue	Vagus and accessory	Raises back of tongue during the first stage of swallowing
Palatopharyngeus	Soft palate	Pharyngeal wall	Vagus and accessory	Shuts off nasopharynx during second stage of swallowing
Uvular	Posterior nasal spine and palatine aponeurosis	Into uvula to form its chief bulk or content	Vagus and accessory	Shortens and raises uvula

Table 2.4 Suprahyoid Muscles

Muscle	*Origin*	*Insertion*	*Nerve*	*Action*
Mylohyoid (anterior belly digastric)	Inner surface of mandible	Upper border of hyoid bone	Trigeminal	Elevates tongue and floor of mouth; depresses jaw when hyoid bone is in fixed position
Digastric (anterior belly)	Intermediate tendon by loop of fascia to hyoid bone	Lower border of mandible	Trigeminal	Raises hyoid bone if jaw is in fixed position; depresses jaw if hyoid bone is in fixed position
Geniohyoid	Mental spine of mandible	Hyoid bone	Cervical (C1 and C2) through hypoglossal	Draws hyoid bone forward; depresses mandible when hyoid bone is in fixed position
Stylohyoid	Stylohyoid process of temporal bone	Body of hyoid at grater cornu	Facial	Elevates hyoid and tongue base
Hyoglossus	Greater cornu of hyoid	Into tongue sides	Hypoglossal	Tongue depression
Genioglossus	Upper genial tubercle of mandible	Hyoid, inferior tongue, and tip	Hypoglossal	Protrusion and depression
Styloglossus	Anterior border of styloid process	Into side of tongue	Hypoglossal	Elevates up and back
Palatoglossus	Anterior surface of soft palate	Dorsum and side of tongue	Glossopharyngeal, vagus, and accessory	Narrows fauces and elevates posterior tongue

hypoglossal (XII) nerve, innervates the styloglossus, which draws the tongue up and back during swallowing (Sloan et al. 1964; Splaingard et al. 1988). The glossopharyngeal and accessory nerves also cause the palatoglossus to raise the back of the tongue and lower the muscular palate. The styloglossus and palatoglossus raise the back of the tongue and lower the sides of the soft palate.

The vagus nerve (cranial nerve X) and the spinal accessory nerve (XI) innervate the muscular pharynx, whose superior, middle, and inferior constrictor muscles constitute its external circular layer and work together to strip a bolus of food toward the esophagus during swallowing. Three other muscles constitute the internal longitudinal layer of the pharynx: the palatopharyngeus, stylopharyngeus, and salpingopharyngeus. The stylopharyngeus (glossopharyngeal nerve) elevates the pharynx and to some extent the larynx during swallowing, while the salpingopharyngeus (accessory nerve and pharyngeal plexus) draws the lateral walls of the pharynx up (Table 2.5). The palatopharyngeus draws the muscular palate down.

The cricopharyngeal muscle is an important single muscle that lies at the transition level between the pharynx and the esophagus. Functionally, it is separate from both the pharynx and the esophagus and acts as a sphincter, relaxing during passage of the bolus from the pharynx into the esophagus. It has been shown to be innervated by both pharyngeal branches of the vagus and sympathetic fibers from the middle and inferior cervical ganglia.

BEHAVIORAL SEQUENCE OF NORMAL SWALLOWING

Healthy individuals simultaneously perform many acts that involve the sequential steps of chewing and swallowing and depend on highly intricate coordination. Thus, a single bolus of varying texture and size can be chewed and swallowed while the person carries on a conversation, and at the same time a beverage may be imbibed while one holds various portions of the more solid food in the mouth. With relaxation of the pharyngeal constrictors, a sword can be passed from the pharynx through the cricopharyngeal muscle, and, with effort, one can swallow solids while standing on one's head.

Food introduced into the mouth cannot be prepared for swallowing by being formed into a bolus unless it is mixed with saliva contributed from three pairs of salivary glands. The parotid gland receives parasympathetic nerve supply via the glossopharyngeal nerve from the inferior salivary nucleus, located in the lower brain stem. The submandibular and sublingual glands are innervated by parasympathetic fibers of the facial nerve. Each gland has single or multiple excretory ducts opening into the mouth.

The usual conditions associated with normal swallowing are a moist cavity, open nostrils, and a closed mouth. The steps involved are illustrated in Figure 2.4. As a bolus is masticated, the tongue tip is elevated to occlude the anterior oral cavity at the alveolar ridge, and the bolus is compressed against the hard palate. This is a preparatory position in which the posterior portion of the

Table 2.5 Muscles of the Pharynx

Muscle	*Origin*	*Insertion*	*Nerve*	*Action*
Palatopharyngeus	Extends from soft palate to pharyngeal wall	Posterior border of thyroid cartilage and pharyngeal aponeurosis	Pharyngeal plexus and accessory	Narrows oropharynx; elevates pharynx; shuts off nasopharynx
Stylopharyngeus	Medial side of root of styloid process	Superior and inferior borders of thyroid cartilage	Glossopharyngeal	Raises and dilates pharynx
Salpingopharyngeus	Pharyngeal end of auditory tube	Blends with palatopharyngeus	Pharyngeal plexus and accessory	Raises nasopharynx; draws lateral pharyngeal walls up

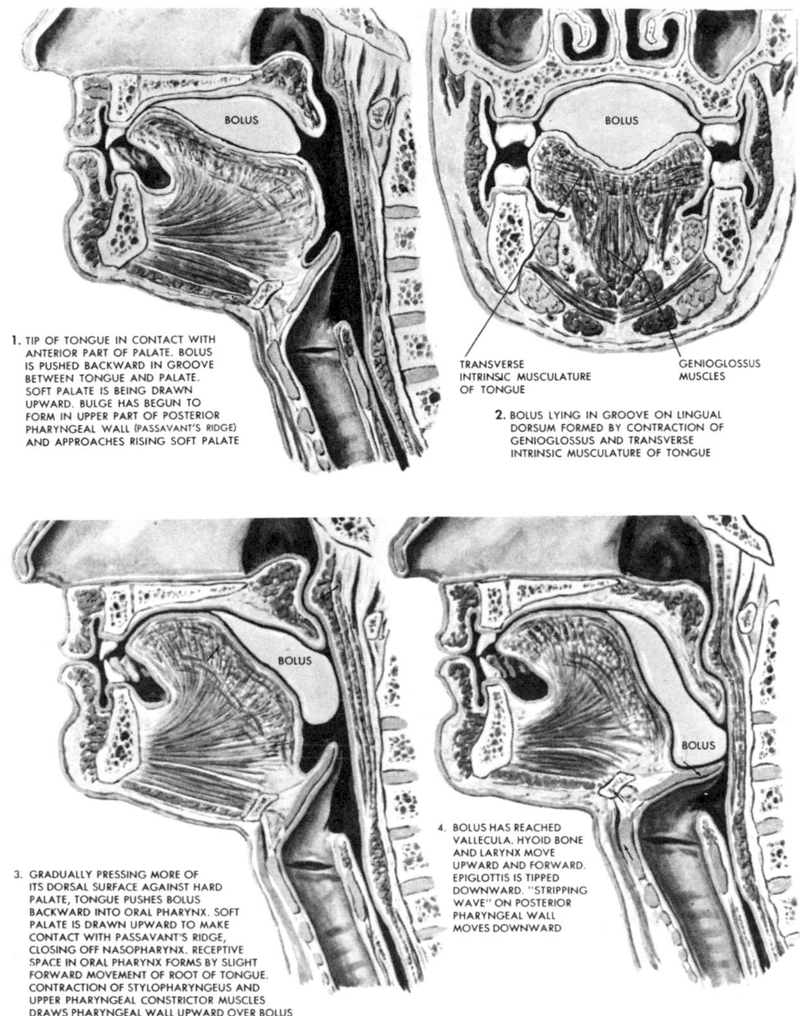

Figure 2.4 Sequential presentation of the steps involved in the normal swallow. (© Copyright 1959, CIBA Pharmaceutical Company, Division of CIBA-GEIGY Corporation. Reprinted with permission from The Ciba Collection of Medical Illustrations, illustrated by F H Netter, M.D. All rights reserved.)

tongue has maneuvered the bolus into position. As pharyngeal swallowing begins, the anterior portion of the tongue is retracted and depressed, mastication then ceases, and respiration is inhibited. Retraction of the tongue and its elevation against the hard palate force the bolus into the upper part of the pharynx. The palatopharyngeal folds are pulled medially to form a slit through which properly masticated food can pass. The levator and tensor veli palatini muscles

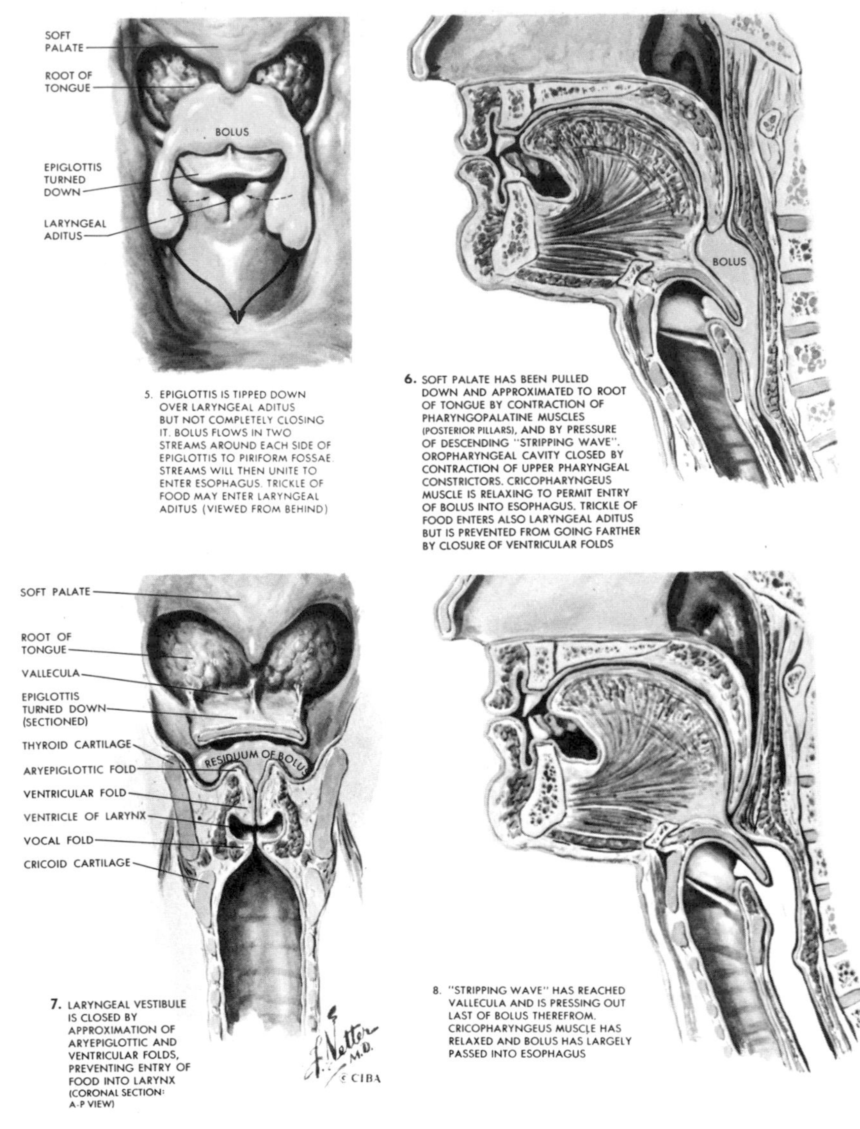

B

Figure 2.4 (*continued*)

help elevate the soft palate and block the nasopharyngeal opening. The tongue moves posteriorly to drive the bolus into the pharynx while the entire larynx is pulled upward and forward. This action causes the epiglottis at the back of the tongue to depress and protect the airway. Food is directed to either side of the epiglottis. Further airway protection is provided when respiration has ceased,

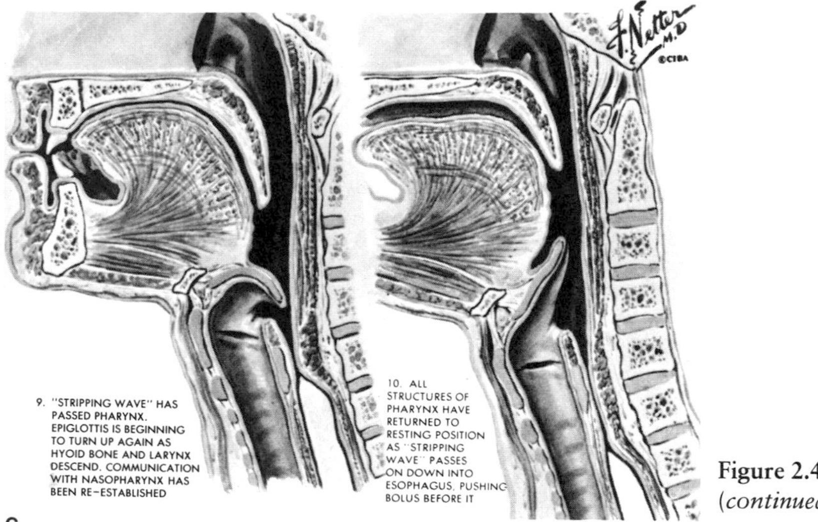

Figure 2.4 (*continued*)

allowing the apposed vocal cords to close off the trachea (Doty and Bosma 1956; Donner et al. 1985). In preparation for propulsion of food toward the esophagus, the cricopharyngeal muscle relaxes and the bolus is propelled into the esophagus. In the esophagus, the bolus is carried toward the stomach by gravity and peristalsis.

The following five sequential steps of pharyngeal swallow (Donner and Siegel 1965) are outlined in Figure 2.5:

1. Tongue movements that initiate the act of swallowing require concomitant contraction of mylohyoid, geniohyoid, and digastric muscles in the floor of the mouth.
2. The styloglossus and hyoglossus muscles force the root of the tongue against the soft palate and posterior pharyngeal wall.
3. The levator and tensor veli palatini muscles elevate the muscular palate with additional shortening and dorsal thickening until approximation against the posterior pharyngeal muscle prevents nasopharyngeal regurgitation.
4. The middle and inferior pharyngeal constrictor muscles narrow the hypopharynx and contribute to the peristaltic movements involving the posterior pharyngeal wall, which generally occur between the level of Passavant's cushion and the cricopharyngeal sphincter.
5. Dorsal and downward tilting of the epiglottis is brought about by the muscular elevation of the larynx and contraction of the floor of the mouth, with concomitant elevation and posterior movement of the hyoid bone.

The food bolus is prevented from passing through the laryngeal vestibule by the contraction of intrinsic laryngeal muscles that shorten and widen the ary-

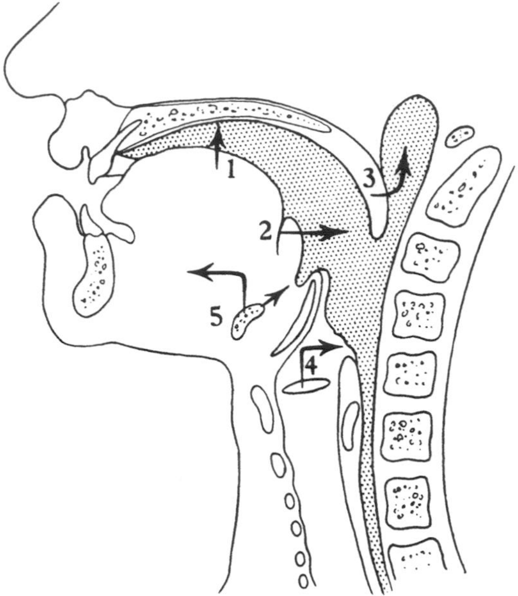

Figure 2.5 Summary of the five important physiologic events involved in the normal swallow. (Reprinted with permission from MW Donner, American Journal of Roentgenology (Vol 94) © 1965.)

tenoepiglottic folds and vocal and vestibular folds, producing an airtight soft stopper for the subglottic region. The laryngeal ventricles are obliterated at this point, while the epiglottis moves downward and backward as a result of approximation of the thyroid cartilage to the hyoid bone. Epiglottic depression does not completely close the laryngeal aditus, which results in the insertion of small particles of the bolus into that opening for a short distance.

A liquid bolus is usually split by the epiglottis, traveling on each side of the larynx through the piriform recesses to rejoin behind the cricoid cartilage (see Figure 2.4). The epiglottis acts as a ledge, checking the descent of the bolus and obviating early closure of the larynx. Protection of the larynx during swallowing is effected by closure of the vocal folds and contraction of the sphincteric girdle of muscle that surrounds the laryngeal vestibule (Sasaki 1977, 1980). Contraction of the sphincteric girdle occurs without elevation of the larynx. The larynx may be closed at any stage during swallowing but is always closed when the last of the bolus leaves the pharynx, at which point material entering the vestibule of the larynx is squeezed out. The hood formed by the epiglottis bending downward over the entrance to the larynx prevents the deposition of bolus residue, and negative pharyngeal pressure associated with reinflation of the airway carries any residue upward, trapping it in the valleculae.

Esophageal tasks require an ordered pattern of function that depends on coordinated activities in three distinct zones: esophageal inlet, esophageal outlet, and body of the esophagus. The inlet consists of visceral striated muscle that maintains the lumen in a closed position and is integrated with the tongue and hypopharynx. In the esophageal outlet, the lumen is closed by specialized muscle that is distinguished from the body of the esophagus and separates it from the stomach. Swallowing initiates a moving contraction that is ring-like and sweeps rapidly through the upper striated portion and less rapidly through the lower smooth muscle portion (Dodds 1976; Castell 1980).

FUNCTIONAL ASSESSMENT OF NEUROGENIC DYSPHAGIA

Patients with neurogenic dysphagia involving the oral stage of feeding may present with complaints of oral spill at the lips (drooling), difficulty chewing, and difficulty in initiating swallow. Patients may complain of excess saliva volume when its volume is actually normal or diminished. Bolus preparation may be impaired by deficient salivation, and patients may also report having a dry mouth, with the implication of deficiency of saliva or increase in its viscosity. Some of these individuals have diminution in neurosecretory function, which can be demonstrated by quantitative assessment of salivary secretions, with and without pharmacologic stimulation. If muscles of lingual manipulation are weak or excessively fatigable, patients may report arduous efforts with the bolus in the oral cavity or often mistakenly complain of poorly fitting dentures and pay numerous visits to the dentist. Patients may restrict their diets to pureed food or may be noted to be exerting excessive effort at vigorous chewing in order to conform with the time constraints implicit in social dining. Frequent small meals associated with avoidance of certain foods that cannot readily be particulated for pharyngeal swallowing may make feeding easier but may fail to maintain daily nutritional requirements. Although weight loss is common, it is not always found with dysphagia, based on the fact that some patients consume excessive quantities of high-calorie, swallow-ready foods, such as ice cream.

Family, friends, or caregivers may observe voluntary compensation measures for oral dysphagia, such as craniocervical flexion, followed by slow extension of the neck to control the transfer of the food bolus at the junction of the mouth and pharynx. Occasionally, patients may use fingers to push the food bolus toward the pharynx. They also use fingers to place the bolus on the molar teeth when muscles of the tongue are weakened and exhibit vertical as opposed to rotary chewing. Some patients prefer to drink liquids through a straw, thereby using suckle feeding to overcome impairments associated with the oral stage of dysphagia. However, such compensation measures may become inadequate with increasing nuclear or supranuclear weakness of the facial nerve, which may result in difficulty with straw feeding, as well as in drooling and loss of food out of the mouth as a result of impaired lip closure. Patients with abnormal face and tongue performance may report retention of food in the buccal area, clinically referred to as "squirreling" behavior. Finally, we must mention those neurologic patients with cognitive dysfunction who simply do not know what to do with the food placed in front of them, or even food placed in their mouths. In such cases, patients are unlikely to report symptoms of dysphagia, and caregivers must be relied on to provide pertinent feeding history. Milder forms of cognitive dysfunction may lead to improper bolus sizing and inappropriate speaking, breathing, or both during feeding.

Neurogenic dysphagia involving the pharyngeal stage of swallowing can be more hazardous if the swallow fails to empty the pharynx of the bolus, with or without subsequent bolus penetration into the larynx. Fortunately, there is effective physiologic compensation for pharyngeal dysphagia for many patients with this disability. This compensation may mask the clinical abnormality so that it can be detected only by videoradiography. Repeat swallowing may be used to clear retained material in the pharyngeal recesses. Tilting the head forward or to the side may facilitate swallowing, and some patients discover that manual pressure against one side of the neck helps them to swallow, particularly in the case of asymmetric pharyngeal weakness. However, even after careful history-taking in patients with neurogenic pharyngeal dysphagia, the clinician may fail to identify patients who have adapted their feeding style to neuromuscular compensations within the pharynx. In such cases, it will be the radiologist who informs the clinician that a patient has neurogenic dysphagia that requires further neurologic evaluation (Robbins et al. 1987). Why should the clinician be concerned about patients with compensated neurogenic dysphagia (Buchholz et al. 1985)? The information is more than academic, for decompensation may occur abruptly. For example, patients who have compensated neurogenic dysphagia who then suffer a second lesion on the contralateral side (as in stroke or metastatic tumor) or progression of their neurologic lesions (as in amyotrophic lateral sclerosis) may become acutely symptomatic and at risk for bronchopulmonary complications.

Symptoms of decompensation from neurogenic pharyngeal dysphagia are alarming to both patient and clinician. The passage of solids through the pharynx may be delayed, with retention of the food bolus in the pharyngeal recesses and subsequent leakage into the laryngeal vestibule, which may lead to frequent throat clearing and a wet-sounding voice (Curtis and Crain 1987). Nasal regurgitation of liquids may be noted, especially in compromising positions such as bending over to drink from a water fountain. The liquids may be retained in the pharynx or aspirated, resulting in coughing or choking episodes, laryngospasm, or pneumonia. Like ingested liquids, oral and pharyngeal secretions are retained in the valleculae and piriform recesses (Curtis 1986; Curtis et al. 1989). Patients sense an accumulation of phlegm or mucus, as if there were an overproduction of secretions, but the real problem is a swallowing impairment. Laryngeal penetration may cause coughing, choking, stridor, and pneumonia. Sensory impairment of the larynx and airways may result in a life-threatening situation in which airway penetration occurs without respiratory response, leading to recurrent pneumonia (Kaplan 1960). Symptoms of retained secretions during sleep include drooling onto the pillow and awakening with choking. Individuals known to have compensated neurogenic dysphagia who show changes in feeding habits or difficulty handling secretions during sleep should be seriously considered for re-examination by videofluoroscopy. In addition, such individuals

Table 2.6 Afferent Controls Involved in Swallowing

Sensory Function	*Innervation*
General sensation, anterior two-thirds of the tongue	Lingual nerve, trigeminal (V)
Taste, anterior two-thirds of the tongue	Chorda tympani, facial (VII)
Taste and general sensation, posterior one-third of the tongue	Glossopharyngeal (IX)
Mucosa of valleculae	Internal branch of superior laryngeal nerve (vagus)
Primary afferent	—
Secondary afferent	Glossopharyngeal (IX)
Tonsils, pharynx, soft palate	Pharyngeal branch of vagus (X)
Pharynx, larynx, viscera	Glossopharyngeal (IX) Vagus (X)

should have endoscopic evaluation to observe intrinsic motor disorders of the larynx, pharynx, or esophagus, such as vocal fold paresis, transverse shift (curtain movement) of the pharyngeal constrictor wall, and structural deficits such as a web, inflammation, or neoplasm of the esophagus. Such structural abnormalities of the lower pharynx or esophagus can become quite extensive without clinical symptoms and can secondarily complicate the course of neurogenic dysphagia. (See Chapter 7 for a discussion of the clinical evaluation for dysphagia.)

STEREOTYPED PHARYNGEAL SWALLOW BEHAVIORS: MEDULLA OF THE BRAIN STEM

Pharyngeal swallow is initiated by sensory impulses transmitted as a result of stimulation of receptors on the fauces, tonsils, soft palate, base of the tongue, and posterior pharyngeal wall. These sensory impulses reach the medulla primarily through the seventh, ninth, and tenth cranial nerves, and the efferent function is mediated through the ninth, tenth, and twelfth cranial nerves (Table 2.6, Table 2.7, and Figure 2.6). Cricopharyngeal sphincter relaxation occurs at the time when the bolus reaches the posterior pharyngeal wall before reaching this sphincter (Palmer 1976; Schultz et al. 1979). There is some controversy over the origin of the cricopharyngeal resting tone, which may not rely solely on the sympathetic nervous system but may depend more heavily on vagal input for both contraction and relaxation. Reference is made in the literature to a swallowing center in the medulla at the level of the obex of the fourth ventricle (Figure 2.7). This is probably an oversimplification. Based on presently available evidence, it is more likely that modulation of oral and pharyngeal swallowing and its voluntary and involuntary behaviors receive major contributions from neural activity in supramedullary structures, such as pons, mesencephalon, and limbic and cerebral cortex.

Table 2.7 Efferent Controls Involved in Swallowing

Efferent/Stage	*Innervation*
Oral	
Masticatory, buccinator, floor of mouth	Trigeminal (V)
Lip sphincter	Facial (VII)
Tongue	Hypoglossal (XII)
Pharyngeal	
Constrictors and stylopharyngeus	Glossopharyngeal (IX)
Palate, pharynx, larynx	Vagus (X)
Tongue	Hypoglossal (XII)
Esophageal	
Esophagus	Vagus (X)

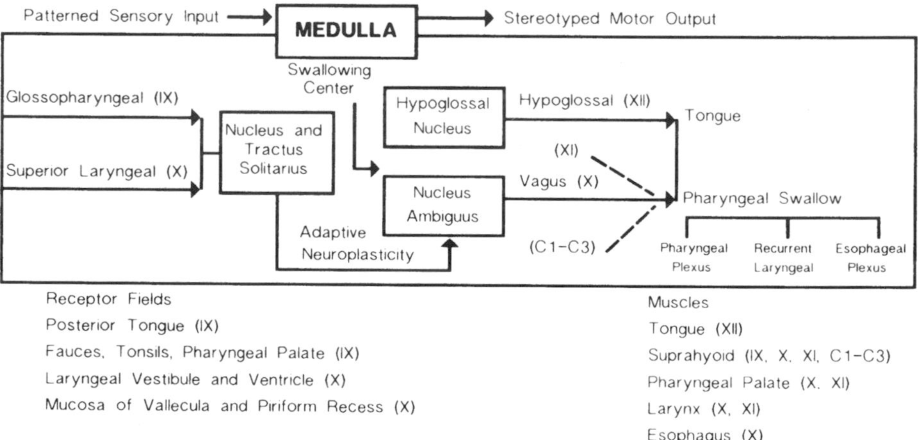

Figure 2.6 Conceptualization of the components of pharyngeal swallow as sensory-cued, stereotyped behaviors.

The brain stem coordinates efferent impulse flow by way of the trigeminal, vagus, and hypoglossal cranial nerves to the muscles of the oropharynx by way of the tenth cranial nerve to the muscles of the hypopharynx, by way of the fifth and twelfth cranial nerves to the extrinsic muscles of the larynx, and by way of the tenth cranial nerve to the intrinsic muscles of the larynx and esophagus. The cervical esophagus may receive two vagal efferent supplies from nerves within the neck: one from the recurrent laryngeal and another from the pharyngoesophageal nerve that rises proximal to the nodose ganglion or from an esophageal branch of the superior laryngeal nerve (SLN). Such double innerva-

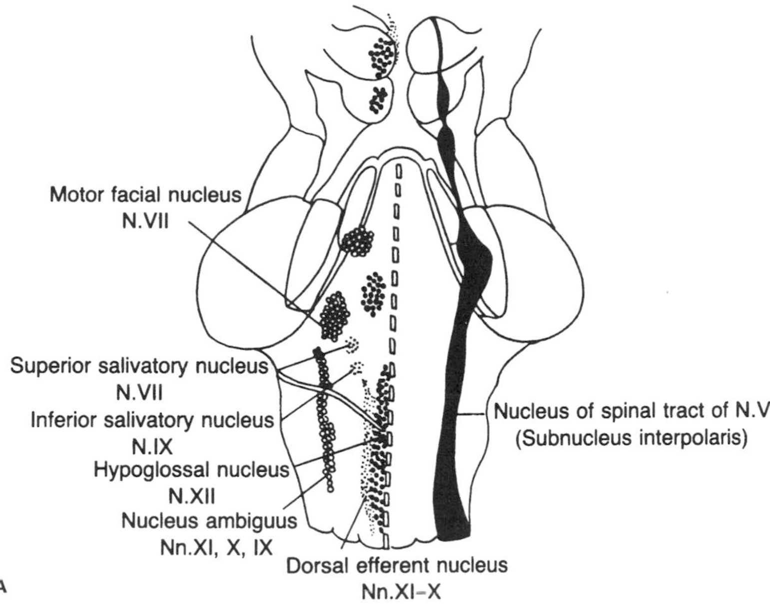

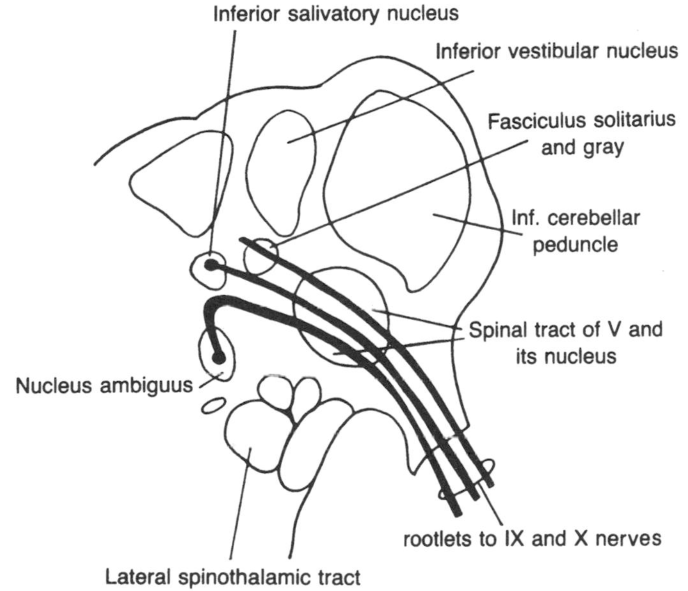

Figure 2.7 A. Longitudinal section through the medulla showing relationships of the vagus nerve to the surrounding structures (modified from Crosby). B. Cross-section at the level of the medulla showing relationship of the vagus nerve to the surrounding structures (modified from Crosby). (Reprinted with permission from M Rontal, E Rontal. Lesions of the vagus nerve: diagnosis, treatment, and rehabilitation. Laryngoscope 1977;87:72.)

tion of the cervical esophagus in humans has not been proved but might provide a margin of safety to prevent esophageal distension and reflux.

Sequentially timed discharges from the medulla result in movement of a bolus through successive levels of the esophageal musculature. Esophageal smooth muscle contractions have a sequential behavior by which proximal activity inhibits the next most distal portion of the esophagus successively (Sanchez et al. 1953; Donner 1974; Ekberg and Nylander, 1982). Esophageal distention is signaled on visceral afferent nerves passing in the upper five or six thoracic sympathetic roots—presumably to the thalamus and inferior postcentral gyrus—where they may give rise to symptoms described as pressure, burning, gas, aching, and so forth. When such symptoms are described as pain, the referral patterns are based on sensory impulses from tissues innervated by somatic nerves that cross the corresponding spinal levels.

Fibers originating in the nucleus ambiguus innervate the pharyngeal, laryngeal, and upper esophageal striated muscles. The nucleus ambiguus also innervates the heart, lungs, and gastrointestinal tract smooth muscle (Rontal and Rontal 1977). It carries afferents for taste, pharyngeal sensation, and sensation from some regions of skin around the external ear. Rootlets emerging from the medulla form the peripheral vagus, which exits the skull through the jugular foramen. Above the nodose ganglion, the vagus nerve sends branches to the pharyngeal plexus, which supplies the mucosa and musculature of the pharynx, larynx, and upper esophagus.

The very important branch of the vagus, the SLN, is sensory to the laryngeal mucosa and motor to the cricothyroid muscle. The vagus terminates as the recurrent laryngeal nerve (RLN) that loops around the aorta and returns to the larynx and hypopharynx (Figure 2.8). The RLN supplies muscles intrinsic to the larynx and is thought not to supply the cricopharyngeus, which apparently derives its innervation from the pharyngeal plexus.

The neural control systems that subserve pharyngeal swallow are initiated by the action of cranial nerve afferents, but isolated central activation is not possible even though voluntary components exist. It appears that afferent impulses competent to initiate swallowing must conform to highly codified stimulus patterns that enter the nucleus solitarius of the brain stem by way of its fasciculus and are relayed into the reticular formation where connections exist to motoneurons lying in the nuclei of the fifth, seventh, and twelfth cranial nerves and the nucleus ambiguus. These neurons are interesting in that they lack recurrent collaterals or monosynaptic connections with cranial nerve efferents.

The motoneurons of interest in the neuroregulation of the pharyngeal swallow and speech include the salivatory nuclei on either side of the genu of the seventh cranial nerve and the dorsal motor nucleus of the vagus, which innervates the esophageal smooth muscle in humans. Experiments to date show that sectioning of the tenth cranial nerve distal to the recurrent laryngeal branch produces degeneration in the nucleus ambiguus as well as in the dorsal motor nucleus. Many neurons in the nucleus of the twelfth cranial nerve participate in swallowing and speech. Histologic studies in patients with bulbar poliomyelitis

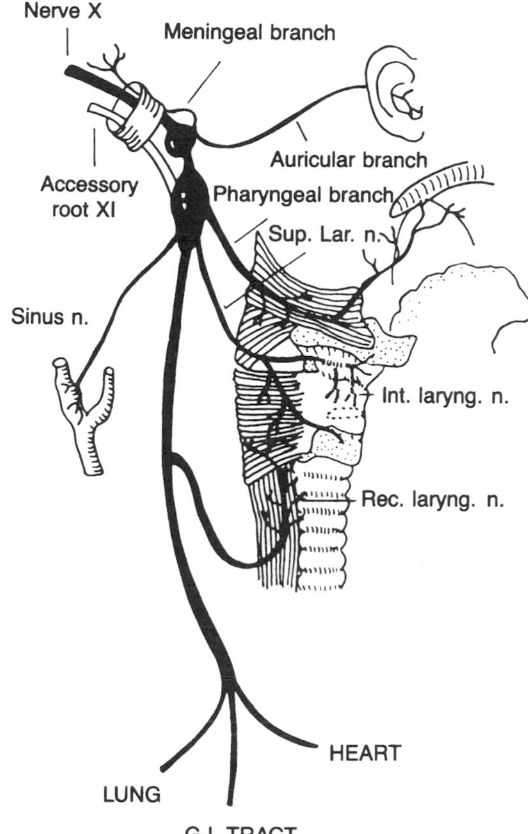

Figure 2.8 Course of the peripheral vagus nerve on exit from the jugular foramen. (Reprinted with permission from M Rontal, E Rontal. Lesions of the vagus nerve: diagnosis, treatment, and rehabilitation. Laryngoscope 1977;87:72.)

reveal loss of neurons in rostral nucleus ambiguus in those who had pharyngeal dysphagia, whereas those with laryngeal dysarthria were found to have cell loss in the caudal portions (Baker et al. 1950; Bosma 1976). These effects would be explained by representation of palatopharyngeal and esophageal musculature in the rostral magnocellular part of the nucleus. Comparative studies have revealed great adaptability of human palatopharyngeal and laryngeal musculature, reflecting progressive evolutionary refinement of the controlling interneuronal network.

The neuroregulatory brain stem mechanisms for pharyngeal swallow exist within the medullary reticular formation 1.5 mm from the midline on either side of the obex of the fourth ventricle (see Figure 2.7). On each side of the midline is a site that communicates with the opposite side through cross-connections running behind the obex. As a result, bilateral symmetry of pharyngeal swallow is achieved. Each half of the medullary reticular formation exerts ipsilateral inhibition and excitation on appropriate motoneurons, with the exception of the lower constrictor muscles, whose excitation is strictly contralateral.

Pharyngeal swallow involves a sequence of excitation and inhibition produced by several motoneuronal pools on each side of the brain stem (Baker et al. 1950). The chronologic synergy of muscular contraction of the esophagus and stomach can be reproduced electrically by stimulation of the internal branch of the SLN. From an electrophysiologic standpoint, pharyngeal swallow is probably the most complex behavioral pattern that can be evoked by electrical stimulation of a sensory branch of a cranial nerve. Since pharyngeal swallow occurs in humans, who congenitally have no brain tissue rostral to the mesencephalon (anencephaly), and in experimental animals, whose brain is intact, at least caudally from the motor nucleus of the tenth cranial nerve, its control appears not to depend unequivocally on cerebral structures or on the cerebellum (Bosma 1963). It appears also that some form of bolus is necessary to sustain repetitive swallowing, a fact that highlights the importance of peripheral afferent stimuli.

Experimental unilateral destruction of the medulla eliminates swallowing in the ipsilateral musculature, except for the crossed constrictor pathway previously described. The responsiveness of the contralateral side to afferent input for the side of the lesion is still normal, however. For example, destruction of the left lateral medulla does not prevent right-sided swallowing if the left SLN is stimulated. This has immediate clinical relevance, especially in the case of unilateral destructive lesions to the brain stem (Doty et al. 1967). As previously outlined, voluntary efforts in the absence of reflex initiation from peripheral stimuli will not result in swallowing. The peripheral stimuli include water, light touch, and chemical stimulation. If we were to seek a principal point from which swallowing is most likely to be initiated, it would normally lie in the palatal area innervated by the maxillary branch of the fifth cranial nerve, although this may vary among species. For example, in cats and dogs the principal effective area is the upper pharynx, innervated by the ninth cranial nerve.

The neural organization of swallowing has been largely elucidated by recording the electrical activity of involved muscles, beginning with onset of contraction in the mylohyoid and including concurrent activity in muscles innervated by the fifth cranial nerve and those of the posterior tongue, superior constrictor, palatopharyngeus, palatoglossus, stylohyoid, and geniohyoid. These initiators constitute what has been called the leading complex (Doty and Bosma 1956). Because the constrictors form a continuous sheet of striated muscle, an overlapping firing sequence is observed beginning with the superior constrictor (the principal muscle), the middle constrictor, and the inferior constrictor, with distinct rostral (thyropharyngeus) and caudal (cricopharyngeus) components. The superior constrictor is active at the same time as the leading complex activity. A reconstruction of firing patterns leads to the conclusion that inhibition would probably be found to surround or bracket (in a time sense) the excitation of swallowing (Doty and Bosma 1956).

From the standpoint of peripheral innervation, elicitation of swallowing may occur as a result of activity in the maxillary branch of the trigeminal, glossopharyngeal, or SLN. It has been suggested that small fibers giving rise to a superficial plexus of beaded terminals on the pharyngeal surface of the epiglottis may be the type of nerve ending that is most likely to be activated in the initiation of swallowing. Many complex endings also exist on the oral side of the soft palate or uvula, although anatomic complexity and overlap make it difficult to identify elements specifically at this point. In addition to sensory endings, there are proprioceptors whose relevance to swallowing has not been clarified (Bosma 1957a; Bosma 1976). It is important that there probably are not more than 2,000 motoneurons on both sides to innervate about 12,000 constrictor muscle fibers, and that this low innervation ratio of the pharyngeal musculature implies neural control comparable in precision with that of the ocular muscles.

VOLUNTARY AND STEREOTYPED ORAL FEEDING BEHAVIORS: CEREBRAL CORTEX AND LIMBIC CORTEX SYSTEMS

To better understand the supranuclear (rostral to the brain stem) organization of oral feeding behaviors, it is necessary to deal in more detail with the central afferent systems, motoneuron pools, and efferent systems (Figure 2.9).

The convergent afferent systems include the maxillary branch of the fifth cranial nerve and the ninth and tenth cranial nerves. These lead to the descending or spinal trigeminal system and the fasciculus and nucleus solitarius. The ninth and tenth cranial nerves admix considerably in terms of source and modality. The magnocellular part of nucleus solitarius receives input from the sensorimotor cortex and the ventromedial thalamus. Some fibers of the ninth and tenth cranial nerves project to the lateral cuneate nucleus (lateral portion of posterior spinal column), serving as a relay to the ventroposteromedial nucleus of the thalamus and limbic cortical system.

The reflexes produced as a result of the afferent, central, and efferent systems for oral feeding behaviors may be divided into brain stem systems (see Figure 2.10), sensory-cued stereotyped (limbic cortical systems) (Figure 2.11), and sensory-guided discriminatory behaviors (sensorimotor neocortical systems) (Figure 2.12). As previously mentioned, the neuronal activities resulting in the oral phase of swallow also overlap with those responsible for phonation, coughing, and speech. Normal oral feeding appears to involve not only brain stem reflex initiation by way of several types of peripheral excitation, but also a central facilitation of its limbic and cortical sensorimotor pathways.

The highly integrated activities of oral swallow depend on a combination of voluntary and involuntary control of the position of lips, teeth, jaw, cheeks, and tongue, all partly mediated by the fifth cranial nerve–innervated muscles that control both the mandible and the masseter. These muscles are involved in the control of leverage, stabilization, and centering of the movable parts of the buccal cavity. Therefore, mastication depends primarily on the fifth cranial nerve, whereas the muscles of the lips and cheeks depend on motor functions of the seventh cranial nerve. All of the extrinsic muscles of the tongue depend on the motor function of the twelfth cranial nerve, except for the palatoglossus (ele-

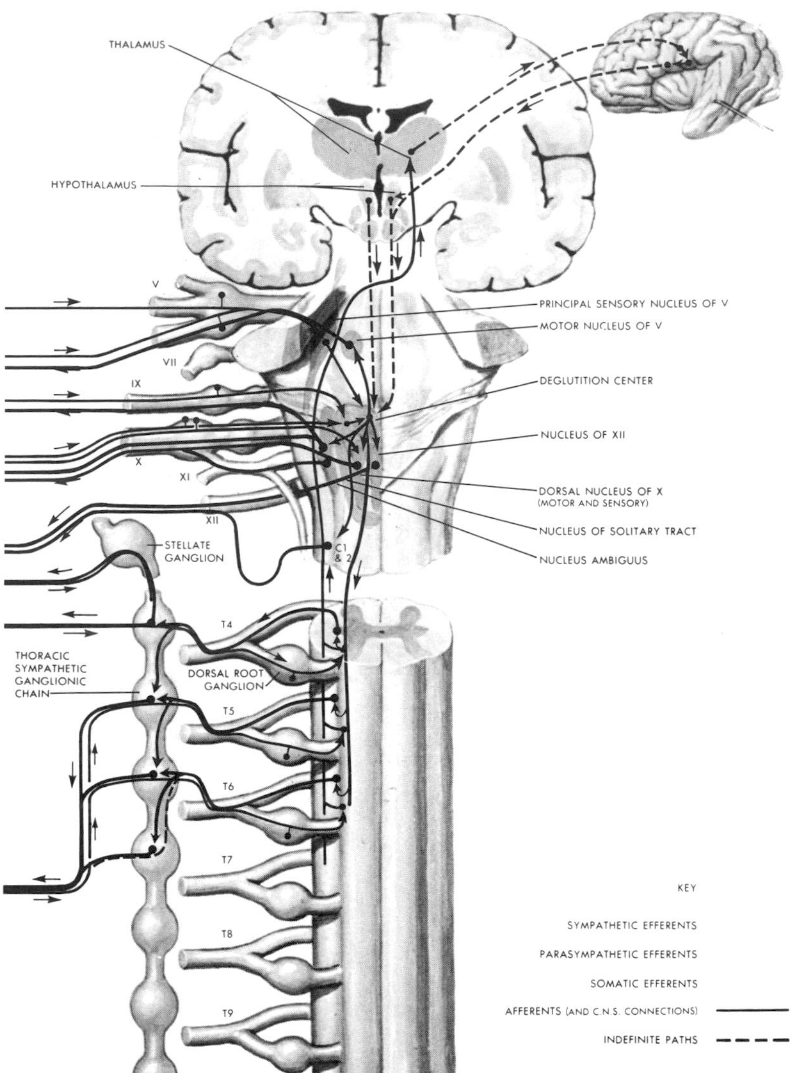

Figure 2.9 Summary of the nervous control of deglutition. (© Copyright 1959, CIBA Pharmaceutical Company, Division of CIBA-GEIGY Corporation. Reprinted with permission from The Ciba Collection of Medical Illustrations, illustrated by FH Netter, M.D. All rights reserved.)

vator of the tongue root), which is innervated by the tenth cranial nerve (Stone and Shawker 1988). All of the intrinsic tongue muscles are innervated by the twelfth cranial nerve. All of the muscles of the soft palate are innervated primarily by the tenth cranial nerve, except the tensor veli palatini, which is innervated by the fifth cranial nerve. The stylopharyngeus, a longitudinal muscle, has the

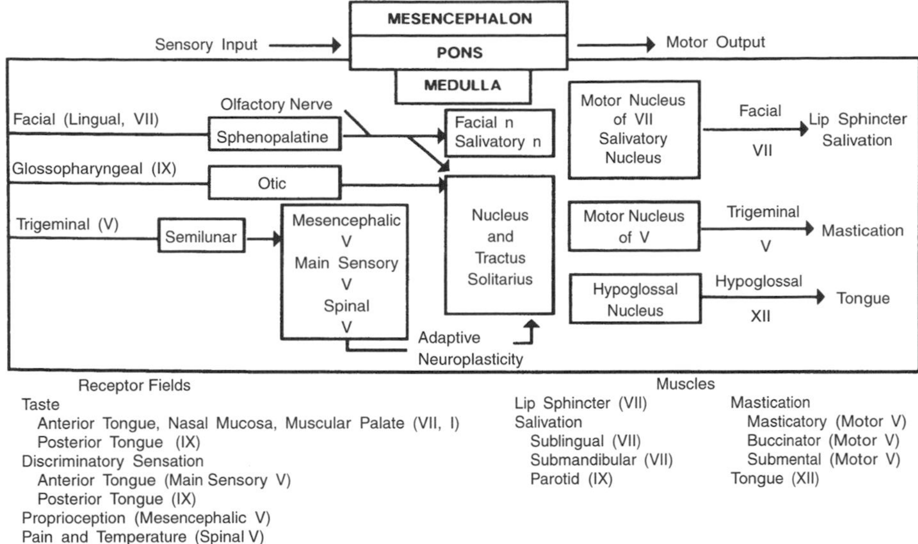

Figure 2.10 The brain stem receives afferent information and produces efferent responses from a number of cranial nerves. This sequence of activity is capable of both sensory-guided, discriminatory behaviors and sensory-cued, stereotyped behaviors.

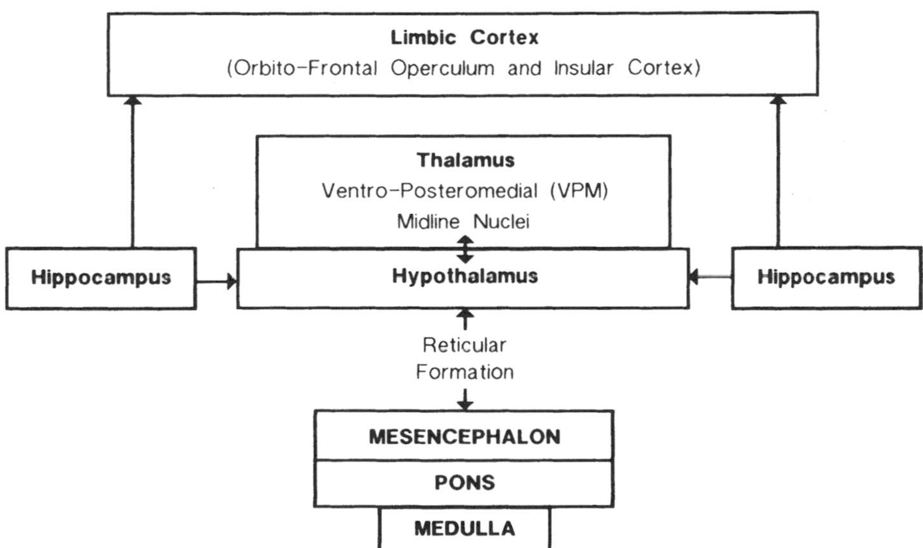

Figure 2.11 Conceptualization of learned components of oral swallow as sensory-cued, stereotyped behaviors from the limbic system.

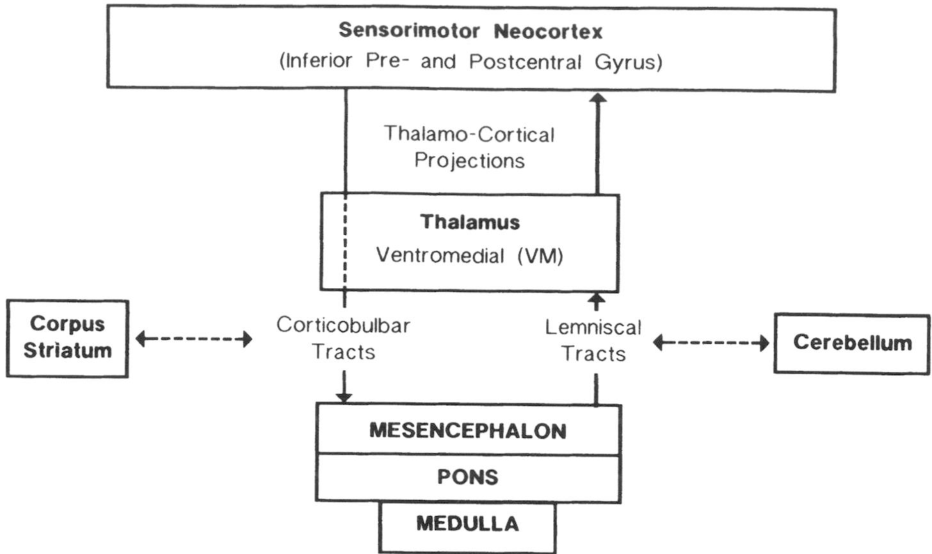

Figure 2.12 Conceptualization of voluntary components of oral swallow as sensory-guided, discriminatory behaviors from the neocortex.

function of widening the pharynx and is innervated by the ninth cranial nerve, whereas the palatopharyngeus is innervated primarily by the tenth cranial nerve. The maxillary and mandibular sensory divisions of the fifth cranial nerve are primarily involved in providing sensation pertaining to the lips, palate, teeth, inner mouth, and proprioceptive aspects of the muscles of mastication. The gag reflex as well as nasal regurgitation depends on the function or dysfunction of the glossopharyngeal and vagus nerves, whose muscles of innervation have been discussed previously.

The neural structures and organization of oral feeding swallowing behaviors result in more than one basic type of pattern—for example, that found in infancy, and more mature patterns developing later in childhood, adolescence, and adulthood. A fundamental description of the neuroregulation of oral feeding behaviors requires a somewhat artificial isolation of the neural organization. Actually, movements of the palate and oral swallowing are probably closely related to those occurring in speech and respiration. Earlier evolutionary patterns such as swallowing of air by amphibia may be regained by adult humans—for example, victims of poliomyelitis. Such movements require some voluntary control of the inferior constrictor with pumping tongue movements, suggestive of glossopharyngeal breathing (Bosma 1963).

Because of the widespread ramifications and functional significance of the vagus nerve (tenth), lesions in the vagal system may have far-reaching deleterious effects on coughing, swallowing, breathing, and phonation, elements of each of which are interrelated at various vagal levels. Although the details of anatomic and physiologic complexity are beyond the scope of this discussion, it is essential that the reader grasp the major pattern of vagal distribution. The afferent side of swallowing behaviors can be stimulated by voluntary movements of the tongue and larynx. This is subserved to some extent by supranuclear corticobulbar fibers of the sensorimotor neocortical system, some of which provide ipsilateral and others bilateral innervation to the motor outflow of the nucleus ambiguus. It also should be noted that swallowing behaviors associated with phonation or vocal fold adduction can be initiated through pathways associated with the limbic cortical systems.

The voluntary components of sensory-guided discriminatory behaviors of oral swallow probably have their origin in neocortex (inferior precentral and postcentral gyrus) (see Figure 2.12). They operate primarily on striated muscles but involve the development of "automatisms" that still may be subject to voluntary monitoring and control by mechanisms associated with the limbic cortex (orbitofrontal operculum and insular cortex) (see Figure 2.11). These include the sensory-cued stereotyped motor behaviors or habits of mouth control and chewing, which are largely distinguishable from individual to individual. Many of the neural mechanisms for oral feeding behaviors are dependent on a combination of brain stem and supranuclear pathways of complex reflexes that have variable expression at different stages of development and evolution. Examples include cough and gag, the rooting and sucking of infancy, and the biting reflexes dependent on masseteric stretch. At the limbic cortex, the inferior portion of the precentral gyrus of the insula produces oral and pharyngeal swallowing on electrical stimulation. This swallowing behavior results from efferent connections to the hypothalamus and thence to the obex of the fourth ventricle at the caudal medulla.

The sensorimotor neocortex and limbic cortex in primates and many other species produce a combination of chewing and swallowing movements that affect many structures of the neck, palate, tongue, and pharynx. These behaviors are usually bilaterally represented. The direct stimulation of sensorimotor and limbic systems elicits swallowing that follows paths through the ventromedial thalamus and hypothalamus, respectively (see Figure 2.11). It is interesting that gagging depends on the spatiotemporal pattern of afferent action integrated at the level of the medulla through the same set of pharyngeal or palatoreceptors that evoke respiration in the limbic and sensorimotor cortical systems. This pluripotential nature of afferent activity is a hallmark of the complex neural organization under discussion, with special emphasis on linking swallowing with speech and respiration.

SUMMARY

The neuroplasticity of the adult nervous system acknowledges the well-established observation that feeding is a continuously adaptive behavior in which optimal performance can be assessed only in relation to the character, volume, and density of the ingested food, in association with factors such as craniocervical posture (Keogh 1957; Cotman and Nadler 1978; Buchholz et al. 1985). The term *adaptive plasticity* has been proposed to describe observations that conditioned reflexive behaviors emanating from the pontomedullary area of the brain stem appear to have the capacity to change over time when challenged by the environment. For example, if such adaptations occur by finding the appropriate inborn synaptic network, adaptive neuroplasticity will tend to mask clinical symptoms of neurogenic dysphagia. For some patients there is increased liability of sudden decompensation caused by progression of neurologic illness, intercurrent nonspecific events such as stress, alcohol, and minor trauma, or a combination of these.

Recent investigations show that the mature brain is intrinsically labile; although some neural functions, such as respiration, are reflexive and require minimal learning and experience, others, such as feeding behaviors (oral and pharyngeal swallow), have provided a substrate exquisitely receptive to programming (Bach-y-Rita 1980; Goldberger and Murray 1988). The scientific basis for the rehabilitation of dysphagia that results from lesions of the nervous system is based on the hypothesis that the fundamental neuroplastic process responsible for feeding can be reprogrammed to enhance function by training and environmental change. For some behaviors, such as respiration, function may return spontaneously with minimal outside interventions; for others, such as feeding, rehabilitation associated with special training routines is usually necessary. However, as we gain a deeper understanding of the fundamental process of neuroplasticity, our ability to predict outcomes, evaluate improvement or regression, and devise new training strategies for dysphagia rehabilitation after nervous system damage is likely to improve (Finger and Stein 1982).

REFERENCES

Ardran GM, Kemp FH. The mechanism of swallowing. Proc R Soc Med 1951;44:1038.

Ardran GM, Kemp FH. Protection of laryngeal airway during swallowing. Br J Radiol 1952;25:406.

Bach-y-Rita P. Recovery of Function: Theoretical Considerations for Brain Injury Rehabilitation. Baltimore: University Park, 1980.

Baker AB, Matzke HA, Brown JR. Poliomyelitis; bulbar poliomyelitis; a study of medullary function. Arch Neurol Psychiatry 1950;63:257.

Bosma JF. Deglutition: pharyngeal stage. Physiol Rev 1957a;37:275.

Bosma JF. Studies of the pharynx. I. Poliomyelitic disabilities of the upper pharynx. Pediatrics 1957b;19:1053.

Bosma JF. Oral and pharyngeal development and function. Physiol Rev 1963;37:275.

Bosma JF. Sensorimotor Examination of the Mouth and Pharynx. In Y Kawamura (ed), Frontiers of Oral Physiology. Basel, Switzerland: Karger 1976;78.

Buchholz DW, Bosma JF, Donner MW. Adaptation compensation and decompensation of the pharyngeal swallow. Gastrointest Radiol 1985;10:235.

Castell DO. Esophageal manometric studies: a perspective of their physiological and clinical relevance. J Clin Gastroenterol 1980;2:91.

Cotman CW, Nadler JV. Reactive Synaptogenesis in the Hippocampus. In CW Cotman (ed), Neuronal Plasticity. New York: Raven, 1978;227.

Curtis DJ. Radiographic anatomy of the pharynx. Dysphagia 1986;2:51.
Curtis DJ, Crain MC. Aerosol regurgitation as a laryngeal sensitizing event explaining acute laryngospasm. Dysphagia 1987;2:93.
Curtis DJ, Cruess DF, Willgross ER. Abnormal bolus swallowing in the erect position. Dysphagia 1989;2:46.
Dodds WJ. Instrumentation and methods for intraluminal esophageal manometry. Arch Intern Med 1976;136:515.
Donner MW. Swallowing mechanisms and neuromuscular disorders. Semin Roentgenol 1974;9:273.
Donner MW, Bosma JF, Robertson DL. Anatomy and physiology of the pharynx. Gastrointest Radiol 1985;10:196.
Donner M, Siegel C. The evaluation of neuromuscular disorders by cinefluorography. AJR Am J Roentgenol 1965;94:299.
Doty RW, Bosma JF. Electromyographic analysis of reflex deglutition. J Neurophysiol 1956;19:44.
Doty RW, Richmond WH, Storey AT. Effect of medullary lesions on coordination of deglutition. Exp Neurol 1967;17:91.
Ekberg O, Nylander G. Cineradiography of the pharyngeal stage of deglutition in 150 individuals without dysphagia. Br J Radiol 1982;55:253.
Finger S, Stein DG. Brain Damage and Recovery: Research and Clinical Perspectives. Orlando, FL: Academic, 1982.
Goldberger ME, Murray M. Patterns of Sprouting and Implications for Recovery of Function. In S Waxman (ed), Advances in Neurology. 1988;361.
Hamilton WJ, Harrison RJ. Anatomy of the Mouth, Pharynx, and Esophagus. In J Ballantyne, J Groves (eds), Diseases of the Ear, Nose, and Throat. London: Butterworth, 1971.
Kaplan HM. Anatomy and Physiology of Speech: McGraw-Hill Series in Speech. New York: McGraw-Hill, 1960.
Keogh CA. The neurology and function of the pharynx and its powers of compensation. Ann Otol Rhino Laryngol 1957;66:1.
Palmer ED. Disorders of the cricopharyngeus muscle: a review. Gastroenterology 1976;71:510.
Robbins JA, Sufit R, Rosenbek J, et al. A modification of the modified barium swallow. Dysphagia 1987;2:83.
Rontal M, Rontal E. Lesions of the vagus nerve: diagnosis, treatment, and rehabilitation. Laryngoscope 1977;87:72.
Sanchez GC, Kramer P, Ingelfinger FJ. Motor mechanisms of the esophagus, particularly its distal portion. Gastroenterology 1953;25:321.
Sasaki CT. Paralysis of the larynx and pharynx. Surg Clin North Am 1980;60:1079.
Sasaki CT, Suzuki M, Horiuchi M, et al. The effect of tracheostomy on the laryngeal closure reflex. Laryngoscope 1977;87:1428.
Schultz A, Niemtzow P, Jacobs S, Naso F. Dysphagia associated with cricopharyngeal dysfunction. Arch Phys Med Rehabil 1979;60:381.
Sinclair WJ. The pharyngeal plexus in initiation of swallowing in man. Am J Physiol 1961;221:1260.
Sloan RF, Brummet SW, Westover JL, et al. Recent cinefluorographic advances in palatopharyngeal roentgenography. AJR Am J Roentgenol 1964;92:977.
Splaingard ML, Hutchins B, Sulton LD, Gouri C. Aspiration in rehabilitation patients: videofluoroscopy vs bedside clinical assessment. Arch Phys Med Rehabil 1988;69:637.
Stone M, Shawker TH. An ultrasound examination of tongue movement during swallowing. Dysphagia 1988;1:78.

3

Neurologic Disorders of Swallowing

David W. Buchholz

The process of swallowing can be divided into three phases: oral, pharyngeal, and esophageal. Difficulty swallowing is referred to as *dysphagia*. Neurogenic dysphagia is difficulty swallowing caused by a neurologic disorder. As a rule, when a neurologic disorder causes difficulty swallowing, it does so by impairing motor and sensory functions of the oral and pharyngeal phases of swallowing. The esophageal phase tends to be relatively spared by neurologic disorders, but even when esophageal function is compromised by neurologic disorders, esophageal dysfunction is less likely to be symptomatic than concomitant oral or pharyngeal dysfunction. Although to a large extent neurogenic dysphagia equates with oral/pharyngeal dysphagia, it is important to distinguish the two. Oral/pharyngeal dysphagia also may result from oral or pharyngeal structural problems including strictures, webs, tumors, diverticula, and edema.

The function of the swallowing tract is to safely transport material through the oral cavity, pharynx, and esophagus to the stomach. In neurogenic dysphagia there may be ineffective transport of swallowed material along its intended course, so that material is delayed or retained along the way. Also, swallowed material may go out of bounds into the nasopharynx or larynx. Misdirection into the larynx and farther down into the respiratory tract is a major source of morbidity and mortality from neurogenic dysphagia.

This chapter is divided into four sections. The first section is a discussion of the clinical features of neurogenic dysphagia. In the second section, specific neurologic disorders that cause dysphagia are described. The third section covers evaluation of neurogenic dysphagia. Finally, there is a brief review of management of neurogenic dysphagia, although most of the specifics of this topic are covered in greater detail elsewhere in this book (see Chapters 9 and 10).

CLINICAL FEATURES OF NEUROGENIC DYSPHAGIA

There are three modes of presentation of neurogenic dysphagia. The first is in a patient with an identified neurologic disorder who develops obvious symptoms or complications of dysphagia (Table 3.1). Examples of this mode of presentation of neurogenic dysphagia include a patient who presents with an obvious brain stem stroke and overt dysphagia, or a patient with the diagnosis of motor neuron disease (MND) in whom dysphagia becomes a clearcut problem as the disease advances.

Table 3.1 Symptoms and Complications of Neurogenic Dysphagia

Oral/pharyngeal symptoms
Drooling
Impaired chewing
Difficulty initiating swallowing
Nasal regurgitation
Coughing
Choking
Food sticking in the throat
Difficulty managing secretions
Throat clearing
Wet voice
Esophageal symptoms
Food sticking in the chest
Regurgitation
Heartburn
Chest discomfort
Complications
Dehydration
Malnutrition
Laryngospasm
Bronchospasm
Aspiration pneumonia
Asphyxia
Loss of pleasure

The prandial symptoms of neurogenic oral/pharyngeal dysphagia include drooling, impaired chewing, difficulty initiating swallow, nasal regurgitation, coughing, choking, and food sticking in the throat. Between meals there may be difficulty managing secretions, often manifested as frequent throat clearing, wet voice, coughing, or choking. When a neurologic disorder produces esophageal dysphagia, the symptoms may include food sticking in the chest, regurgitation, heartburn, and chest discomfort, although neurogenic esophageal dysfunction may also cause or contribute to symptoms localized to the pharynx.

Among the complications of neurogenic dysphagia are dehydration, malnutrition, laryngospasm, bronchospasm, aspiration pneumonia, and asphyxia (Horner et al. 1988a; Horner et al. 1988b; Martin et al. 1994; Schmidt et al. 1994; Teasell et al. 1994).

Too often overlooked among the complications of neurogenic dysphagia is loss of pleasure, related to not only the patient's personal eating experience but also the social activity of dining. The essence of effectively managing neurogenic dysphagia is to be vigilant for its symptoms, which enables intervention and avoidance of complications.

Table 3.2 Findings of Videofluorographic Swallowing Studies in Neurogenic Dysphagia

Oral leakage anteriorly or posteriorly
Poor bolus formation in the mouth
Reduced tongue movement
Nasal regurgitation
Decreased pharyngeal contraction
Retention of barium in the valleculae or piriform sinuses
Diminished displacement of the epiglottis, hyoid bone, or larynx
Laryngeal penetration or aspiration
Abnormal opening of the pharyngoesophageal segment

The second mode of presentation of neurogenic dysphagia is in the patient with overt neurogenic dysphagia who does not have an established neurologic diagnosis. In this scenario the problem of dysphagia itself is recognizable by virtue of the symptoms and complications detailed above, but the underlying neurologic disorder is not readily identified. A common problem contributing to this scenario is the tendency among many physicians to focus on the esophagus rather than the oral cavity or pharynx when confronted with dysphagia. In this way, physicians tend to not even consider the possibility of a neurologic disorder that may be causing oral/pharyngeal impairment. Another frequent diagnostic mistake is to overemphasize structural findings (such as prominent anterior cervical osteophytes) or esophageal findings (such as reflux or dysmotility), even though these findings are often incidental and asymptomatic.

The solution to these diagnostic errors is twofold: (1) Clinicians need to be aware of the symptoms of oral/pharyngeal as opposed to those of esophageal dysphagia (see Table 3.1) and the fact that most cases of oral/pharyngeal dysphagia are neurogenic; (2) A videofluorographic swallowing study (VSS) should be obtained whenever the cause of dysphagia is not entirely clear. The symptoms of neurogenic oral/pharyngeal dysphagia are helpful in pointing to an underlying neurologic disorder as opposed to a structural lesion or an esophageal problem, but VSS is more sensitive and specific than a patient's history in detecting neurogenic motor and sensory dysfunction of the oral cavity and pharynx as well as coincident non-neurologic problems.

VSS of a patient with neurogenic dysphagia usually demonstrates not only decreased or poorly timed movement of oral, pharyngeal, and laryngeal structures during swallowing but also abnormal movement or collection of barium (Table 3.2) (Bosma 1953; Silbinger et al. 1967; Bosma and Brodie 1969; Grunebaum and Salinger 1971; Donner 1974; O'Connor and Ardran 1976; Jones and Donner 1988; Chen et al. 1990; Stroudley and Walsh 1991; Chen et al. 1992; Kidd et al. 1993). There may be anterior or posterior oral leakage; poor bolus formation in the mouth; reduced tongue movement; nasal regurgitation; decreased pharyngeal contraction; retention of barium in the valleculae or

Table 3.3 Reasons for "Silent" Neurogenic Dysphagia

Compensatory processes
Voluntary
Avoiding difficult-to-swallow items
Cutting food into smaller pieces
Taking smaller boluses
Chewing more thoroughly
Eating more slowly
Washing down solids with liquids
Double swallowing
Throat clearing or coughing
Tilting or turning the head while eating
Involuntary
Reduced laryngeal cough reflex
Cognitive impairment

piriform sinuses; diminished displacement of the epiglottis, hyoid bone, or larynx; laryngeal penetration or aspiration; and abnormal opening of the pharyngoesophageal segment. Esophageal findings of VSS in neurogenic dysphagia tend to be nonspecific abnormalities, such as esophageal dysmotility or reflux, that do not clearly indicate the presence of an underlying neurologic disorder and may, in fact, be unrelated.

As much as VSS is useful in revealing neurogenic oral/pharyngeal dysfunction and pointing to the presence of an underlying neurologic disorder, VSS is relatively nonspecific in pointing to the particular disorder. There are exceptions to this general rule (see Evaluation of Neurogenic Dysphagia). Neurologic investigation is needed to make a specific neurologic diagnosis when neurogenic dysphagia is suggested by VSS.

The third mode of presentation of neurogenic dysphagia is when a patient with or without a clear neurologic diagnosis harbors substantial oral/pharyngeal dysfunction that is "silent," or at least "quiet," despite being potentially dangerous. There are three basic reasons for silent or quiet dysphagia: (1) compensatory processes, both voluntary and involuntary; (2) reduced laryngeal cough reflex; and (3) cognitive impairment (Table 3.3).

Compensatory processes for neurogenic dysphagia include both voluntary behavioral modifications during eating as well as involuntary adjustments in oral/pharyngeal performance during swallowing (Buchholz et al. 1985). The alterations of diet and eating methods that characterize voluntary compensation include avoiding difficult-to-swallow items, cutting food into smaller pieces, taking smaller boluses, chewing more thoroughly, eating more slowly, washing down solids with liquids, double swallowing, throat clearing or coughing during meals, and tilting or turning the head while eating.

These compensatory behaviors serve to reduce the overt symptoms of dysphagia (see Table 3.1), thereby rendering dysphagia relatively quiet or even silent. In this situation, the compensatory behaviors themselves are the symptoms of neurogenic dysphagia and must be diligently sought in the course of a careful dysphagia history. Even though these are voluntary, compensatory strategies, patients may be unaware that they may have adopted these strategies, at least to the extent that they may not volunteer a history of these behaviors unless they are specifically asked about them. Relative unawareness of changes in eating behavior is especially likely in patients with slowly progressive neurologic disorders (for example, MND or myopathy) in whom the changes have been acquired gradually. Also, there is a tendency to regard altered eating behavior in elderly individuals as being secondary to aging, and these subtle clues of neurogenic dysphagia are even more likely to be overlooked in the elderly. Recognizing the symptoms of voluntary compensation and realizing that these symptoms may reflect neurogenic oral/pharyngeal dysphagia is the first step toward proactive management of dysphagia to effectively intervene and avoid potentially catastrophic complications.

Involuntary compensation refers to automatic adjustments in oral/pharyngeal motor performance that minimize the functional impact of a neurologic disorder. This process may represent the phenomenon of adaptive neuroplasticity—a process that is not well understood but may play a similar role, for example, in recovery from stroke or traumatic brain injury (Finger and Stein 1982; Cotman 1985; Wolpaw 1985; Bach-y-Rita 1988). It is possible that involuntary compensation can be enhanced by swallowing rehabilitation techniques (Bartolome and Neumann 1993; Neumann 1993; Neumann et al. 1995a).

The laryngeal cough reflex is not only an important mechanism of protecting the respiratory tract but also a major source of neurogenic dysphagia symptoms. Triggering of the cough reflex by penetration of food or secretions into the larynx accounts for coughing or choking, which often signals the presence of neurogenic dysphagia. When the cough reflex is not triggered in response to laryngeal contamination, dysphagia, including aspiration, becomes quiet or silent (Linden and Siebans 1983; Horner and Massey 1988; Kahrilas 1989; Linden et al. 1993).

There are several reasons for reduction of the laryngeal cough reflex. Some neurologic disorders, such as brain stem stroke, can directly disrupt either the afferent limb of the reflex (laryngeal sensation), the efferent limb (coughing), or both. Other mechanisms account for reduction of the cough reflex that is seen with neurologic disorders that do not directly disrupt the reflex. These mechanisms probably involve desensitization of the cough reflex by means of either centrally mediated adaptation in the face of persistent stimulation of the reflex or damage to local sensory receptors as a result of chronic laryngeal inflammation. Many other superimposed factors can impair the laryngeal cough reflex, including endotracheal intubation, tracheostomy, medications (sedatives and anesthetics), and decreased level of arousal (Hochman et al. 1965; Taylor and Towey 1971; Cleaton-Jones 1976; Rubin et al. 1977; Sasaki et al. 1977; Huxley 1978; Bishop et al. 1984; Greenberg 1984).

The final reason why neurogenic dysphagia may be relatively silent is cognitive impairment. Individuals with neurogenic dysphagia may also have mental retardation or dementia. These individuals have limited ability to recognize, understand, and communicate their difficulty eating. This and the other barriers to the recognition of neurogenic dysphagia can be overcome if the clinician observes the patient eating, carefully questions not only the patient but also his or her companions and caregivers, and keeps in mind the tendency for dysphagia to be quiet or silent for a number of reasons.

CAUSES OF NEUROGENIC DYSPHAGIA

The act of swallowing is highly complex and requires exquisite organization at many levels of the nervous system, as discussed in Chapter 2. Another way of looking at this is to say that there are many vulnerable target sites within the nervous system, both centrally and peripherally, at which neurologic disorders may strike and thereby cause neurogenic dysphagia.

Neurologic disorders can result in oral/pharyngeal dysphagia if there is involvement of the central efferent pathway for swallowing, including parts of the cerebral cortex, basal ganglia, subcortical structures (such as the hypothalamus and midbrain central gray matter), corticobulbar tracts, and brain stem structures, including multiple lower cranial nerve nuclei and the ventral and dorsal medullary swallowing centers. Generally speaking, brain stem disease is more likely to be associated with dysphagia than cortical or subcortical disease. When a neurologic disorder is localized above the brain stem, oral/pharyngeal dysphagia is more likely to occur and to be more severe if the disorder is distributed bilaterally rather than unilaterally.

Central nervous system (CNS) disorders can also result in oral/pharyngeal dysphagia by involving afferent systems, including the trigeminal nuclear complex, nucleus tractus solitarius, ascending pathways in the brain stem and subcortex, subcortical structures such as the thalamus, and the cerebral cortex. Peripheral nervous system disorders associated with oral/pharyngeal dysphagia have potential target sites including the lower cranial nerves, neuromuscular junctions, and striated muscle fibers in the oral cavity, tongue, pharynx, and larynx.

Understanding the potential target sites for neurologic disorders causing esophageal dysphagia is made easier by dividing the esophagus into two parts, proximal and distal, each with distinct neuromuscular features (Buchholz 1996). Remarkably, despite this anatomic and physiologic distinction, there is seamless coordination of proximal and distal esophageal function, indicating the role of centrally mediated integration of proximal and distal esophagomotor performance, even as the neural control of the esophagus shifts from predominantly central control proximally to predominantly peripheral control distally.

The proximal esophagus (upper one-third to one-half) consists of striated muscle and has neural control generally similar to the striated muscle of the pharynx, except that the role of cortical input to the esophagus is less clear. The distal esophagus (lower one-half to two-thirds) consists of smooth muscle, and the contribution, if any, of cortical and subcortical structures to brain stem control of the distal esophagus is poorly understood. Central regulation of the distal esophagus arises from the dorsal vagal nuclei and a pattern generator in the medulla. Impulses are carried by the vagus nerves to a complex network of intrinsic neurons, the myenteric plexus, which coordinate contraction of smooth muscle fibers to generate orderly distal esophageal peristalsis. In addition to vagal (parasympathetic) input, sympathetic nerve fibers also control activity of the myenteric plexus and other specialized intramural neurons in the distal esophagus.

From a clinical standpoint, these unique features of neurologic control of the distal esophagus provide additional targets for neurologic disorders to strike, including the autonomic nerve fibers and myenteric plexus, and thereby cause neurogenic esophageal dysphagia.* On the other hand, the relative lack of cortical and subcortical control of the proximal and, even more so, the distal esophagus renders the esophagus less vulnerable than the oral cavity or pharynx in the face of CNS disorders.

Before surveying the specific neurologic disorders that can cause dysphagia, it is worth noting that there are only limited data reliably distinguishing the characteristics of dysphagia produced by any one of these disorders as compared to others. In other words, current knowledge suggests that the clinical and videofluorographic features of dysphagia largely overlap among patients with, for example, stroke, traumatic brain injury, Parkinson's disease (PD), MND, and myopathy. The relative nonspecificity of neurogenic dysphagia is understandable when compared to other functional impairments arising from neurologic disorders. Hemiparesis, for instance, may appear much the same in patients with stroke, multiple sclerosis, or brain tumor, and it is only by thoroughly evaluating the patient that a specific neurologic diagnosis can be made, whether the presenting problem is hemiparesis or dysphagia. On occasion, certain clinical and videofluorographic findings tend to point more in one specific diagnostic direction than another, and examples of these findings are mentioned in the discussion of specific neurologic disorders.

The following review of causes of neurogenic dysphagia is intended to be illustrative but not exhaustive (Table 3.4). Given that any neurologic disorder associated with motor or sensory impairment of the oral cavity, pharynx, or esophagus can potentially cause dysphagia, an encyclopedic effort would be necessary to include every possible item. The disorders discussed below are roughly sequenced in terms of the hierarchy of the nervous system from central to peripheral.

Stroke

Stroke is probably the most common cause of neurogenic dysphagia (Kuhlemeier 1991). Of the approximately 500,000 new strokes annually in the

*Somewhat arbitrarily, disorders of the myenteric plexus, such as achalasia, are regarded as gastroenterologic rather then neurologic.

Table 3.4 Causes of Neurogenic Dysphagia

Stroke
Traumatic brain injury
Cerebral palsy
Dementia, including Alzheimer's disease
Parkinson's disease
Progressive supranuclear palsy
Huntington's disease
Wilson's disease
Torticollis
Motor neuron disease
Multiple sclerosis
Neoplasms and other structural disorders
Poliomyelitis and postpolio syndrome
Infectious disorders
Guillain-Barré syndrome and other polyneuropathies
Myasthenia gravis
Myopathy
Iatrogenic oral/pharyngeal dysphagia
Age-related changes
Psychogenic dysphagia

United States (American Heart Association 1991), one-fourth to one-half result in at least temporary dysphagia (Groher and Bukatinan 1986; Wade and Hewer 1987; Horner et al. 1988a; Chen et al. 1990; Palmer and DuChane 1991), and dysphagia is a major cause of post-stroke morbidity related to respiratory complications and malnutrition (Veis and Logemann 1985; Hewer and Wade 1987; Horner et al. 1988b; Gresham 1990).

Large hemispheral ischemic strokes are caused most frequently by either internal carotid artery atherosclerosis or cardiac embolism, usually involving the middle cerebral artery territory. The typical symptoms are contralateral hemiparesis and, if the stroke is in the dominant (usually left) hemisphere, dysphasia. According to conventional neurologic teaching, bilateral, but not unilateral, hemispheral strokes can also cause dysphagia, presumably by interrupting the corticobulbar pathways that connect the cortical and brain stem centers for swallowing. While it is clear that bilateral hemispheral strokes are associated with a higher incidence and greater severity of dysphagia than unilateral strokes (Horner et al. 1988a; Celifarco et al. 1990; Teasell 1994), there are data to suggest that unilateral hemispheral strokes can also cause dysphagia (Meadows 1973; Robbins and Levine 1988; Logemann et al. 1993; Robbins et al. 1993; Teasell 1994). Moreover, there appear to be differences between the impact of left versus right hemispheral strokes on oral and pharyngeal swallowing performance. It has been reported that left-sided lesions tend to predominantly impair the oral phase and that right-sided strokes are more likely to compromise pharyngeal function and result in aspiration (Robbins and Levine 1988; Robbins et al. 1993). There is virtually no information about esophageal dysfunction secondary to hemispheral stroke (Fischer et al. 1965).

Lacunar strokes are caused by the occlusion of deep penetrating arterioles by lipohyalinosis, a process associated with hypertension. This process is sometimes referred to as *small vessel disease* (as opposed to *large vessel disease* related to atherosclerosis). Lacunar strokes tend to be small, multiple, and bilateral, and they often involve periventricular regions including the internal capsules (the anterior limbs of which carry the corticobulbar tracts) and basal ganglia. The relationship between lacunar strokes and dysphagia is unclear.

There is limited understanding of the relationship between periventricular signal abnormalities demonstrated by magnetic resonance imaging (MRI) in elderly individuals and the issue of lacunar strokes. Specifically, it is unclear whether or not these MRI findings represent ischemic damage (due to lacunar strokes) and to what extent these findings may be responsible for either "normal" changes in oral and pharyngeal function in asymptomatic elderly subjects or clinically relevant findings among elderly patients with dysphagia (Baum and Bodner 1983; Sonies et al. 1984; Börgstrom and Ekberg 1988b; Tracy et al. 1989; Levine et al. 1991; Alberts et al. 1992; Buchholtz 1992; Robbins et al. 1992; Robbins et al. 1995).

Brain stem strokes can result from atherosclerosis, cardiac embolism, or small vessel disease. Brain stem strokes cause dysphagia when the corticobulbar tracts, nuclei tracti solitarii, trigeminal nuclear complexes, nuclei ambigui, hypoglossal nuclei, or medullary swallowing centers are involved (Horner et al. 1991; Teasell et al. 1994; Aviv et al. 1996; Chua and Kong 1996). Since the brain stem is densely packed with many other tracts and nuclei, brain stem strokes resulting in dysphagia tend also to cause impairment of other functions such as eye movements, voice, balance, and limb movements. On occasion brain stem stroke is very discreet, and dysphagia may be the sole or primary consequence (Buchholz 1993). Despite its high sensitivity, MRI may fail to demonstrate a tiny brain stem stroke, even though the stroke has caused severe dysphagia (Buchholz 1993). Failure to recognize brain stem stroke, often because of diagnostic insistence on other brain stem deficits and over-reliance on negative MRI findings, is a common oversight among patients seen at a tertiary referral center for undiagnosed dysphagia (Buchholz et al. 1995b).

A common form of brain stem stroke resulting in pharyngeal dysphagia is lateral medullary infarction (Wallenberg's syndrome), usually secondary to vertebral artery occlusion. Accompanying symptoms and signs vary but often include vertigo, dysarthria, Horner's syndrome (ipsilateral ptosis and miosis), ataxia, and numbness and weakness of the ipsilateral face and contralateral body. Studies have demonstrated that lateral medullary infarction, which is a unilateral event, produces bilateral pharyngeal dysfunction (Neumann et al. 1994; Neumann et al. 1995b). This finding implies that the musculature on each side of the pharynx depends on intact input from both sides of the medulla in order to function normally. Remarkably, even though the dorsal vagal nucleus is often involved in lateral medullary infarction, there are, to the author's knowledge, no data regarding esophageal dysphagia secondary to brain stem stroke.

The diagnosis of stroke is mainly clinical and should be suspected whenever there is acute onset of neurologic dysfunction related to a definable vascular territory. Confirmation and localization of stroke may be assisted by MRI (Kim et al. 1987), which often reveals additional, clinically silent strokes that may contribute to the impact of a new stroke in terms of dysphagia. Other tests, such as carotid artery and cardiac and blood studies, may be indicated to determine the cause of stroke so that therapy can be targeted to prevent its recurrence.

It is important to recognize stroke-related dysphagia for several reasons. First, appropriate swallowing evaluation and management can be undertaken to avoid dysphagia complications. Keeping in mind that post-stroke dysphagia is both common and often relatively silent, clinicians caring for stroke patients should be on the lookout for dysphagia clues, such as dysphonia, overt difficulty managing secretions or food, reduced level of consciousness, and an abnormal gag reflex (Horner et al. 1988a; Horner et al. 1988b; Horner and Massey 1988; Alberts et al. 1992; Leder 1996).* Stroke patients with these signs should be considered for VSS before eating, to help guide management decisions about tube feeding, dietary modification, and swallowing rehabilitation.

A second reason for the importance of recognizing dysphagia in the wake of stroke is that misguided diagnostic efforts can thereby be avoided. For instance, if a patient presents with acute post-stroke dysphagia, but it is not appreciated that a stroke has occurred, the patient may be subjected to diagnostic procedures, such as esophagoscopy, that are not only unnecessary but also potentially risky in the post-stroke setting. A third reason for recognizing post-stroke dysphagia is that making the diagnosis of stroke as the cause of acute dysphagia opens the door to acute stroke interventions, including tissue plasminogen activator, that can improve stroke outcome. Finally, correctly diagnosing stroke as the cause of dysphagia provides the opportunity to implement stroke prevention measures including risk factor reduction and anti-platelet or anticoagulant medication. Fortunately, most patients with post-stroke dysphagia spontaneously improve within days to months, and this favorable prognosis points even more strongly to the need for appropriate interim stroke and dysphagia care.

Traumatic Brain Injury

Traumatic injury to the brain, brain stem, or cranial nerves can give rise to dysphagia, and many of the principles regarding post-stroke dysphagia, including the potential for recovery, apply to post-traumatic dysphagia (Winstein

*Correlation of the gag reflex and intact swallowing is weak, such that a patient with a profound neurogenic dysphagia may have a normal or increased gag reflex, whereas approximately one-third of normal individuals have an absent or diminished gag reflex (Davies et al. 1995).

1983; Ylvisaker and Logemann 1986; Lazarus and Logemann 1987; Tepid et al. 1987; Lazarus 1989; Brown et al. 1992). One difference is that traumatic brain injury tends to be more diffusely localized than stroke, and cognitive impairment is more likely to be a confounding factor in rehabilitation efforts (Hutchins 1989; Mackay and Morgan 1993).

Cerebral Palsy

Cerebral palsy (CP) is a syndrome that arises from damage to the developing brain early in life, and the chronic neurologic problems that arise may include oral/pharyngeal dysphagia. Dysphagia in CP is often characterized by persistent primitive reflexes that are normal in infants but maladaptive later in life. For example, a persistent bite reflex, suckle-swallow reflex, or asymmetric tonic neck reflex can contribute to dysphagia in patients with CP (Ogg 1975; Ottenbacher et al. 1983). Also, patients with CP may have other neurologic deficits, such as impaired tongue movement or instability of the lower jaw, that add to difficulty eating (Parrott et al. 1992; Casas et al. 1994; Kenny et al. 1994; Mirrett et al. 1994; Rogers et al. 1994). Mental retardation may be present, and, as in the case of dementia with traumatic brain injury, can complicate management of CP-related dysphagia. Swallowing therapy techniques have been suggested—for example to decrease muscle hypertonicity (Morris 1982; Gisel 1994; Gisel et al. 1996)—and difficulty eating among patients with CP may be alleviated with assistant devices including customized utensils and supports for the trunk, neck, and head (Helfrich-Miller et al. 1993).

Dementia (Including Alzheimer's Disease)

Dementia is global cognitive impairment, and it is not usually associated with motor or sensory impairment of the oral cavity or pharynx. Nonetheless, dementia is a highly prevalent cause of difficulty eating, because it interferes with essential functions related to eating, such as food preparation in the kitchen and on the plate, transport of food from the plate to the mouth, and voluntary bolus preparation and transport within the oral cavity (Volicer et al. 1989, Horner et al. 1994).

The most common cause of dementia is Alzheimer's disease; other causes include multiple strokes, traumatic brain injury, hydrocephalus, brain tumor, and a myriad of metabolic disturbances. There is yet no specific diagnostic test for Alzheimer's disease, and it remains a diagnosis of exclusion. The workup of dementia should include complete blood counts, chemistry panel, thyroid screening, vitamin B_{12} level, serologic test for syphilis, and computed tomographic (CT) scanning or MRI of the brain. Depression should be considered, since it can masquerade as dementia (pseudodementia), and cognitive impairment as a side effect of medication should not be overlooked.

The deficits of Alzheimer's disease relate in part to deficient function of cholinergic neurons, and agents that enhance cholinergic function, such as tacrine, may be somewhat helpful. A major dilemma in managing patients with dementia is whether gastrostomy is indicated and, if so, when. It is difficult to know when the potential benefits of gastrostomy, including better nutrition and fewer care demands, outweigh the loss of pleasure of eating, one of the few pleasures that may be left for a patient with advanced dementia (Norbert et al. 1980; Horner et al. 1994). Two other factors complicating decisions about gastrostomy in patients with dementia are that, contrary to common belief, gastrostomy may actually increase the risk of aspiration pneumonia (Feinberg et al. 1996) and ethical considerations may argue against inappropriate prolongation of life by means of gastrostomy (Weir and Grostin 1990; Sullivan 1993).

Parkinson's Disease

PD involves progressive degeneration of neurons in a number of subcortical and brain stem regions, especially the dopamine-producing neurons of the substantia nigra in the midbrain. PD initially presents as some combination of rest tremor, reduced limb movements, gait impairment (slow, stooped, shuffling, and unstable), and monotonic, hypophonic speech. PD gradually progresses, and dysphagia often arises later as a result of both oral/pharyngeal and esophageal dysfunction (Leiberman et al. 1980; Schneider et al. 1985; Robbins et al. 1986; Croxson and Pye 1988; Edwards et al. 1991; Stroudley and Walsh 1991; Edwards et al. 1992; Bird et al. 1994; Bine et al. 1995; Ali et al. 1996; Leopold and Kagel 1996; Nilsson et al. 1996). Esophageal dysphagia in PD (Gibberd et al. 1974; Blonsky et al. 1975; Bramble et al. 1978; Qualman et al. 1984; Kempster et al. 1989; Castell et al. 1994; Johnston et al. 1995a; Johnston et al. 1995b) may reflect involvement of the dorsal vagal nuclei, the esophageal myenteric plexus, or both, and oral/pharyngeal dysphagia in PD could be related to either basal ganglia or brain stem degeneration. Aspiration pneumonia is a leading cause of death in advanced PD (Hoehn and Yahr 1967). Many of the symptoms of PD, but less so dysphagia, respond well to treatment with dopaminergic agonists (Bushmann et al. 1989; Li et al. 1994; Fonda and Schwarz 1995; Fuh et al. 1995).

Progressive Supranuclear Palsy

Progressive supranuclear palsy (PSP) is a "Parkinson's-plus" syndrome that resembles PD but has additional features because of more widespread neuronal degeneration in multiple systems and is less responsive to dopaminergic treatment. Oral/pharyngeal dysphagia is a common but not an initial symptom of PSP (Sonies 1992; Johnston et al. 1995b; Neumann et al. 1995c).

Huntington's Disease

Huntington's disease (HD) is an autosomal dominant neurodegenerative disorder characterized by progressive psychiatric disturbances, dementia, and involuntary movements (especially chorea) commencing in adulthood. The genetic defect involves a repeating trinucleotide sequence that can be detected with a blood test. Dysphagia is a typical feature of HD that often results in terminal respiratory complications (Edmonds 1966; Leopold and Kagel 1985). Oral/pharyngeal dysfunction is the predominant mechanism of dysphagia in HD, but esophageal dysfunction has also been described (Kagel and Leopold 1992). Swallowing therapy using compensatory techniques has been reported to be beneficial (Kagel and Leopold 1992).

Wilson's Disease

Wilson's disease is an inherited disorder of copper metabolism that damages the brain and liver. Neurologic problems include psychiatric disturbances, tremor, rigidity, dysarthria, and pharyngeal dysphagia (Gulyas and Salazar-Grueso 1988). The diagnosis of Wilson's disease can be confirmed by the detection of Kayser-Fleischer corneal rings, elevated serum and urinary copper levels, and decreased serum ceruloplasmin. Chelation therapy (medication that extracts copper from bodily tissues) is effective in reducing organ damage related to copper deposition; therefore, it is important not to miss the diagnosis of Wilson's disease.

Torticollis

Torticollis refers to involuntary contraction of muscles around the head and neck resulting in abnormal posture of the head, usually tilting toward one side and rotating to the other. It is a form of dystonia, a term that refers to abnormal, sustained muscle contraction. Dystonias and dyskinesias (involuntary movement disorders in general) are regarded as extrapyramidal disorders arising from dysfunction of the basal ganglia and, perhaps, brain stem. Dystonias and dyskinesias often have spontaneous onset, but they may also be precipitated by treatment with dopamine antagonists. An example of this is tardive dyskinesia involving the mouth, which results from treatment with antipsychotic medications (neuroleptics), antiemetic agents, or metoclopramide (see Iatrogenic Dysphagia below). Focal dystonias such as torticollis cause oral/pharyngeal dysphagia by either postural effects (interference with the normal anatomic relationships of the swallowing tract) or neurogenic impairment (abnormal muscle contraction in the oral cavity or pharynx) (Kakigi et al. 1983; Logemann 1988; Riski et al. 1990; Horner et al. 1992; Horner et al. 1993). Focal dystonias can be effectively treated for several months at a time following chemodenervation by injection of botulinum toxin, which blocks neuromuscular transmission, into the excessively contracting muscles. Ironically, botulinum toxin injection can lead to dysphagia (Comella et al. 1992; Holzer and Ludlow 1996; Tuite and Lang 1996) (see Iatrogenic Dysphagia below).

Motor Neuron Disease

MND is also known as amyotrophic lateral sclerosis. MND causes degeneration of motor neurons in the brain, brain stem, and spinal cord. Recent evidence has indicated that motor neuron loss occurs as a result of excitotoxicity related to excessive action of glutamate, an excitatory neurotransmitter. An anti-glutamate agent, riluzole, is effective in slowing the progression of MND with bulbar features such as dysphagia (Bensimon et al. 1994), and riluzole is now available for routine clinical use.

Unfortunately, despite riluzole, MND remains relentlessly progressive and usually leads to death, often as a result of dysphagia complications, within 5 years of symptom onset. The presentation of MND is highly variable because it may involve muscles innervated by the brain stem, the spinal cord, or both, and because there may be upper motor neuron features, lower motor neuron features, or both. Upper motor neuron features include spasticity, incoordination, and increased reflexes, whereas lower motor neuron features include muscle wasting, fasciculations, and decreased reflexes.

Dysphagia in MND (Bosma and Brodie 1969; Lebo et al. 1976; Dworkin and Hartman 1979; Meyer et al. 1985; Robbins 1987; Wilson et al. 1990; Kasarskis et al. 1996; Strand et al. 1996) may relate to either upper motor neuron dysfunction (which causes the clinical syndrome of pseudobulbar palsy), lower motor neuron dysfunction (which causes bulbar palsy), or a mixture of the two.* There are minimal data regarding the esophagus in MND (Smith et al. 1957). It is not unusual for previously undiagnosed MND to be the cause of progressive oral/pharyngeal dysphagia, often accompanied by dysphonia or dysarthria, among patients referred to a tertiary center for evaluation of unexplained dysphagia. In the early stages of MND presenting with dysphagia, there may be few, if any, signs in the limbs, and test results consistent with MND (such as denervation demonstrated by electromyography [EMG] or muscle biopsy) may also be absent.

Multiple Sclerosis

In multiple sclerosis (MS) there is immune-mediated demyelination of nerve fibers in the brain and spinal cord that can result in dysphagia (Daly et al. 1962; Boucher and Hendrix 1991) if the corticobulbar tracts or brain stem pathways that mediate swallowing are involved. MS typically produces a variety of subacutely fluctuating neurologic deficits, but it can also be gradually progressive. When dysphagia occurs in MS it is rarely an isolated, presenting symptom. In addition to dysfunction of the oral cavity and pharynx, abnormal taste sensation has also been reported in MS (Catalanotto et al. 1984). Information about the esophagus in MS is scant (Daly et al. 1962).

The diagnosis of MS is based on a combination of (1) clinical evidence of CNS deficits that are multifocal in space and time and (2) laboratory studies including MRI, cerebrospinal fluid (CSF) examination (revealing abnormal antibody production), and evoked potentials. Attacks of MS may be shortened by

*For further discussion of the distinction between pseudobulbar and bulbar palsy, see the section entitled Evaluation of Neurogenic Dysphagia.

treatment with high-dose intravenous corticosteroids, and beta-interferon may help reduce the frequency and severity of relapses or slow progression in some cases.

Neoplasms and Other Structural Disorders

Primary brain tumors more commonly cause oral/pharyngeal dysphagia than has been generally recognized (Newton et al. 1994). This is true even with unilateral hemispherical tumors (Newton et al. 1994), which lends support to similar findings in stroke patients indicating that, contrary to conventional neurologic teaching, unilateral hemispheral lesions can cause dysphagia. Esophageal dysfunction has been reported in a case of CNS lymphoma (Benjamin et al. 1982).

Intrinsic brain stem tumors, including gliomas, may produce oral/pharyngeal dysphagia as a result of invasion of brain stem nuclei and tracts involved in swallowing (Frank et al. 1989; Straube and Witt 1990). Extrinsic tumors within the posterior fossa, such as meningiomas and acoustic neuromas, may compress the brain stem or cranial nerves. Tumors at the base of the skull, including chordomas and nasopharyngeal carcinomas, often compress or invade cranial nerves, commonly in association with local pain. Strictly unilateral pharyngeal, laryngeal, or lingual dysfunction is suggestive of lower cranial nerve involvement by a tumor at the base of the skull. Diagnosis of a tumor causing dysphagia is usually made by MRI or CT scanning with enhancement. Treatment modalities include surgery, radiation, and chemotherapy.

Neoplastic meningitis occurs because of the tendency of certain tumors, especially adenocarcinomas, small cell carcinomas, and lymphomas, to metastasize to the meninges, where the neoplastic cells infiltrate and compress cranial nerves. Patients with neoplastic meningitis typically present with a combination of multiple cranial nerve deficits (including oral/pharyngeal dysphagia), altered mental status, and headache. The diagnosis of neoplastic meningitis is established by MRI (which may demonstrate meningeal thickening and enhancement) and CSF examination revealing abnormal cytopathology. Even when treated with radiation therapy or chemotherapy, neoplastic meningitis has a poor outcome.

Non-neoplastic structural disorders can involve the brain stem or cranial nerves and thereby cause oral/pharyngeal dysphagia. Examples include syringobulbia (cavitation of the central brain stem) (Bleck and Shannon 1984; Fernandez et al. 1986), Arnold-Chiari malformation (congenital downward displacement of the cerebellum, which may cause brain stem compression) (Achiron and Kuritzky 1990; Pollack et al. 1992; Elta et al. 1996; Ikusaka et al. 1996), and aneurysm of the basilar artery (Massey et al. 1984). As in the case of tumors, diagnosis of these structural disorders is usually made by MRI, and surgical treatment may be indicated.

Poliomyelitis and Postpolio Syndrome

Acute paralytic poliomyelitis is a viral infection that predominantly affects lower motor neurons and, in 105% or more of cases, involves the brain stem, leading to problems such as dysphagia (Baker et al. 1950). Acute polio is rare today, but there are approximately 250,000 polio survivors in the United States alone, and 20% complain of residual dysphagia (Lueck et al. 1952; Bosma and Brodie 1969; Halstead et al. 1985).

Postpolio syndrome (PPS) refers to some combination of progressive fatigue, weakness, muscle wasting, and pain, typically presenting decades after acute polio (Speier et al. 1985). Approximately 60% of patients with polio in the remote past meet these diagnostic criteria for PPS (Windebank et al. 1991), and there has been enormous confusion as to what this means.

To understand the basis for confusion surrounding PPS, it is necessary to distinguish between PPS and progressive postpolio muscular atrophy (PPMA). PPMA is a very rare disorder that causes painless, progressive muscle wasting and weakness in patients with a remote history of polio (Cornil 1875; Mulder et al. 1972). It is thought to occur as a result of gradual loss of axon terminals of the motor neurons that survived acute polio and that, in the recovery process, sprouted axons to reinnervate muscle fibers that had lost their nerve input. After decades, these surviving motor neurons may be unable to sustain their abnormally large numbers of axons; therefore, the terminals of some of the axons disintegrate (Dalakas et al. 1986).

The primary confusion regarding PPS stems from the failure to distinguish it from PPMA. Only a tiny fraction of patients with PPS have PPMA, and the majority of patients with PPS have either (1) subjective complaints of progressive symptoms without objective findings of progressive neuromuscular disease or (2) some other problem, unrelated to polio, to account for their progressive symptoms (Windebank et al. 1996). Too often there is a tendency to label postpolio patients who have progressive symptoms as victims of PPS rather than performing thorough evaluation that may lead to effective treatment of the actual problem.

This point holds true for dysphagia and PPS (Buchholz 1987a; Coelho and Ferrante 1988; Buchholz and Jones 1991a; Buchholz and Jones 1991b; Sonies and Dalakas 1991; Jones et al. 1992; Buchholz 1994a; Ivanyi et al. 1994). Patients with past histories of polio who have new or progressive dysphagia should be carefully studied for the possibility of coincident (and potentially treatable) structural or esophageal dysfunction as well as to guide swallowing therapy (Buchholz and Marsh 1986; Silbergleit et al. 1991).

Infectious Disorders

Chronic meningitis resulting from infection by fungi, mycobacteria, or parasites produces a clinical picture, including dysphagia secondary to lower cranial nerve dysfunction, similar to that of neoplastic meningitis. Spirochetal diseases, such as syphilis and Lyme disease, may result in dysphagia not only by causing chronic meningitis, but also by involving the brain or brain stem (Cook 1953). Diagnosis is made by blood tests looking for specific antibodies and by CSF examination.

Diphtheria is a bacterial infection of the throat that is associated with acute lower cranial nerve dysfunction, including oral/pharyngeal dysphagia. Botulism, usually from consumption of preformed botulinum toxin in contaminated food, produces generalized muscle weakness secondary to impaired neuromuscular transmission. Viral encephalitis, especially rabies, may involve the brain stem and corticobulbar tracts, causing dysphagia in addition to the usual features of headache, fever and abnormal mental status.

Guillain-Barré Syndrome and Other Polyneuropathies

The immune-mediated demyelination of peripheral and cranial nerves that characterizes Guillain-Barré syndrome may cause subacute weakness and sensory loss involving the oral cavity, pharynx, and larynx, as well as the limbs (Chen et al. 1996). Spontaneous recovery is the rule, but it can be enhanced by treatment with plasmapheresis or intravenous immunoglobulin; aggressive supportive care, often including temporary mechanical ventilation and tube feeding, is essential.

Aside from Guillain-Barré syndrome, most polyneuropathies affect axons in a length-dependent fashion, such that any resulting weakness is predominantly in the distal limbs. It is uncommon for cranial nerves, which are relatively short, to be affected by most polyneuropathies to the extent that there is symptomatic pharyngeal weakness. In other words, it is unlikely for polyneuropathy from common causes such as diabetes or alcohol abuse to be associated with oral/pharyngeal dysphagia.

On the other hand, polyneuropathies often preferentially involve small unmyelinated nerve fibers that mediate autonomic functions, such as the small vagal branches that innervate the myenteric plexus and regulate distal esophageal motility. As a consequence, small fiber polyneuropathies, such as those associated with diabetes or amyloidosis, may substantially impair distal esophageal function and cause esophageal dysphagia (Gilat and Spiro 1968; Mandelstam et al. 1969; Silber 1969; Vix 1969; Vela and Balart 1970; Stewart 1976; Hollis et al. 1977; Russell et al. 1983; Burakoff et al. 1985; Channer et al. 1985; Loo et al. 1985a; Loo et al. 1985b; Richter et al. 1985; Westin et al. 1986; Borgström et al. 1988; Vannini et al. 1989).

Myasthenia Gravis

Under normal circumstances the contraction of skeletal muscle fibers is triggered when nerve terminals release acetylcholine that traverses the synapse of the neuromuscular junction and binds to receptors on muscle membranes. In myasthenia gravis (MG), abnormal antibodies damage acetylcholine receptors, and therefore neuromuscular transmission is defective. The result is weakness that tends to worsen with sustained or repetitive effort. Common sites of involvement include not only the extraocular muscles (producing ptosis and diplopia) and proximal limbs, but also the tongue, palate, and pharynx (leading to oral/pharyngeal dysphagia) (Edwards and Murray 1957; Murray 1962; Carpenter et al. 1979).

The diagnosis of MG is supported by anti-acetylcholine receptor antibodies in the serum, decremental response to repetitive nerve stimulation (an EMG technique), and positive clinical response to anticholinesterase medication (drugs that potentiate acetylcholine by inhibiting the enzyme that degrades it). Treatment of MG includes anticholinesterase medication, immunosuppressant agents (corticosteroids and others), and thymectomy (surgical removal of the thymus gland, the source of abnormal antibody production).

Myopathy

Myopathy is a generic term for muscle disease, and it tends to present as limb weakness, but muscles of the face, oral cavity, pharynx, or esophagus may additionally or even selectively be involved. Inflammatory myopathies are characterized by immune-mediated damage to skeletal muscle fibers; these diseases include polymyositis, dermatomyositis, inclusion body myositis, and sarcoidosis (Hardy et al. 1967; O'Hara et al. 1967; Grunebaum and Salinger 1971; Metheny 1978; Dietz et al. 1980; Jacob et al. 1983; Cunningham and Lowry 1985; Kagen et al. 1985; Horowitz et al. 1986; Vencovsky et al. 1988; Darrow et al. 1992; Riminton et al. 1993; Shapiro and Martin 1996). Among the supportive diagnostic findings are elevated muscle enzymes (creatine kinase and aldolase), EMG findings of small motor potentials and irritability, and muscle biopsy evidence, including inflammatory cell infiltration and muscle fiber degeneration. Inflammatory myopathy is an especially important consideration in cases of undiagnosed neurogenic dysphagia, because immunosuppressant treatment with corticosteroids, intravenous immunoglobulin, and other agents can be highly effective.

Noninflammatory myopathies include late-onset muscular dystrophies such as myotonic dystrophy and oculopharyngeal muscular dystrophy. Although both of these disorders are hereditary, there may not be a recognized family history. Both pharyngeal (Casey and Aminoff 1971; Duranceau et al. 1978; Swick et al. 1981; Dobrowski et al. 1986; Kiel 1986; Buckler et al. 1989; Johnson et al. 1992; Hillarp et al. 1994; Salvesen and Brautaset 1996) and esophageal (Kelle 1964; Bray et al. 1965; Harvey et al. 1965; Hughes et al. 1965; Pierce et al. 1965; Siegal et al. 1966; Roberts and Bamforth 1968; Weitzner 1969; Simpson and Kilnani 1975; Bender 1976; Eckardt et al. 1986; Castell et al. 1995; Stübgen 1996) dysfunction have been reported. Genetic therapy may some day be available. Myopathy may also be associated with endocrine diseases such as hyperthyroidism, hypothyroidism, and Cushing's syndrome (corticosteroid excess, which may be endogenous or related to corticosteroid therapy), and dysphagia may result (Christensen 1967; Meshkinpour et al. 1979; Wright and Penner 1979; Eastwood et al. 1982; Branski et al. 1984). It is worthwhile to check thyroid function tests as a routine part of the workup of unexplained neurogenic dysphagia.

Table 3.5 Mechanisms and Causal Treatments Associated with Iatrogenic Oral/Pharyngeal Dysphagia

Mechanisms	*Causal Treatments*
Medication-related	
Sedation and suppression of brain stem control of swallowing	Benzodiazepines
Extrapyramidal reactions	Neuroleptics
Impairment of neuromuscular transmission	Botulinum toxin
Myopathy	Corticosteroids
Altered salivation	Anticholinergics
Decreased laryngeal cough reflex	Topical anesthetics
Postsurgical	
Denervation of the pharyngeal plexus from the pharyngeal constrictors	Anterior cervical fusion
Brain stem contusion or ischemia; cranial nerve damage	Posterior fossa surgery
Stroke	Coronary artery bypass grafting

Iatrogenic Oral/Pharyngeal Dysphagia

Iatrogenic (treatment-related) oral/pharyngeal dysphagia arises from a variety of mechanisms (Table 3.5) (Buchholz 1995). Putting aside the problems related to surgical treatment of head and neck cancer, both medications and other surgical procedures can cause neurogenic dysfunction of the oral cavity and pharynx. To consider the possibility that a patient's medication may be causing or contributing to dysphagia and to reduce or eliminate the offending agent are among the easiest and most important aspects of managing neurogenic dysphagia, but are also among the most frequently overlooked.

Sedative medications that decrease level of arousal or directly suppress brain stem functions (including control of swallowing) can exacerbate dysphagia in a patient with underlying neurologic disease, and also cause oral/pharyngeal dysfunction in an otherwise normal patient (Wyllie et al. 1986; Buchholz et al. 1995a). It has been demonstrated that, in the case of benzodiazepines, this effect is reversible, such that benzodiazepine-induced dysphagia resolves when the medication is removed (Buchholz et al. 1995a).

Dopamine antagonists, including neuroleptics (antipsychotic agents), antiemetics, and metoclopramide, can cause extrapyramidal reactions (involuntary movement disorders), including tardive dyskinesia and lingual or laryngeal dystonia (Massengil and Nashold 1969; Flaherty and Lahmeyer 1978; McDanal 1981; Menuck 1981; Craig and Richardson 1982; Samie et al. 1987; Gregory et al. 1992). Neuromuscular transmission can be depressed by systemic medications, such as aminoglycoside antibiotics, but the most common example of dysphagia caused by neuromuscular blockade is inadvertent pharyngeal weakness resulting from injection of botulinum toxin into dystonic muscles around the neck for relief of torticollis and other focal dystonias (Comella et al. 1992; Holzer and Ludlow 1996; Tuite and Lang 1996).

Myopathy is a common side effect of medications such as corticosteroids, lipid-lowering agents, amiodarone, colchicine, and L-tryptophan (Kuncl and Wiggins 1988). Anticholinergic side effects of medications, such as tricyclic antidepressants and antihistamines, include decreased salivation that may impair bolus preparation (Hughes et al. 1987; Kaplan and Baum et al. 1993). Increased salivation, which may exacerbate difficulty managing secretions in the face of neurogenic oral/pharyngeal dysphagia, can result from drugs including clonazepam, clozapine (Bazemore et al. 1995), bethanechol, and anticholinesterases. It may be that the perception of increased salivation associated with clonazepam, a benzodiazepine, represents benzodiazepine-induced depression of swallowing regulation (Buchholz 1995; Buchholz et al. 1995a) leading to decreased salivary clearance, rather than being due to increased salivary production. Topical anesthetics for procedures such as esophagoscopy temporarily suppress the laryngeal cough reflex and predispose patients to silent dysphagia. Laryngeal dysfunction is also associated with general anesthesia, endotracheal intubation, and tracheostomies (Hochman et al. 1965; Taylor and Towey 1971; Cleaton-Jones 1976; Rubin et al. 1977; Sasaki et al. 1977; Huxley et al. 1978; Bishop et al. 1984; Greenburg 1984; de Larminat et al. 1995).

A variety of forms of surgery in and around the neck have been associated with postoperative neurogenic oral/pharyngeal dysphagia. These procedures include carotid endarterectomy (Ekberg et al. 1989), ventral rhizotomy for spasmodic torticollis (Horner et al. 1992), transhiatal esophagectomy (Ong et al. 1978; Hambraeus et al. 1987; Heitmiller and Jones 1991; Buchholz et al. 1993; Hirano et al. 1993), and anterior cervical fusion (Buchholz et al. 1992). This problem may result, at least in part, from unintentional disconnection of the nerve fibers of the pharyngeal plexus from the muscle fibers of the pharyngeal constrictors, secondary to intraoperative traction and manipulation (Buchholz et al. 1995a). In some cases the weakness that results from denervation gradually resolves because of successful reinnervation, and, in some cases, recovery does not occur or is incomplete.

Surgery involving the posterior fossa (Schröter et al. 1995) or base of the skull (Levine 1988; Fenton et al. 1996) may result in damage to cranial nerves and brain stem structures, leading to dysphagia. When posterior fossa surgery is complicated by dysphagia, the problem may reflect intraoperative contusion or ischemia of the brain stem rather than damage to individual cranial nerves (Buchholz 1995; Schröter-Morasch et al. 1995). Patients undergoing surgery around the posterior fossa or base of skull should be managed postoperatively with a high degree of suspicion of dysphagia, and evidence of oral/pharyngeal impairment should provoke restriction of eating pending further evaluation, including VSS.

Perioperative stroke is not uncommon with certain cardiac surgery (Ricotta et al. 1995), and it may involve the brain stem and therefore present with dysphagia, sometimes without other brain stem deficits. The patient who awakens with dysphagia after coronary artery bypass grafting or cardiac valve replacement is too often misdiagnosed as having a problem related to endotracheal intubation, and the diagnosis of stroke is too often overlooked, especially if other brain stem deficits are not obvious or if brain MRI does not demonstrate a brain stem stroke (Buchholz 1993).

Radiation therapy to the head and neck for cancer can result in either radiation-induced nerve damage or vascular and fibrotic changes of the muscles and other soft tissues of the oral cavity and pharynx (Ekberg and Nylander 1983; Dejaeger and Goethals 1995). In these cases it is very difficult to distinguish the neurogenic aspect of the problem from the mechanical, restrictive component.

AGE-RELATED CHANGES

Changes in oral/pharyngeal performance in "normal" elderly subjects as well as symptomatic elderly individuals have been detected by some studies but not others (Ekberg and Nylander 1982; Baum and Bodner 1983; Sonies et al. 1984; Ekberg and Wahlgreen 1985; Borgström and Ekberg 1988a; Börgstrom and Ekberg 1988b; Sheth and Diner 1988; Tracy et al. 1989; Logemann 1990; Donner and Jones 1991; Ekberg and Feinberg 1991; Feinberg and Ekberg 1991; Feinberg et al. 1992; Robbins et al. 1992; Dejaeger et al. 1994; Jaradeh 1994; Shaker and Lang 1994; Wood et al. 1994; Robbins et al. 1995; Shaw et al. 1995). Despite evidence of alterations in oral and pharyngeal function in healthy older people, these individuals are asymptomatic with regard to swallowing and are able to eat unrestricted diets safely and pleasurably (Tracy et al. 1989; Robbins et al. 1992). When an elderly person develops oral/pharyngeal dysphagia it is because of medical (usually neurologic) illness, not aging alone. Most neurologic disorders of swallowing have a higher incidence among the elderly. Additionally, older individuals are more likely to have concurrent medical problems that may worsen the impact of neurogenic dysphagia. Dysphagia in an elderly person should be thoroughly evaluated, as in any patient, and should not be attributed to aging.

Psychogenic Dysphagia

Most often when a patient has symptoms of neurogenic dysphagia but no definable neurologic disorder, the inability to make a specific neurologic diagnosis reflects our limited diagnostic capabilities, and the patient does have a neurologic disorder even though we cannot ascertain it. On occasion, however, a patient complaining of symptoms consistent with neurogenic dysphagia may not have a neurologic disorder and may instead be suffering from psychological or emotional problems that are manifesting as dysphagia. This syndrome is termed "psychogenic dysphagia" (Buchholz et al. 1994). In other words, psychogenic dysphagia is difficulty swallowing, usually in a manner suggestive of neurogenic dysphagia, resulting from psychological or emotional factors as opposed to a neurologic disorder or any other physical process.

It is important to distinguish between psychogenic dysphagia and the globus symptom. Globus, also known as globus hystericus, is the sensation of a lump in the throat, typically unassociated with swallowing. Ironically, even though most physicians tend to think of globus as being a symptom of psychological or emotional problems, globus usually has a physical basis such as gastroesophageal reflux or esophageal dysmotility.

Psychogenic dysphagia is a diagnosis of exclusion, meaning that it should not be regarded as a probable diagnosis unless thorough evaluation has excluded a neurologic disorder or some other physical condition as the cause of the patient's symptoms. Nonetheless, there are certain clinical and videofluorographic features that are characteristic of psychogenic dysphagia. Patients with psychogenic dysphagia typically are otherwise physically healthy and have no known neurologic disorder. Psychogenic oral/pharyngeal dysphagia symptoms often have peculiar temporal patterns, such as fluctuating between minimal and severe symptoms. Complications of psychogenic dysphagia may include weight loss (raising the possibility that in some cases psychogenic dysphagia is a form of eating disorder) but not aspiration pneumonia. There may or may not be a background of other psychological or emotional problems.

Physical examination is normal in psychogenic dysphagia except that some patients demonstrate orolingual apraxia. This finding may also be revealed by VSS. Patients with psychogenic dysphagia sometimes behave as if they cannot swallow when they are asked to do so during VSS. In the process, they may perform complex and coordinated but nonpropulsive tongue movements that superficially appear to represent difficulty initiating swallowing but actually reveal intact orolingual sensorimotor function (Barofsky et al. 1996). The other key finding of VSS in psychogenic dysphagia is normal pharyngeal performance once the involuntary phase of swallowing is triggered. It is possible but unlikely for a neurologic disorder to cause strictly oral phase impairment, and, when that is the case, the oral phase impairment does not have the characteristics of psychogenic dysphagia as described above.

It has been suggested that when a patient has symptoms of neurogenic dysphagia but normal VSS findings, pharyngeal manometry may be able to detect pharyngeal dysfunction that may relate to the patient's symptoms (Olsson et al. 1995; Buchholz and Neumann 1996), but this is controversial. Thorough neurologic investigation should be conducted before concluding that a patient has psychogenic dysphagia. While it is essential not to overlook a neurologic disorder or some other physical problem causing oral/pharyngeal dysphagia, it is also important to consider the possibility of psychogenic dysphagia in patients with the characteristics described above; only then is there a chance to address the psychological or emotional problems that underlie the patient's complaints.

EVALUATION OF NEUROGENIC DYSPHAGIA

A careful history is the most valuable source of information leading to recognition of neurogenic dysphagia and identification of the specific underlying neurologic disorder is a careful history (Buchholz 1987b; Castell and Donner 1987). In recognizing neurogenic dysphagia, one must search for not only overt symptoms and complications of oral/pharyngeal dysphagia (see Table 3.1) but also the subtle behavioral clues of voluntary compensation in the face of dysphagia (see Table 3.3). The temporal pattern of symptoms is the most powerful indicator of the specific neurologic disorder causing neurogenic dysphagia. Acute onset, with subsequent improvement, usually means stroke, whereas MND and myopathy cause gradually progressive dysphagia.

Distinguishing between bulbar palsy and pseudobulbar palsy is a key step in establishing a specific neurologic diagnosis of neurogenic dysphagia. Bulbar and pseudobulbar palsy are clinical syndromes, not diseases, and bulbar and pseudobulbar palsy each are associated with specific diseases. Hence, distinguishing between bulbar and pseudobulbar palsy helps to distinguish among the many potential neurologic disorders associated with neurogenic dysphagia. The primary clinical features of both bulbar and pseudobulbar palsy are dysphagia and dysarthria. Bulbar palsy is the expression of a neurologic disorder involving the motor unit (that is, either the lower motor neurons in the medulla, cranial nerves, neuromuscular junctions, or muscles supplied by these neurons). Since bulbar palsy is a lower motor neuron syndrome, its features often include not only weakness of muscles supplied by the medulla but also muscle atrophy, fasciculations, and decreased reflexes (jaw jerk and gag reflex). Neurologic disorders that cause bulbar palsy include MND (when lower motor neurons of the medulla are involved), polio, Guillain-Barré syndrome, MG, and polymyositis.

Pseudobulbar palsy results from a neurologic disorder above the medulla. It is an upper motor neuron syndrome; hence, patients tend to have not only weakness of the face, tongue, pharynx, and larynx but also specific impairment of voluntary functions (that is, incoordination out of proportion to weakness), spasticity, and increased jaw jerk and gag reflex. Patients with pseudobulbar palsy often have slow, strained, effortful speech, and the palate may appear to move poorly with voluntary functions such as phonation but hyperactively when the gag reflex is triggered. Other common clinical features of pseudobulbar palsy include emotional lability and upper motor neuron signs in the limbs, including hyperreflexia, spasticity, and extensor plantar responses (Babinski's signs). Common causes of pseudobulbar palsy include bilateral hemispheral strokes, traumatic brain injury, MS, and MND (when upper rather than lower motor neurons are predominantly affected).

Further characterization of a specific neurologic disorder depends on other historic and physical findings that add up to a diagnostic pattern. For instance, myopathy is suggested by proximal limb weakness, and PD is usually (but not always) associated with bradykinesia, tremor, and shuffling gait. In any case of

Table 3.6 Evaluation of Neurogenic Dysphagia When There is No Specific Neurologic Diagnosis

Blood studies
- Complete blood counts
- Chemistry panel
- Creatine kinase
- Vitamin B_{12}
- Thyroid screening
- Anti-acetylcholine receptor antibodies
- Serologic test for syphilis

Brain magnetic resonance imaging with enhancement
Electromyography, nerve conduction studies, and repetitive nerve stimulation
Muscle biopsy*
CT of the base of the skull*
Cerebrospinal fluid examination*

*These studies are not indicated in every case but may be appropriate depending on other findings.

neurogenic dysphagia, when the neurologic diagnosis is unclear, neurologic consultation should be obtained.

VSS is useful for both evaluation and management of neurogenic dysphagia, although it is generally not very helpful in determining the specific neurologic disorder causing dysphagia. Occasionally, certain distinctive patterns of VSS findings point to certain underlying neurologic disorders. Difficulty initiating swallow is characteristic of the syndrome of pseudobulbar palsy and the various neurologic disorders that cause it. PD may cause lingual rest tremor. Intrinsic brain stem disease, such as brain stem stroke, may be associated with impaired triggering of the pharyngeal phase of swallowing, despite barium in the pharynx. Strictly unilateral pharyngeal weakness is consistent with unilateral lower cranial nerve involvement by, for example, a tumor at the base of the skull. Psychogenic dysphagia should be considered when there are complex and coordinated but nonpropulsive lingual movements during attempted swallowing, followed by normal pharyngeal performance (Barofsky et al. 1996).

Another purpose for performing VSS in evaluating neurogenic dysphagia is to look for coincident (and potentially treatable) structural or esophageal problems that may be contributing to dysphagia (Buchholz and Marsh 1986). The esophagus must be fully evaluated by fluorography in every case of neurogenic oral/pharyngeal dysphagia. Caution is advised regarding overinterpretation of the significance of anterior cervical osteophytes, for these are rarely symptomatic in terms of dysphagia (Zerhouni et al. 1987; Valadka et al. 1995; Bridger et al. 1996).

When no specific neurologic diagnosis accounts for neurogenic dysphagia, there are a number of additional studies that should routinely be considered (Table 3.6) (Buchholz 1994c). Evaluation of any type of dysphagia, including neurogenic dysphagia, is a multidisciplinary effort. Various specialties may offer valuable input into the diagnosis and treatment of a patient with neurogenic

Table 3.7 Factors Suggesting Unsafe Eating and Indicating Potential Need for Tube Feeding

Progressive or unstable neurologic disorder
Decreased level of consciousness
Decreased pulmonary reserve
Difficulty managing secretions
Coughing and choking episodes
Wet voice
Aspiration pneumonia
Laryngospasm or bronchospasm
Videofluorographic evidence of laryngeal penetration or aspiration, especially without coughing

dysphagia, including otolaryngology, gastroenterology, surgery, swallowing therapy (speech/language pathology and others), physical medicine and rehabilitation, pulmonary medicine, nutrition, dentistry, psychiatry, and psychology.

MANAGEMENT OF NEUROGENIC DYSPHAGIA

Often the foremost issue in managing neurogenic dysphagia is whether a patient needs tube feeding, either temporarily (nasogastric tube feeding) or permanently (gastrostomy or jejunostomy). The need for tube feeding is straightforward when a patient is unable to eat and drink enough to maintain adequate nutrition and hydration. The more difficult circumstance is determining the appropriateness of tube feeding when eating may be unsafe. The factors that suggest unsafe eating and argue for tube feeding are listed in Table 3-7. Other key issues in the management of neurogenic dysphagia include the following: (1) if possible, treatment of the neurologic disorder causing dysphagia (see Causes of Neurogenic Dysphagia); (2) avoidance of medications that contribute to oral/pharyngeal impairment (see Iatrogenic Dysphagia); (3) treatment of coincident esophageal or structural problems (see Chapters 5 and 11); (4) swallowing therapy (see Chapters 9–11); and (5) surgical management of dysphagia (see Chapter 14). Finally, the psychological consequences of neurogenic dysphagia, especially anxiety and depression, are potentially treatable conditions that deserve thoughtful attention.

REFERENCES

Achiron A, Kuritzky A. Dysphagia as the sole manifestation of adult type I Arnold-Chiari malformation. Neurology 1990;40:186.

Alberts MJ, Horner J, Gray L, Brazer SR. Aspiration after stroke: lesion analysis by brain MRI. Dysphagia 1992;7:170.

Ali GN, Wallace KL, Schwartz R, et al. Mechanisms of oral-pharyngeal dysphagia in patients with Parkinson's disease. Gastroenterology 1996;110:383.
American Heart Association. 1992 Heart and Stroke Facts. Dallas: American Heart Association, 1991.
Aviv JE, Martin JH, Sacco RL, et al. Supraglottic and pharyngeal sensory abnormalities in stroke patients with dysphagia. Ann Otol Rhinol Laryngol 1996;105:92.
Bach-y-Rita P. Recovery of Function: Theoretical Considerations for Brain Injury Rehabilitation. Baltimore: University Park, 1988.
Baker AB, Matzke A, Brown JR. Bulbar poliomyelitis: a study of medullary function. Arch Neurol Psychiatry 1950;63:257.
Barofsky I, Ravich W, Buchholz D, Jones B. Oral findings on video swallowing study in neurogenic and psychogenic dysphagia. Presented at the Society of Gastrointestinal Radiologists 25th Annual Meeting, Bermuda, 1996.
Bartolome G, Neumann S. Swallowing therapy in patients with neurologic disorders causing cricopharyngeal dysfunction. Dysphagia 1993;8:146.
Baum BJ, Bodner L. Aging and oral motor function: evidence for altered performance among older persons. J Dent Res 1983;62:2.
Bazemore PH, Tonkonogy J, Ananth R, Colby J. Clozapine treatment and an unusual type of dysphagia. Dysphagia 1995;10:62.
Bender MD. Esophageal manometry in oculopharyngeal dystrophy. Am J Gastroenterol 1976;65:215.
Benjamin SB, Eisold J, Gearhardt DC, Castell DO. Central nervous system lymphoma presenting as dysphagia. Dig Dis Sci 1982;27:155.
Bensimon G, Lacomblez L, Meininger V. ALS/Riluzole Study Group: a controlled trial of riluzole in amyotrophic lateral sclerosis. N Engl J Med 1994;330:585.
Bine JE, Frank EM, McDade HL. Dysphagia and dementia in subjects with Parkinson's disease. Dysphagia 1995;10:160.
Bird MR, Woodward MC, Gibson EM, et al. Asymptomatic swallowing disorders in elderly patients with Parkinson's disease: a description of findings on clinical examination and videofluoroscopy in sixteen patients. Age Ageing 1994;23:251.
Bishop M, Weymuller EA, Fink BR. Laryngeal effects of prolonged intubation. Anesth Analg 1984;63:335.
Bleck TP, Shannon KM. Disordered swallowing due to a syrinx: correction by shunting. Neurology 1984;34:1497.
Blonsky ER, Logemann JA, Boshes B, Fisher HB. Comparison of speech and swallowing function in patients with tremor disorders and in normal geriatric patients: a cinefluorographic study. J Gerontol 1975;30:299.
Borgström PS, Ekberg O. Pharyngeal dysfunction in the elderly. J Med Imaging 1988a;2:74.
Borgström PS, Ekberg O. Speed of peristalsis in pharyngeal constrictor musculature: correlations to age. Dysphagia 1988b;2:140.
Borgström PS, Olsson R, Sundkvist G, Ekberg O. Pharyngeal and oesophageal function in patients with diabetes mellitus and swallowing complaints. Br J Radiol 1988;61:817.
Bosma JF. Studies of the disabilities of the pharynx resultant from poliomyelitis. Ann Otol Rhinol Laryngol 1953;64:529.
Bosma JF, Brodie DR. Disabilities of the pharynx in amyotrophic lateral sclerosis as demonstrated by cineradiography. Radiology 1969;92:97.
Boucher RM, Hendrix RA. The otolaryngologic manifestations of multiple sclerosis. Ear Nose Throat J 1991;70:224.
Bramble MG, Cunliffe J, Dellipiani AW. Evidence for a change in neurotransmitter affecting oesophageal motility in Parkinson's disease. J Neurol Neurosurg Psychiatry 1978;41:709.
Branski D, Levy J, Globus M, et al. Dysphagia as a primary manifestation of hyperthyroidism. J Clin Gastroenterol 1984;6:437.

Bray GM, Kaarsoo M, Ross RT. Ocular myopathy with dysphagia. Dysphagia 1965;15:678.
Bridger AG, Stening WA, Bridger GP. Cervical osteophytes—an unusual cause of dysphagia. Aust N Z J Surg 1996;66:261.
Brown GE, Nordloh S, Donowitz AJ. Systematic desensitization of oral hypersensitivity in a patient with a closed head injury. Dysphagia 1992;7:138.
Buchholz D. Dysphagia in Post-Polio Patients. In LS Halstead, DO Wiechers (eds), Research and Clinical Aspects of the Late Effects of Poliomyelitis. New York: March of Dimes, 1987a.
Buchholz D. Neurologic evaluation of dysphagia. Dysphagia 1987b;1:187.
Buchholz D. Periventricular white matter changes and oropharyngeal swallowing in normal individuals [editorial]. Dysphagia 1992;7:148.
Buchholz D, Jones B. Dysphagia occurring after polio. Dysphagia 1991a;6:165.
Buchholz D, Barofsky I, Edwin D, et al. Psychogenic oropharyngeal dysphagia: report of 26 cases. Dysphagia 1994;9:267.
Buchholz D, Jones B, Neumann S, Ravich W. Benzodiazepine-induced pharyngeal dysphagia: report of two possible cases. Dysphagia 1995a;10:142.
Buchholz D, Neumann S. Comments on selected recent dysphagia literature. Dysphagia 1996;11:217.
Buchholz D, Neumann S, Jones B, Ravich W. Neurogenic dysphagia: results of swallowing center evaluation of 228 cases. Dysphagia 1995b;10:137.
Buchholz DW. Clinically-probable brainstem stroke presenting primarily as dysphagia and nonvisualized by MRI. Dysphagia 1993;8:235.
Buchholz DW. Editorial: postpolio dysphagia. Dysphagia 1994a;9:99.
Buchholz DW. Neurogenic Dysphagia. In T Bayless (ed), Current Therapy in Gastroenterology and Liver Disease (4th ed). St. Louis: Mosby, 1994b.
Buchholz DW. Neurogenic dysphagia: what is the cause when the cause is not obvious? Dysphagia 1994c;9:245.
Buchholz DW. Oropharyngeal dysphagia due to iatrogenic neurological dysfunction. Dysphagia 1995;10:248.
Buchholz DW. Esophageal dysfunction due to neurological disorders. Dysphagia 1996;11:30.
Buchholz DW, Bosma JF, Donner MW. Adaptation, compensation and decompensation of the pharyngeal swallow. Gastrointest Radiol 1985;10:235.
Buchholz DW, Jones B. Post-polio dysphagia: alarm or caution? J Orthop 1991b;14:1303.
Buchholz DW, Jones B, Ravich, WJ. Dysphagia following anterior cervical fusion [abstract]. Presented at Dysphagia Research Society, First Annual Meeting, Milwaukee, 1992.
Buchholz DW, Jones B, Ravich WJ. Dysphagia following anterior cervical fusion. Dysphagia 1993;8:390.
Buchholz DW, Marsh BR. Multifactorial dysphagia: looking for a second, treatable cause. Dysphagia 1986;1:88.
Buckler RA, Pratter MR, Chad DA, Smith TW. Chronic cough as the presenting symptom of oculopharyngeal muscular dystrophy. Chest 1989;95:921.
Burakoff R, Rubinow A, Cohen AS. Esophageal manometry in familial amyloid polyneuropathy. Am J Med 1985;79:85.
Bushmann M, Dobmeyer SM, Leeker L, Perlmutter JS. Swallowing abnormalities and their response to treatment in Parkinson's disease. Neurology 1989;39:1309.
Carpenter R, McDonald T, Howard F. The otolaryngologic presentation of myasthenia gravis. Laryngoscope 1979;89:922.
Casas MJ, Kenny DJ, McPherson KA. Swallowing/ventilation interactions during oral swallow in normal children and children with cerebral palsy. Dysphagia 1994;9:40.
Casey E, Aminoff M. Dystrophica myotonia presenting with dysphagia. Br Med J 1971;2[Suppl]:443.

Castell DO, Donner MW. Evaluation of dysphagia: a careful history is crucial. Dysphagia 1987;2:65.

Castell JA, Castell DO, Duranceau CA, Topart P. Manometric characteristics of the pharynx, upper esophageal sphincter, esophagus and lower esophageal sphincter in patients with oculopharyngeal muscular dystrophy. Dysphagia 1995;10:22.

Castell JA, Li Q, Gideon RM, et al. Esophageal dysfunction in Parkinson's disease. Gastroenterology 1994;106:A60.

Catalanotto FA, Dore-Duffy P, Donaldson J, et al. Quality specific taste changes in multiple sclerosis. Ann Neurol 1984;16:611.

Celifarco A, Gerard G, Faegenburg D, Burakoff R. Dysphagia as the sole manifestation of bilateral strokes. Am J Gastroenterol 1990;85:610.

Channer KS, Jackson PC, O'Brien I, et al. Oesophageal function in diabetes mellitus and its association with autonomic neuropathy. Diabet Med 1985;2:378.

Chen MY, Ott DJ, Peele VN, Gelfand DW. Oropharynx in patients with cerebrovascular disease: Evaluation with videofluoroscopy. Radiology 1990;176:641.

Chen MYM, Donofrio PD, Frederick MG, et al. Videofluoroscopic evaluation of patients with Guillain-Barré syndrome. Dysphagia 1996;11:11.

Chen MYM, Peele VN, Donalt D, et al. Clinical and videofluoroscopic evaluation of swallowing in 41 patients with neurologic disease. Gastrointest Radiol 1992; 17:95.

Christensen J. Esophageal manometry in myxedema. Gastroenterology 1967;52:1130.

Chua KSG, Kong KH. Functional outcome in brain stem stroke patients after rehabilitation. Arch Phys Med Rehabil 1996;77:194.

Cleaton-Jones P. The laryngeal-closure reflex and nitrous oxide analgesia. Anesthesiology 1976;45:569.

Coelho CA, Ferrante R. Dysphagia in post-polio sequelae: report of three cases. Arch Phys Med Rehabil 1988;69:634.

Comella CL, Tanner CM, DeFoor-Hill L, Smith C. Dysphagia after botulinum toxin injections for spasmodic torticollis. Neurology 1992;42:1307.

Cook RE. Progressive bulbar palsy due to syphilis. Am J Syphilis Gonorrhea Venereal Diseases 1953;37:161.

Cornil L. Sur un case de paralysie generale spinale anterieure subaigue, suivi d'autopsie. Gaz Med (Paris) 1875;4:127.

Cotman CW. Synaptic Plasticity. New York: Guilford, 1985.

Craig TJ, Richardson MA. Swallowing, tardive dyskinesia, and anticholinergics. Am J Psychiatry 1982;139:1083.

Croxson SCM, Pye I. Dysphagia as the presenting feature in Parkinson's disease. Geriatr Med 1988;8:16.

Cunningham J, Lowry L. Head and neck manifestations of dermatomyositis-poliomyositis. Otolaryngol Head Neck Surg 1985;93:673.

Dalakas MC, Elder G, Hallett M, et al. A long-term follow-up study of patients with post-poliomyelitis neuromuscular symptoms. N Engl J Med 1986;314:959.

Daly DD, Code CF, Anderson HA. Disturbances of swallowing and esophageal motility in patients with multiple sclerosis. Neurology 1962;12:250.

Darrow DH, Hoffman HT, Barnes GJ, Wiley CA. Management of dysphagia in inclusion body myositis. Arch Otolaryngol Head Neck Surg 1992;118:313.

Davies AE, Kidd D, Stone, SP, MacMahon J. Pharyngeal sensation and gag reflex in healthy subjects. Lancet 1995;345:487.

de Larminat V, Montravers P, Dureuil B, Desmonts J-M. Alteration in swallowing reflex after extubation in intensive care unit patients. Crit Care Med 1995;23:486.

Dejaeger E, Goethals P. Deglutition disorder as a late sequel of radiotherapy for a pharyngeal tumor. Am J Gastroenterol 1995;90:493.

Dejaeger E, Pelemans W, Bibau G, Ponette E. Manofluorographic analysis of swallowing in the elderly. Dysphagia 1994;9:156.

Dietz F, Logemann JA, Sahgal V, Schmid FR. Cricopharyngeal muscle dysfunction in the differential diagnosis of dysphagia in polymyositis. Arthritis Rheum 1980;23:491.

Dobrowski JM, Zajtchuk JT, LaPiana FG, Hensley SD. Oculopharyngeal muscular dystrophy: clinical and histopathological correlations. Otolaryngol Head Neck Surg 1986;95:131.

Donner MW. Swallowing mechanism and neuromuscular disorders. Semin Roentgenol 1974;3:273.

Donner MW, Jones B. Aging and Neurological Disease. In B Jones, MW Donner (eds), Normal and Abnormal Swallowing: Imaging in Diagnosis and Therapy. New York: Springer, 1991.

Duranceau CA, Letendre J, Clermont RJ, et al. Oropharyngeal dysphagia in patients with oculopharyngeal muscular dystrophy. Can J Surg 1978;21:326.

Dworkin JP, Hartman DE. Progressive speech deterioration and dysphagia in amyotrophic lateral sclerosis: case report. Arch Phys Med Rehabil 1979;60:423.

Eastwood GL, Braverman LE, White EM, Vander Salm TJ. Reversal of lower esophageal sphincter hypotension and esophageal aperistalsis after treatment for hypothyroidism. J Clin Gastroenterol 1982;4:307.

Eckardt VF, Nix W, Kraus W, Bohl J. Esophageal motor function in patients with muscular dystrophy. Gastroenterology 1986;90:628.

Edmonds C. Huntington's chorea, dysphagia and death. Med J Aust 1966;53:273.

Edwards JW, Murray JP. Barium swallow examination in myasthenia gravis. Br J Radiol 1957;30:263.

Edwards LL, Pfeiffer RF, Quigley EMM, et al. Gastrointestinal symptoms in Parkinson's disease. Mov Disord 1991;6:151.

Edwards LL, Quigley EMM, Pfeiffer RF. Gastrointestinal dysfunction in Parkinson's disease. Neurology 1992;42:726.

Ekberg O, Bergqvist D, Takolander R, et al. Pharyngeal function after carotid endarterectomy. Dysphagia 1989;4:151.

Ekberg O, Feinberg MJ. Altered swallowing function in elderly patients with dysphagia: radiographic findings in 56 patients. AJR Am J Roentgenol 1991;156:1181.

Ekberg O, Nylander G. Cineradiography of the pharyngeal stage of deglutition in 150 individuals without dysphagia. Br J Radiol 1982;55:255.

Ekberg O, Nylander G. Pharyngeal dysfunction after treatment for pharyngeal cancer with surgery and radiotherapy. Gastrointest Radiol 1983;8:97.

Ekberg O, Wahlgreen L. Pharyngeal dysfunctions and their interrelationship in patients with dysphagia. Acta Radiol 1985;26:659.

Elta GH, Caldwell CA, Nostrant TT. Esophageal dysphagia as the sole symptom in Type I Chiari malformation. Dig Dis Sci 1996;41:512.

Feinberg MJ, Ekberg O. Videofluoroscopy in elderly patients with aspiration: importance of evaluating both oral and pharyngeal stages of deglutition. AJR Am J Roentgenol 1991;156:293.

Feinberg MJ, Ekberg O, Segall L, Tully J. Deglutition in elderly patients with dementia: findings of videofluorographic evaluation and impact on staging and management. Radiology 1992;183:811.

Feinberg MJ, Knebl J, Tully J. Prandial aspiration and pneumonia in an elderly population followed over 3 years. Dysphagia 1996;11:104.

Fenton JE, Brake H, Shirazi A, et al. The management of dysphagia in jugular foramen surgery. J Laryngol Otol 1996;110:144.

Fernandez F, Leno C, Commbarros O, Berciano J. Cricopharyngeal dysfunction due to syringobulbia. Neurology 1986;36:1635.

Finger S, Stein DG. Brain Damage and Recovery: Research and Clinical Perspectives. New York: Academic, 1982.

Fischer RA, Ellison GW, Thayer WR, et al. Esophageal motility in neuromuscular disorders. Ann Intern Med 1965;63:229.

Flaherty JA, Lahmeyer HW. Laryngeal-pharyngeal dystonia as a possible cause of asphyxia with haloperidol treatment. Am J Psychiatry 1978;135:1414.
Fonda D, Schwarz J. Parkinsonian medication one hour before meals improves symptomatic swallowing: a case study. Dysphagia 1995;10:165.
Frank Y, Schwartz SB, Epstein NE, Beresford HR. Chronic dysphagia, vomiting and gastroesophageal reflux as manifestations of a brainstem glioma: a case report. Pediatr Neurosci 1989;15:265.
Fuh J-L, Lee R-C, Wang S-J, et al. Swallowing abnormalities in Parkinson's disease. Neurology 1995;45:(Suppl 4):A338.
Gibberd FB, Gleeson JA, Gossagfe AAR, Wilson RSE. Oesophageal dilatation in Parkinson's disease. J Neurol Neurosurg Psychiatry 1974;37:938.
Gilat T, Spiro HM. Amyloidosis and the gut. Am J Dig Dis 1968;13:619.
Gisel EG. Oral-motor skills following sensorimotor intervention in the moderately eating-impaired child with cerebral palsy. Dysphagia 1994;9:180.
Gisel EG, Applegate-Ferrante BA, Benson J, Bosma JF. Oral-motor skills following sensorimotor therapy in two groups of moderately dysphagic children with cerebral palsy: aspiration vs nonaspiration. Dysphagia 1996;11:59.
Greenberg DJ. The incidence of aspiration in patients with tracheostomies. Anesth Analg 1984;63:1142.
Gregory RP, Smith PT, Rudge P. Tardive dyskinesia presenting as severe dysphagia. J Neurol Neurosurg Psychiatry 1992;55:1203.
Gresham SL. Clinical assessment and management of swallowing difficulties after stroke. Med J Aust 1990;153:397.
Groher ME, Bukatinan R. The prevalence of swallowing disorders in two teaching hospitals. Dysphagia 1986;1:3.
Grunebaum M, Salinger H. Radiological findings in polymyositis-dermatomyositis involving the pharynx and upper oesophagus. Clin Radiol 1971;22:97.
Gulyas AE, Salazar-Grueso EF. Pharyngeal dysmotility in a patient with Wilson's disease. Dysphagia 1988;2:230.
Halstead LS, Wiechers DO, Rossi CD. Late Effects of Poliomyelitis: A National Survey. In LS Halstead, DO Wiechers (eds), Late Effects of Poliomyelitis. Miami, Symposia Foundation, 1985.
Hambraeus GM, Ekberg O, Fletcher R. Pharyngeal dysfunction after total and subtotal oesophagectomy. Acta Radiol 1987;28:409.
Hardy WE, Tulgan H, Haidak G, Budnitz J. Sarcoidosis: a case presenting with dysphagia and dysphonia. Ann Intern Med 1967;66:353.
Harvey JC, Sherbourne DH, Siegel CI. Smooth muscle involvement in myotonic dystrophy. Am J Med 1965;39:810.
Heitmiller RF, Jones B. Transient diminished airway protection following transhiatal esophagectomy. Am J Surg 1991;162:422.
Helfrich-Miller KR, Rector KL, Straka JA. Dysphagia: its treatment in the profoundly retarded patient with cerebral palsy. Arch Phys Med Rehabil 1993;74:178.
Hewer RL, Wade DJ. Dysphagia in acute stroke. Br Med J 1987;295:411.
Hillarp B, Ekberg O, Jacobsson S, Nylander G, Åberg M. Myotonic dystrophy revealed at videoradiography of deglutition and speech in adult patients with velopharyngeal insufficiency: presentation of four cases. Cleft Palate Craniofac J 1994;31:125.
Hirano M, Tanaka S, Fujita M, Fujita H. Vocal cord paralysis caused by esophageal cancer surgery. Ann Otol Rhinol Laryngol 1993;102:182.
Hochman RA, Martin JT, Devine KD. Anesthesia and the larynx. Surg Clin North Am 1965;45:1031.
Hoehn MM, Yahr M. Parkinsonism: onset, progression and mortality. Neurology 1967;17:427.
Hollis JB, Castell DO, Braddon RL. Esophageal function in diabetes mellitus and its relation to peripheral neuropathy. Gastroenterology 1977;73:1098.

Holzer SES, Ludlow CL. The swallowing side effects of botulinum toxin type A injection in spasmodic dysphonia. Laryngoscope 1996;106:86.

Horner J, Alberts M, Dawson D, Cook G. Swallowing in Alzheimer's disease. Alzheimer's Dis Assoc Disord 1994;8:1.

Horner J, Buoyer FG, Alberts MJ, Helms MJ. Dysphagia following brain-stem stroke: clinical correlates and outcome. Arch Neurol 1991;48:1170.

Horner J, Massey EW. Silent aspiration following stroke. Neurology 1988;38:317.

Horner J, Massey EW, Brazer SR. Aspiration in bilateral stroke patients. Neurology 1988a;40:1686.

Horner J, Massey EW, Riski JE, et al. Aspiration following stroke: clinical correlates and outcome. Neurology 1988b;38:1359.

Horner J, Riski JE, Ovelmen-Levitt J, Nashold BS. Swallowing in torticollis before and after rhizotomy. Dysphagia 1992;7:117.

Horner J, Riski JE, Weber BA, Nashold BS. Swallowing, speech and brainstem auditory-evoked potentials in spasmodic torticollis. Dysphagia 1993;8:29.

Horowitz M, McNeil JD, Maddern GJ, et al. Abnormalities of gastric and esophageal emptying in polymyositis and dermatomyositis. Gastroenterology 1986;90:434.

Hughes CV, Baum BJ, Cox PC, et al. Oropharyngeal dysphagia: a common sequel of salivary gland dysfunction. Dysphagia 1987;1:173.

Hughes DTD, Swann JC, Gleeson JA, Lee FI. Abnormalities in swallowing associated with dystrophica myotonica. Brain 1965;88:1037.

Hutchins B. Establishing a dysphagia family intervention program for head-injured patients. J Head Trauma Rehabil 1989;4:64.

Huxley EJ, Viroslav J, Gray WR, Pierce AK. Pharyngeal aspiration in normal adults and patients with depressed consciousness. Am J Med 1978;64:565.

Ikusaka M, Iwata M, Sasaki S, Uchiyama S. Progressive dysphagia due to adult Chiari I malformation mimicking amyotrophic lateral sclerosis. J Neurol Neurosurg Psychiatry 1996;60:357.

Ivanyi B, Phoa SSKS, de Visser M. Dysphagia in post-polio patients: a videofluorographic follow-up study. Dysphagia 1994;9:96.

Jacob H, Berkowitz D, McDonald E, et al. The esophageal motility disorder of polymyositis: a prospective study. Arch Intern Med 1983;143:2262.

Jaradeh S. Neurophysiology of swallowing in the aged. Dysphagia 1994;9:218.

Johnson ER, McKenzie SW, Rosenquist CJ, et al. Dysphagia following stroke: quantitative evaluation of pharyngeal transit times. Arch Phys Med Rehabil 1992;73:419.

Johnston BJ, Castell JA, Colcerh A, et al. Component of swallowing function in Parkinson's disease (PD) and progressive supranuclear palsy (PSP). Gastroenterology 1995a;108:A124.

Johnston BT, Li Q, Castell JA, Castell DO. Swallowing and esophageal function in Parkinson's disease. Am J Gastroenterol 1995b;90:1741.

Jones B, Buchholz DW, Ravich WJ, Donner MW. Swallowing dysfunction in the postpolio syndrome: a cineradiographic study. AJR Am J Roentgenol 1992;158:283.

Jones B, Donner MW. Examination of the patient with dysphagia. Radiology 1988;167:319.

Kagel MC, Leopold NA. Dysphagia in Huntington's disease: a 16-year retrospective. Dysphagia 1992;7:106.

Kagen LJ, Hochman RB, Strong EW. Cricopharyngeal obstruction in inflammatory myopathy (polymyositis/dermatomyositis). Arthritis Rheum 1985;28:630.

Kahrilas PJ. The Anatomy and Physiology of Dysphagia. In DW Gelfard, JE Richter (eds), Dysphagia: Diagnosis and Treatment. New York: Igaku-Shoin, 1989.

Kakigi R, Shibasaki H, Kuroda Y, et al. Meige's syndrome associated with spasmodic dysphagia. J Neurol Neurosurg Psychiatry 1983;46:589.

Kaplan MD, Baum BJ. The functions of saliva. Dysphagia 1993;8:225.

Kasarskis EJ, Berryman S, Vanderleest JG, et al. Nutritional status of patients with amyotrophic lateral sclerosis—relation to the proximity of death. Am J Clin Nutr 1996;63:130.
Kelle ML. Dysphagia and motor failure of the esophagus in myotonia dystrophica. Neurology 1964;14:955.
Kempster PA, Lees AJ, Crichton P, et al. Off-period belching due to a reversible disturbance of esophageal motility in Parkinson's disease and its treatment with apomorphine. Mov Disord 1989;4:47.
Kenny DJ, Koheil RM, Greenberg J, et al. Development of multidisciplinary feeding profile for children who are dependent feeders. Dysphagia 1994;9:209.
Kidd D, Lawson J, Nesbit R, MacMahon J. Aspiration in acute stroke: clinical study with videofluoroscopy. Q J Med 1993;86:825.
Kiel DP. Oculopharyngeal muscular dystrophy as a cause of dysphagia in the elderly. J Am Gastroenterol Soc 1986;34:144.
Kim WS, Buchholz D, Kumar AJ, et al. Magnetic resonance imaging for evaluating neurogenic dysphagia. Dysphagia 1987;2:40.
Kuhlemeier KV. Epidemiology and dysphagia. Dysphagia 1994;9:209.
Kuncl RW, Wiggins WW. Toxic myopathies. Neurol Clin 1988;6:593.
Lazarus CL. Swallowing disorders after traumatic brain injury. J Head Trauma Rehabil 1989;4:34.
Lazarus CL, Logemann JA. Swallowing disorders in closed head trauma patients. Arch Phys Med Rehabil 1987;69:79.
Lebo CP, Sang K, Norris FH. Cricopharyngeal myotomy in amyotrophic lateral sclerosis. Laryngoscope 1976;86:862.
Leder SB. Gag reflex and dysphagia. Head Neck 1996;18:138.
Leopold NA, Kagel MC. Dysphagia in Huntington's disease. Arch Neurol 1985;42:57.
Leopold NA, Kagel MC. Prepharyngeal dysphagia in Parkinson's Disease. Dysphagia 1996;11:14.
Levine R, Robbins J, Maser A. Periventricular white matter changes and oropharyngeal swallowing in normal individuals. Dysphagia 1991;7:142.
Levine TM. Swallowing disorders following skull base surgery. Otolaryngol Clin North Am 1988;21:751.
Li Q, Gideon MR, Castell JA, Hurtig H, et al. Manometric evaluation of Sinemet effect on esophageal function in Parkinson's disease. Gastroenterology 1994;106:530.
Lieberman AN, Horowitz L, Redmond P, et al. Dysphagia in Parkinson's disease. Am J Gastroenterol 1980;74:157.
Linden P, Kuhlemeier KV, Patterson C. The probability of correctly predicting subglottic penetration from clinical observations. Dysphagia 1993;8:170.
Linden P, Siebens A. Dysphagia: predicting laryngeal penetration. Arch Phys Med Rehabil 1983;64:281.
Logemann JA. Dysphagia in Movement Disorders. In J Jankovic, E Tolosa (eds), Advances in Neurology 1988;307.
Logemann JA. Effects of aging on the swallowing mechanism. Otolaryngol Clin North Am 1990;23:1045.
Logemann JA, Shanahan T, Rademaker AW, et al. Oropharyngeal swallowing after stroke in the left basal ganglion/internal capsule. Dysphagia 1993;8:230.
Loo FD, Dodds WJ, Doergel KH, Arndorfer RC, Helm JF, Hogan WJ. Multipeaked esophageal peristaltic pressure waves in patients with diabetic neuropathy. Gastroenterology 1985a;88:485.
Loo FD, Soergel KH, Dodds WJ. Reply. Gastroenterology 1985b;89:480.
Lueck W, Galligan J, Bosma JF. Persistent sequelae of bulbar poliomyelitis. J Pediatr 1952;41:549.
Mackay L, Morgan AS. Early swallowing disorders with severe head injuries: relationships between RLA and the progression of oral intake. Dysphagia 1993;8:161.

Mandelstam P, Siegel CI, Lieber A, Siegel M. The swallowing disorder in patients with diabetic neuropathy-gastroenteropathy. Gastroenterology 1969;56:1.
Martin BJW, Corlew MM, Wood H, et al. The association of swallowing dysfunction and aspiration pneumonia. Dysphagia 1994;9:1.
Massengil R, Nashold B. A swallowing disorder denoted in tardive dyskinesia patients. Acta Otolaryngol (Stockh) 1969;68:457.
Massey CE, El Gammal T, Brooks BS. Giant posterior inferior cerebellar artery aneurysm with dysphagia. Surg Neurol 1984;22:467.
McDanal CE. Haloperidol and laryngeal-pharyngeal dystonia. Am J Psychiatry 1981;138:1262.
Meadows JC. Dysphagia in unilateral cerebral lesions. J Neurol Neurosurg Psychiatry 1973;36:853.
Menuck M. Laryngeal-pharyngeal dystonia and haloperidol. Am J Psychiatry 1981;139:304.
Meshkinpour H, Afrasiabi MA, Valenta LJ. Esophageal motor function in Graves' disease. Dig Dis Sci 1979;24:159.
Metheny J. Dermatomyositis: a vocal and swallowing disease entity. Laryngoscope 1978;88:147.
Meyer T, Logemann JA, Jubelt B. Nature of swallowing disorders in amyotrophic lateral sclerosis. J Am Speech Hearing Assoc 1985;276:123.
Mirrett PL, Riski JE, Glascott J, Johnson V. Videofluorographic assessment of dysphagia in children with severe spastic cerebral palsy. Dysphagia 1994;9:174.
Morris S. Program Guidelines for Children with Feeding Problems. Edison, NJ: Childcraft, 1982.
Mulder DW, Rosenbaum RA, Layton DD. Late progression of poliomyelitis or forme fruste amyotrophic lateral sclerosis? Mayo Clin Proc 1972;47:756.
Murray JP. Deglutition in myasthenia gravis. Br J Radiol 1962;35:43.
Neumann S. Swallowing therapy with neurologic patients: results of direct and indirect therapy methods in 66 patients suffering from neurologic disorders. Dysphagia 1993;8:150.
Neumann S, Bartolome G, Buchholz D, Prosiegel M. Swallowing therapy of neurologic patients: correlation of outcome with pretreatment variables and therapeutic methods. Dysphagia 1995a;10:1.
Neumann S, Buchholz D, Jones B, Palmer J. Pharyngeal dysfunction after lateral medullary infarction is bilateral: review of 15 additional cases. Dysphagia 1995b;10:136.
Neumann S, Buchholz D, Wuttge-Hannig A, et al. Bilateral pharyngeal dysfunction after lateral medullary infarction. Dysphagia 1994;9:263.
Neumann S, Reich S, Buchholz D, et al. Progressive supranuclear palsy (PSP): characteristics of dysphagia in 14 patients. Dysphagia 1996;11:164.
Newton HB, Newton C, Pearl D, Davidson T. Swallowing assessment in primary brain tumor patients with dysphagia. Neurology 1994;44:1927.
Nilsson H, Ekberg O, Olsson R, Hindfelt B. Quantitative assessment of oral and pharyngeal function in Parkinson's disease. Dysphagia 1996;11:144.
Norbert A, Norberg B, Bexell G. Ethical problems in feeding patients with advanced dementia. Br Med J 1980;281:847.
O'Connor A, Ardran C. Cinefluorography in the diagnosis of pharyngeal palsies. J Laryngol Otol 1976;90:1015.
O'Hara JM, Szemes G, Lowman RM. The esophageal lesions in dermatomyositis: a correlation of radiographic and pathologic findings. Radiology 1967;89:27.
Ogg HL. Oral-pharyngeal development and evaluation. Phys Ther 1975;55:235.
Olsson R, Castell JA, Castell DO, Ekberg O. Solid-state computerized manometry improves diagnostic yield in pharyngeal dysphagia: simultaneous videoradiography and manometry in dysphagia patients with normal barium swallows. Abdom Imaging 1995;20:230.

Ong GB, Lam KH, Lam PHM, Wong J. Resection for carcinoma of the superior mediastinal segment of the esophagus. World J Surg 1978;2:497.
Ottenbacher K, Bundy A, Short MA. The development and treatment of oral-motor dysfunction: A review of clinical research. Phys Occup Ther Pediatr 1983;3:1.
Palmer JB, DuChane AS. Rehabilitation of swallowing disorders due to stroke. Arch Phys Med Rehabil Clin North Am 1991;2:529.
Parrott LC, Selley WG, Brooks WA, et al. Dysphagia in cerebral palsy: a comparative study of the Exeter dysphagia assessment technique and a multidisciplinary assessment. Dysphagia 1992;7:209.
Pierce JW, Creamer B, MacDermott V. Pharynx and oesophagus in dystrophica myotonica. Gut 1965;6:392.
Pollack IF, Pang D, Kocoshis S, Putman P. Neurogenic dysphagia resulting from Chiari malformations. Neurosurgery 1992;30:709.
Qualman SJ, Haupt HM, Yang P, Hamilton SR. Esophageal Lewy bodies associated with ganglion cell loss in achalasia: similarity to Parkinson's disease. Gastroenterology 1984;87:848.
Richter JE, Wo WC-L, Castell DO. Double-peaked contraction waves—a variant of normal [letter]. Gastroenterology 1985;89:479.
Ricotta JJ, Saggioli GL, Castilone A, Hassett JM. Risk factors for stroke after cardiac surgery: Buffalo Cardiac-Cerebral Study Group. J Vasc Surg 1995;21:359.
Riminton DS, Chambers ST, Parkin PJ, et al. Inclusion body myositis presenting solely as dysphagia. Neurology 1993;43:1241.
Riski JR, Horner J, Nashold BS. Swallowing function in patients with spasmodic torticollis. Neurology 1990;40:1443.
Robbins J. Swallowing in ALS and motor neuron disorders. Neurol Clin 1987;5:213.
Robbins J, Hamilton J, Lof G, Kempster G. Oropharyngeal swallowing in normal adults of different ages. Gastroenterology 1992;103:823.
Robbins J, Levine RL. Swallowing after unilateral stroke of the cerebral cortex: preliminary evidence. Dysphagia 1988;3:11.
Robbins JR, Levine RL, Maser AM, et al. Swallowing after unilateral stroke of the cerebral cortex. Arch Phys Med Rehabil 1993;74:1295.
Robbins JR, Levine RL, Wood JW, et al. Age effects on lingual pressure generation as a risk factor for dysphagia. Gerontology 1995;5:M257.
Robbins J, Logemann JA, Kirshner HS. Swallowing and speech production in Parkinson's disease. Ann Neurol 1986;19:283.
Roberts AH, Bamforth J. The pharynx and esophagus in ocular muscular dystrophy. Neurology 1968;18:645.
Rogers B, Arvedson J, Buck G, Smart P, Msall M. Characteristics of dysphagia in children with cerebral palsy. Dysphagia 1994;9:69.
Rubin J, Brock-Utne JG, Greenberg M, et al. Laryngeal incompetence during experimental "relative analgesia" using 50% nitrous oxide oxygen. A preliminary report. Br J Anaesth 1977;49:1005.
Russell COH, Gannan R, Coatsworth J, et al. Relationship among esophageal dysfunction, diabetic gastroenteropathy, and peripheral neuropathy. Dig Dis Sci 1983;28:289.
Salvesen R, Brautaset NJ. Oculopharyngeal muscular dystrophy in Norway—survey of a large Norwegian family. Acta Neurolog Scand 1996;93:281.
Samie MR, Dannenhoffer MA, Rozek S. Life-threatening tardive dyskinesia caused by metoclopramide. Mov Disord 1987;2:125.
Sasaki CT, Suzuki M, Horiuchi M, Kirchner JA. The effect of tracheostomy on the laryngeal closure reflex. Laryngoscope 1977;87:1428.
Schmidt J, Holas M, Harvorson K, Reding M. Videofluoroscopic evidence of aspiration predicts pneumonia and death but not dehydration following stroke. Dysphagia 1994;9:7.

Schneider JS, Diamond SG, Markham CH. Deficits in orofacial sensorimotor function in Parkinson's disease. Ann Neurol 1985;19:275.

Schröter-Morasch H, Winkler R, Lumenta C. Dysphagia after posterior fossa tumor surgery. Dysphagia 1995;10:139.

Shaker R, Lang IM. Effect of aging on the deglutitive oral, pharyngeal, and esophageal motor function. Dysphagia 1994;9:221.

Shapiro J, Martin S. Inflammatory myopathy causing pharyngeal dysphagia: a new entity. Ann Otol Rhinol Laryngol 1996;105:331.

Shaw DW, Cook IJ, Gabb M, et al. Influence of normal aging on oral-pharyngeal and upper esophageal sphincter function during swallowing. Am J Physiol Gastrointest Liver Physiol 1995;31:G 389.

Sheth N, Diner WC. Swallowing problems in the elderly. Dysphagia 1988;2:209.

Siegel CI, Hendrix TR, Harvey JC. The swallowing disorder in myotonia dystrophica. Gastroenterology 1966;50:541.

Silber W. Diabetes and oesophageal dysfunction. Br Med J 1969;3:688.

Silbergleit AK, Waring WP, Sullivan MJ, Maynard FM. Evaluation, treatment and follow-up results of post-polio patients with dysphagia. Otolaryngol Head Neck Surg 1991;104:333.

Silbiger ML, Pikielney R, Donner MW. Neuromuscular disorders affecting the pharynx: cineradiographic analysis. Invest Radiol 1967;2:442.

Simpson AJ, Kilnani MT. Gastrointestinal manifestations of the muscular dystrophies: a review of roentgen findings. Am J Radiol 1975;125:948.

Smith AW, Mulder D, Code C. Esophageal motility in amyotrophic lateral sclerosis. Mayo Clin Proc 1957;32:438.

Sonies BC. Swallowing and Speech Disturbances. In I Litvan, Y Agid (eds), Progressive Supranuclear Palsy: Clinical and Research Approaches. New York: Oxford University Press, 1992.

Sonies BC, Dalakas MC. Dysphagia in patients with the post-polio syndrome. N Engl J Med 1991;324:1162.

Sonies BC, Tone M, Shawker T. Speech and swallowing in the elderly. Gerodontology 1984;3:115.

Speier JL, Owen RR, Knapp M, Canine JK. Occurrence of Post-Polio Sequelae in an Epidemic Population. In LS Halstead, DO Wiechers (eds), Late Effects of Poliomyelitis. Miami: Symposia Foundation, 1985.

Stewart IM, Hosking DJ, Preston BJ, Atkinson M. Oesophageal motor changes in diabetes mellitus. Thorax 1976;31:278.

Strand EA, Miller RM, Yorkston KM, Hillel AD. Management of oral pharyngeal dysphagia symptoms in amyotrophic lateral sclerosis. Dysphagia 1996;11:129.

Straube A, Witt TN. Oculo-bulbar myasthenic symptoms as the sole sign of tumor involving or compressing the brain stem. J Neurol 1990;237:369.

Stroudley J, Walsh M. Radiological assessment of dysphagia in Parkinson's disease. Br J Radiol 1991;64:890.

Stübgen J-P. Limb girdle muscular dystrophy: a radiologic and manometric study of the pharynx and esophagus. Dysphagia 1996;11:25.

Sullivan RJ. Accepting death without artificial nutrition or hydration. J Gen Intern Med 1993;8:220.

Swick HM, Werlin SL, Doods WJ, Hogan WJ. Pharyngoesophageal motor function in patients with myotonic dystrophy. Ann Neurol 1981;10:454.

Taylor PA, Towey RM. Depression of laryngeal reflexes during ketamine anesthesia. Br Med J 1971;2:688.

Teasell RW, Bach D, McRae M. Prevalence and recovery of aspiration poststroke: a retrospective analysis. Dysphagia 1994;9:35.

Tepid DC, Palmer JB, Linden P. Management of dysphagia in a patient with closed head injury: a case report. Dysphagia 1987;1:221.

Tracy JF, Logemann JA, Kahrilas PJ, Jet al. Preliminary observations on the effects of age on oropharyngeal deglutition. Dysphagia 1989;4:90.

Tuite PJ, Lang AE. Severe and prolonged dysphagia complicating botulinum toxin A injections for dystonia in Machado-Joseph disease. Neurology 1996;46:846.

Valadka AB, Kubal WS, Smith MM. Updated management strategy for patients with cervical osteophytic dysphagia. Dysphagia 1995;10:167.

Vannini P, Ciavarella A, Corbelli C, et al. Oesophageal transit time and cardiovascular neuropathy in type 1 (insulin-dependent) diabetes mellitus. Diabetes Res 1989;11:21.

Veis SL, Logemann JA. Swallowing disorders in persons with cerebrovascular accident. Arch Phys Med Rehabil 1985;66:372.

Vela AR, Balart LA. Esophageal motor manifestations in diabetes mellitus. Am J Surg 1970;119:21.

Vencovsky J, Rehak F, Pafko P, et al. Acute cricopharyngeal obstruction in dermatomyositis. J Rheumatol 1988;15:1016.

Vix VA. Esophageal motility in diabetes mellitus. Radiology 1969;92:363.

Volicer L, Seltzer B, Rheaume Y, et al. Eating difficulties in patients with probable dementia of the Alzheimer type. J Geriatr Psychiatry Neurol 1989;2:188.

Wade D, Hewer L. Motor loss and swallowing difficulty after stroke: frequency, recovery and prognosis. Acta Neurol Scand 1987;76:50.

Weir RF, Grostin L. Decisions to abate life-sustaining treatment for non-autonomous patients. JAMA 1990;264:1846.

Weitzner S. Changes in the pharyngeal and esophageal musculature in oculopharyngeal muscular dystrophy. Am J Dig Dis 1969;14:805.

Westin L, Lilja B, Sundkvist G. Esophagus scintigraphy in patients with diabetes mellitus. Scand J Gastroenterol 1986;21:1200.

Wilson PS, Bruce-Lockhart FJ, Johnson AP. Videofluoroscopy in motor neurone disease prior to cricopharyngeal myotomy. Ann R Coll Surg Engl 1990;72:345.

Windebank AJ, Litchy WJ, Daube JR, Iverson RA. Lack of progression of neurologic deficit in survivors of paralytic polio: a 5-year prospective population-based study. Neurology 1996;46:80.

Windebank AJ, Litchy WJ, Duabe JR, et al. Late effects of paralytic poliomyelitis in Olmsted County, Minnesota. Neurology 1991;41:501.

Winstein CJ. Neurogenic dysphagia: frequency, progression and outcome in adults following head injury. Phys Ther 1983;63:1992.

Wolpaw JR. Adaptive plasticity in the spinal stretch reflex: an accessible substrate of memory? Cell Mol Neurobiol 1985;5:147.

Wood JL, Robbins JA, Roecker EB, et al. Age effects on lingual pressure generation and implications for swallowing. Dysphagia 1994;9:270.

Wright RA, Penner DB. Myxedema and upper esophageal dysmotility. Dig Dis Sci 1979;24:159.

Wyllie E, Wyllie R, Cruse RP, et al. The mechanism of nitrazepam-induced drooling and aspiration. N Engl J Med 1986;314:35.

Ylvisaker M, Logemann JA. Therapy for Feeding and Swallowing Following Head Injury. In M Ylvisaker (ed), Management of Head Injured Patients. San Diego: College-Hill, 1986.

Zerhouni EA, Bosma JF, Donner MW. Relationship of cervical spine disorders to dysphagia. Dysphagia 1987;1:129.

4

Mechanical Disorders of Swallowing

Michael E. Groher

Patients with mechanical swallowing disorders evidence difficulty secondary to combinations of deglutitory muscle loss and loss of the motor and sensory innervations to those muscles. The central and most of the peripheral neurologic controls for deglutition are intact. The structures needed to complete the act are not. Even though causes and mechanisms of the neurologic and mechanical groups are different, some of the deglutitory problems are shared. These include sialorrhea (excessive expectoration of fluid resembling saliva), difficulty with mastication, oral and pharyngeal pooling, lengthened swallowing transit times, difficulty channeling food into the esophagus, and aspiration. For the purposes of this and subsequent chapters, aspiration is defined as the residual, unswallowed pharyngeal content that is drawn into the larynx and trachea by inspiration after an attempt at a normal swallow. Aspiration is to be differentiated from spillage of oral contents into the pharynx, larynx, or both without elicitation of swallow, which is called penetration. Most patients with mechanical dysphagia have had oral, pharyngeal, laryngeal, or esophageal structures removed or reconstructed during surgery for cancer. There are, however, other causes that must be considered in the differential diagnosis. The most common of these are considered here.

ACUTE INFLAMMATIONS

Acute inflammatory processes that produce or exacerbate dysphagia are nonspecific reactions to injury of the oropharyngeal tissue. These reactions are secondary to fungal, bacterial, or viral agents, chemical irritants, or traumatic insults.

Acute inflammations of the oropharyngeal tissues alone may not create significant, extended dysphagia. They are particularly significant, however, when superimposed on other, more obvious swallowing disorders such as pseudobulbar dysphagia or the dysphagia seen in elderly debilitated patients. Early recognition and treatment of acute inflammatory reactions can make the difference between success and failure in attempts at oral feeding. They should be ruled out in patients whose mental state or competence interferes with the ability to communicate oral pain and those who evidence unexplainable dysphagia or sudden refusal to eat. Early identification is important because most inflammations can be controlled within a short period of time, and oral nutritional intake can resume.

Herpes Simplex

Viral in origin, a herpetic infection is characterized by round vesicles that break to form shallow ulcers surrounded by a narrow zone of inflammation (DeWeese and Saunders 1973). Typically, they are found on the lips; however, the pharynx and buccal mucosa may be involved. Palatal and pharyngeal ulcers create significant pain and discomfort on swallowing.

Ludwig's Angina

The most typical type of infection to occur in the submandibular space that may compromise swallow is Ludwig's angina. Odontogenic infections such as abscesses, caries, and postextraction infection are implicated in 70–85% of cases of Ludwig's angina (Williams and Guralnick 1943; Patterson et al. 1982). Clinical manifestations of Ludwig's angina include massive swelling and displacement of the tongue. The floor of the mouth also will appear red, swollen, hard, and tender. Posterior extension may result in epiglottitis, with further compromise of the airway. If the patient is able to speak, he or she may have a muffled, "hot potato" voice. The neck exhibits a woody, tender swelling, especially in the suprahyoid region. Patients generally present with complaints of mouth pain, stiff neck, drooling, and dysphagia. Complications of a supramandibular space infection include asphyxia, aspiration pneumonia, lung abscess, and tongue necrosis. Treatment of Ludwig's angina includes airway control, intravenous (IV) antibiotics, or surgical exploration and drainage.

Lingual Tonsillitis

Patients with lingual tonsillitis have symptoms similar to those of other throat infections, except they complain of pain in the medial pharyngeal region. Often they describe a lump in the throat associated with complaints of dysphagia. The mechanism of lingual tonsillitis can be confirmed by indirect mirror examination of the base of the tongue and pharynx.

Epiglottitis

Epiglottitis is an inflammatory disease that affects the supraglottic region and often results in acute respiratory distress because of airway obstruction. It is most commonly seen in children but has more recently been recognized with increasing frequency in adults (Hawkins et al. 1973; Kander and Richards 1977; Sarant 1981; Mayosmith et al. 1986). Patients often complain of sore throat, dysphagia, respiratory difficulty, muffled voice, drooling, and stridor (Schabel et al. 1977; Cohen 1984; Mayosmith et al. 1986). An incorrect initial diagnosis of streptococcal or viral pharyngitis is often made (Cohen 1984). A modified barium swallowing study may reveal abnormal enlargement of supraglottic structures. An epiglottis that is 8 mm or greater in width and aryepiglottic folds greater than 7 mm in width seem to suggest epiglottitis in adults (Schumaker et al. 1984). Maintenance of a competent airway is the most important factor in the treatment of patients with epiglottitis.

Acute Pharyngitis

Acute pharyngitis may be viral or bacterial in origin. The reddened inflammation that it causes in the oropharyngeal region frequently precedes the common cold, leading patients to complain of swallowing difficulty. It often is accompanied by a mild fever without any other complications. The pain and dysphagia subside within 4–6 days.

The most common bacterial form of pharyngitis is streptococcal. The diagnosis is confirmed by laboratory analysis. The patient has an acutely inflamed oropharynx with characteristic white or yellow follicles. Most complain of headache and muscle joint pain and have fevers that reach 103°F. Streptococcal infections respond well to a full course of antibiotics.

Lateral Pharyngeal Space Infections

Infections in the lateral pharyngeal space are classified as anterior or posterior, depending on the location of the infection. Infections of the lateral pharyngeal space may be secondary to primary infection in the tonsil or pharynx. Clinical presentation of symptoms differs between anterior and posterior compartments. When the patient has an anterior compartment infection, he or she may present with dysphagia, trismus, chills, high fever, hardening and swelling of the mandibular arch, systemic toxicity, medial bulging of the lateral pharyngeal wall, and pain (Blomquist and Bayer 1988). Dyspnea occurs infrequently.

An infection involving the posterior compartment is characterized by marked sepsis in the absence of trismus or tonsillar prolapse. Edema and swelling of the epiglottis and larynx may result in dyspnea. Sudden death syndrome, fatal myocarditis, and further complications are associated when the infection spreads to the retropharyngeal space.

Treatment of lateral pharyngeal space infections is similar to that of Ludwig's angina but with a few important differences. Therapeutic management includes antibiotic therapy, surgical drainage, and airway maintenance. Surgical intervention plays a primary role in patient management in lateral pharyngeal space infections rather than a secondary role as in Ludwig's angina (Blomquist and Bayer 1988). In addition, airway control is not required as often and is associated with fewer complications than that in Ludwig's angina.

Retropharyngeal and Prevertebral Space Infections

Retropharyngeal and prevertebral space infections occur between the common pharyngoesophageal wall and the spine. Retropharyngeal space infections arise acutely from an adjacent abscess, most commonly from the lateral pharyngeal space, or after cervical trauma. Prevertebral space infections are most often secondary to chronic disease, such as osteomyelitis, whereas inflammation after trauma is associated with infected hematomas resulting from vertebral fractures. A patient with a retropharyngeal abscess may complain of fever, sore throat, dysphagia, stridor, regurgitation, dyspnea, and stiff neck. The consequences of retropharyngeal space infections include meningitis, mediastinitis, epiglottitis, pneumonia, empyema, spontaneous rupture of the larynx with aspiration and asphyxiation, bronchial erosion, pyopneumothorax, and purulent pericarditis. Treatment for retropharyngeal space infection includes antibiotic therapy and surgical drainage.

Fungal Inflammation

One of the common fungal inflammations is candidiasis (thrush). Most frequently seen on the tongue, the lesions appear as soft, white, slightly elevated plaques (Figure 4.1) (Keyes 1980). If left untreated, the lesions cause associated pain and difficulty swallowing. They are more common in debilitated and immunosuppressed patients, in those who are undergoing extensive antibiotic therapy, and in patients receiving irradiation treatments. *Candida* species are the most common cause of odynophagia and dysphagia in patients with acquired immunodeficiency syndrome (AIDS) (Raufman 1988). Odynophagia may also occur in AIDS patients as a result of Kaposi's sarcoma. Kaposi's sarcoma is most commonly found on the hard palate but may also be found in any part of the oral mucosa (Greenspan and Greenspan 1988). These lesions are differentiated from other white plaques such as leukoplakia because they can be scraped away, leaving a raw, bloody surface (Keyes 1980).

Chemical Agents

Mucosal inflammation may result from exposure to chemicals. The subsequent pain interferes most often with the oropharyngeal stage of swallowing.

Chemical inflammation can result from the prolonged use of phenol (toothache drops). Other drugs that precipitate mucosal burns include aspirin, which causes irritation to the cheek lining; some gargles; and anesthetic throat lozenges when used excessively (Kerr and Ash 1978). The latter reduce oral sensation and invite traumatic lesions in individuals who unknowingly bite their oral mucosa.

Mucosal burns can be red or white, but they represent a change in the normal, pinkish, mucosal lining. More severe inflammations have a whitish slough covering an intensely reddened area. The most severe form of a chemical burn, lye ingestion, can cause severe blistering of the entire digestive tract. The clinician should be aware that patients who undergo chemotherapy can develop painful oral ulcerations that interfere with swallowing. Drugs used in these regi-

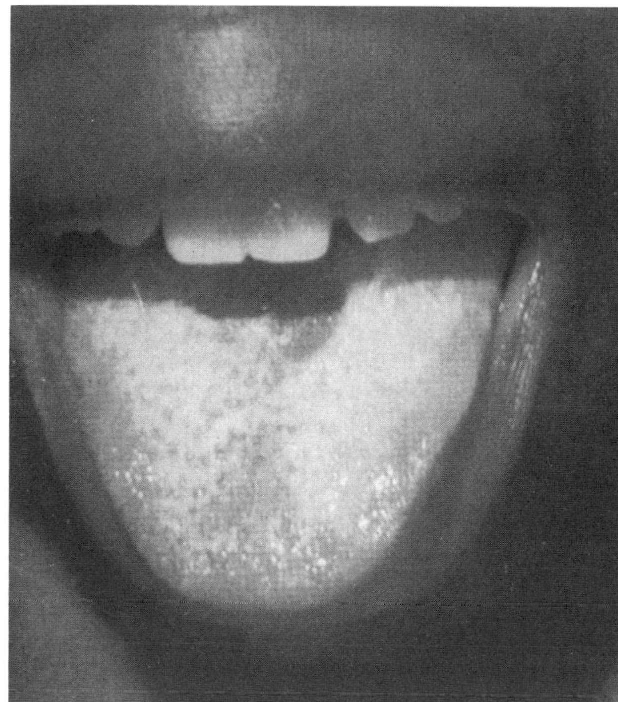

Figure 4.1 Fungal inflammations of the tongue appear as milky-white elevated lesions. (Reprinted with permission from S Dreizen, TE Daly, JB Dranc, et al. Oral complications of cancer radiotherapy. Postgrad Med 1977;61:85.)

mens, such as doxorubicin (Adriamycin), methotrexate, and cyclophosphamide (Cytoxan), can cause oral mucositis (Carl 1980).

TRAUMA

Other than major traumatic tissue losses, such as those resulting from gunshot wounds, more frequently occurring injuries in the oral cavity are fairly benign and generally do not create significant swallowing complaints except when superimposed on other mechanisms of dysphagia. Examples include trauma from a toothbrush and mucosal irritation from ill-fitting dentures. Patients who complain of a poorly fitted denture can localize their pain. Clinical examination will usually reveal a reddened or whitish change in the mucosa at the point of denture contact where the patient has the sensation of most discomfort. Prolonged irritation can cause gingival hyperplasia (Figure 4.2) that results in soft, sometimes flexible masses of tissue that appear markedly inflamed.

Biting the sides of the lip or, more commonly, the cheek because of lost sensation may cause lesions that create some swallowing discomfort. These lesions usually appear as small, irregularly shaped areas covered by a gray necrotic membrane surrounded by inflammation (LaVelle and Proctor 1978).

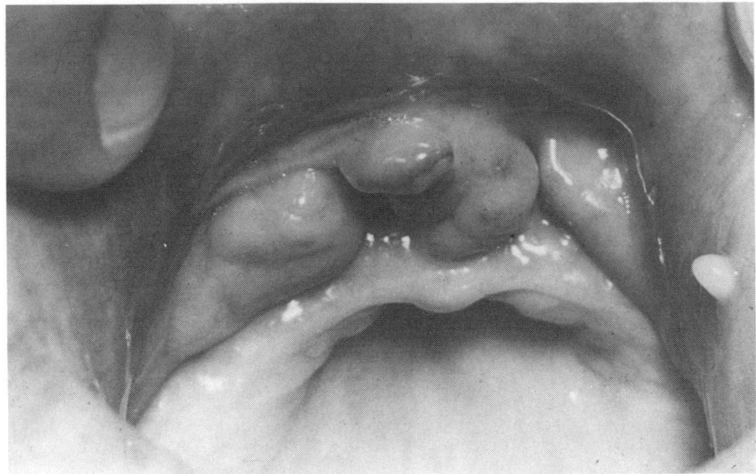

Figure 4.2 Gingival hyperplasia caused by an ill-fitting denture. (Reprinted with permission from DD DeWeese, WH Saunders. Textbook of Otolaryngology [6th ed]. St. Louis: Mosby, 1982.)

MACROGLOSSIA

An abnormally large tongue can interfere with the propulsive action of the bolus. The clinician should consider some of the conditions that may contribute to macroglossia in the differential diagnosis. They include macroglossia secondary to lymphatic obstruction, secondary to surgery or irradiation, hypothyroidism, mongolism, amyloid deposits, and lymphangiomatous or hemangiomatous processes. The speech and swallowing characteristics in a patient with primary amyloidosis affecting the tongue and cervical musculature have been described (Groher and Enderle 1988).

PHARYNGOESOPHAGEAL DIVERTICULUM

A pharyngoesophageal diverticulum, commonly referred to as Zenker's diverticulum in the cervical esophagus, is an abnormal muscular outpouching that forms from either above the cricopharyngeal muscle through Killian's dehiscence or below through Laimer's triangle. The exact mechanism of pouch formation is unknown, although in small percentages of patients it can be associated with esophageal disease, including traction diverticula, varices, achalasia, carcinoma, and hiatal hernia. Speculation that abnormal relaxation of the cricopharyngeal muscle is the source of pouch formation is not substantiated by manometric evaluation (Knuff et al. 1982). Zenker's diverticula are more common in men in the sixth and seventh decades of life. They must become very large to produce dysphagic symptoms. Patients complain of regurgitation of undigested food, foul breath, fullness in the neck, weight loss, and nocturnal cough with aspiration.

MECHANICAL DYSPHAGIA SECONDARY TO CARCINOMA

The largest group of patients with mechanical swallowing disorders has had oral, pharyngeal, laryngeal, or esophageal structures removed, rearranged, or reconstructed secondary to surgery for carcinoma. Most often, combinations of these structures are involved.

Most clinicians are aware of the general rule for predicting significant dysphagic episodes after surgical excision: The removal of less than 50% of an area or organ concerned with deglutition will not interfere seriously or permanently with swallowing function (Conley 1960). A review of the pertinent literature suggests that we must use care when applying this rule.

First, the word *seriously* is nonspecific and can be defined in many different and subjective ways. Second, permanent dysphagia could mean that the patient has persistent dysphagia and cannot tolerate oral feedings, or it could mean that he or she will have difficulty initiating or completing a normal swallow but will tolerate oral feedings with limited success if supplemented by alternative methods. Differences in the permanence of the disorders suggest different treatment approaches and final outcomes. In short, the 50% rule is only a guide, and individual differences should not be overlooked. In fact, individual differences among patients who have had cancerous lesions and subsequent resections may not be related to the amount of the structure removed but rather to factors such as preoperative and postoperative health, psychological reaction to the disability, and ability to learn adaptive swallowing techniques.

The 50% rule also applies if the structure in question is rearranged or if adjacent structures are rearranged (Summers 1974; Weaver and Fleming 1978). Procedures on adjacent structures appear to carry a more negative prognosis for deglutitory recovery than does loss of mobility of those structures (Doberneck and Antoine 1974).

Sessions and coworkers (1979) implied that the 50% rule not be applied randomly to any swallowing structure. They pointed out that the original size of the lesion was not as important a prognosticator of dysphagia as was the area excised, and that resultant dysphagia could be predicted if surgical excision involved either the arytenoid cartilages or the base of the tongue. Logemann and Bytell (1979) analyzed swallowing transit times and motility in three separate groups of patients with head and neck resections. They concluded, "We cannot assume that the patient facing less ablative surgery will have only minimal functional problems in swallowing." Although this conclusion appears to stand alone, the differences in data interpretation once again come from the way in which we define a minimal as opposed to a significant swallowing disorder. In fact, the overall success at oral feeding during and after the study period was not reported in the Logemann and Bytell (1979) data. Therefore, it is difficult to interpret the ultimate significance of dysphagia in those patients who have abnormal videofluoroscopic findings with little ablative surgery.

An additional complication to the loss of structural function is the total or partial loss of sensation or interruption of the neurologic afferent controls in the oropharynx that surgical procedures can precipitate. The use of tissue flaps to close surgical defects interferes with the normal sensation that provides adequate sensory guidance of the bolus needed to effect a normal swallow.

In addition to receiving surgical treatment for lesions, patients may also be candidates for irradiation, chemotherapy, or both in an effort to control the malignancy. There is some disagreement among clinicians whether preoperative or postoperative irradiation predisposes the patient to functional dysphagic complications more than if this treatment were not undertaken.

These disagreements exist because of the different methods of subject selection, small sample sizes that affect statistical evaluation, the type of outcome measure used, and the time when the outcome measure was made. For instance, if one were to judge outcomes in postsurgical glossectomized patients based on patient report alone, swallowing abnormality may not be detected (Baker et al. 1991). Lazarus (1993) compared two groups of postsurgical patients with complaints of dysphagia who had completed radiotherapy within 6 months, and those who had completed their therapy 10 years before the study. He concluded that the effects of radiation therapy for these two groups of patients were similar. Both groups, regardless of tumor site or size, had similar radiographic findings: reduced posterior tongue movement, restricted laryngeal motion, and restricted arytenoid cartilage to epiglottic base motion. After following a mixed group of glossectomized patients, Pauloski et al. (1994) found few differences in oropharyngeal swallowing efficiency at 1 and 12 months postsurgery. However, they noted a decrease in swallowing function at 6 months that was regained at the 12-month measurement. They attributed this temporary decrement of swallowing efficiency to the effects of irradiation. Hamlet and colleagues (1991) studied the effects of irradiation on glossectomized patients with differing lesion sizes and operative closure techniques. Radiographic studies before and shortly after radiation therapy did not delay the recovery of swallowing.

These findings refute the majority of studies that suggest the effects of either preoperative or postoperative irradiation on swallowing are detrimental in mixed groups of patients with head and neck carcinoma (Summers 1974; Weaver and Fleming 1978; Sessions et al. 1979; Beckhardt et al. 1994). Coyle et al. (1995) compared swallowing velocities in two groups of head and neck cancer patients: those who received surgical management only and those who received radiotherapy without surgery. At 6 months, swallowing velocities for patients receiving irradiation were higher than pretherapy velocities. Swallowing velocities were slower at 6 months for surgical patients when compared to their preoperative swallowing measures.

EXPECTED IMPAIRMENT FROM SURGICAL RESECTIONS

Oral Lesions

Cancers in the oral cavity may involve the anterior tongue, floor of the mouth, submental structures, mandible, and maxilla. Often, more than one of these structures is involved. It is not unusual to have parts of the tongue, mandible, and floor of the mouth resected.

In general, patients with resected oral structures have difficulty with mastication, formation and retention of a bolus, and anteroposterior transport. Major resections of parts of the mandible and submental region can significantly alter the relationships among oral, pharyngeal, and laryngeal structures, which results in aspiration before the swallow response because uncontrolled material in the oral phase may enter the pharynx prematurely. Disturbance of the sequential movements involved in swallowing is common and may involve both oral and pharyngeal swallowing mechanics. For instance, loss of the occlusal jaw relationships after mandibulectomy can interfere with mastication in a way that lengthens the oral phase of feeding. This can result not only in delayed and therefore poorly timed propulsion but also in premature attempts at swallowing that cause aspiration, because the delay is not well tolerated by most patients.

Patients with resections that involve the tongue only (simple glossectomy) experience difficulty with bolus transport to the oropharynx. The question of how much this delay in transport permanently interferes with the oral route of feeding remains somewhat controversial; most evidence supports that even patients who lose all of their tongue can swallow.

After reviewing over 700 patients with resected tongue lesions (some had had preoperative irradiation), Frazell and Lucas (1962) reported that 40 of the 168 patients experienced transitory dysphagic complications, and only 13 of the 168 required permanent tube feedings. Other investigators have reported similar success, although most describe periods of transitory postoperative dysphagia that depend partially on the amount of tongue that is resected. Frazell and Lucas (1962) implied that the prognosis for recovery of swallow was better for those who did not have structures other than the tongue resected, such as part of the mandible or the submental region. They concluded that postoperative complications were correlated more positively with preoperative factors such as age and general health, size and position of the primary tumor, invasion of neighboring structures, and status of the regional lymph nodes.

Conley (1960) and Summers (1974) agreed that patients who lose up to one-third of the tongue have only transitory swallowing disorders. These resolve in 2–4 weeks without specific remediation of dysphagia. McConnell and Logemann (1990) also found that the prognosis for swallowing recovery for patients with total glossectomy was good unless it was combined with anterior mandibular resection. When the mandible is resected, patients are unable to elevate the larynx, compromising the function of the pharygoesophageal segment.

The loss of oral stage propulsion combined with the probability of hypopharyngeal dysfunction will predispose the patient to aspiration (McConnell and Logemann 1990). In a study of glossectomies with varying amounts of tissue loss, Hirano and colleagues (1992) found no statistically significant differences in swallowing disability, although those that had removal of the geniohyoid and myohyoid musculature, tongue base resection, or both had poorer dietary levels and extended periods of tube feeding.

Most of these studies looked at the outcome of their patients' swallowing functions in the early postoperative stages. Comparing the immediate postoperative swallowing outcomes and those at a median of 14 months in total and near total glossectomized patients, Weber et al. (1991) found that of the 67% of patients who were on total oral diets after surgery, only 44% were eating orally at 14 months.

Logemann and Bytell (1979) provided a more detailed analysis of the deglutition problems glossectomy patients might encounter 1 week after attempts at oral feeding. They used videofluoroscopy to study 10 patients who had excision of lesions of the floor of the mouth and tongue (10–70% of those structures) with accompanying dissections of the anterior mandible and neck. All had difficulty forming and maintaining a bolus. Oral transit times were delayed, except in the two patients who had longitudinally divided tongue flaps. Eight of the patients were unable to chew because they could not orient material to the molar table. All experienced difficulty with anterior drooling. The swallowing stimuli (thin barium, cookie coated with barium paste, cookie with thin barium) often collected in the anterior and lateral sulci. Oral content of thick consistency was accumulated on the oral palate. Anteroposterior propulsion was disturbed and the bolus frequently spilled into the oropharynx before the patient was ready to initiate a swallow. This was true for all food consistencies used, except for the thin paste, which required less oral effort and was associated with better transport times. Once the bolus was moved posteriorly, all patients could initiate swallow.

Kothary and DeSouza (1973) used cineradiography in their analysis of 25 patients undergoing glossectomy. They found that these patients compensated well for poor lingual propulsion by increasing the use of the buccal musculature, inclining the floor of the mouth, and developing a more prominent forward movement of the pharyngeal musculature. Similar results were reported in 7 of 11 patients with anterior floor of the mouth resections who were studied postoperatively at 3 and 6 months (Fujiu et al. 1995). Fujiu et al. (1995) noted that a more prominent bulge of the pharyngeal musculature was found more often in patients who had larger surgical deficits. They suggested that this anterior movement of the posterior pharyngeal wall was a natural compensation that might be enhanced therapeutically. Encouragement of this movement provides the necessary contact point for the posterior tongue, forcefully propelling the bolus into the pharynx.

Even though these problems with propulsion and transport exist in the early postoperative stages, reports in the literature suggest that patients with tongue resections uncomplicated by surgical involvement of related structures are able to

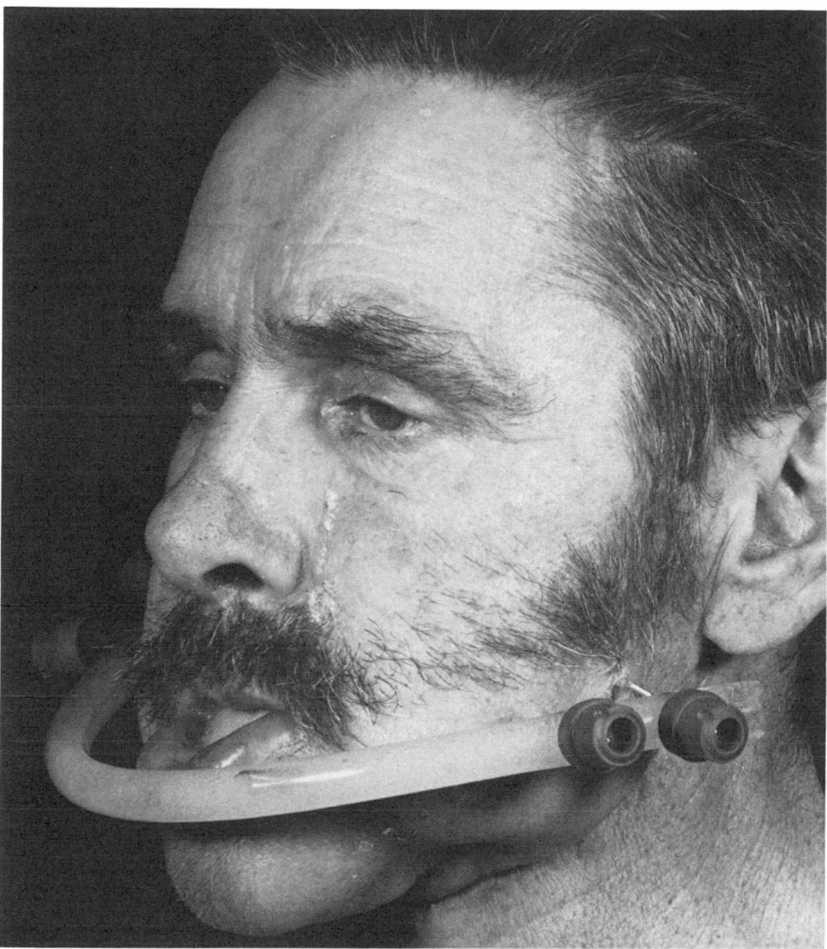

Figure 4.3 Patient after surgery for carcinoma of the anterior floor of the mouth and mandible with a right radical and left suprahyoid resection including the tongue. A right trapezius myocutaneous flap was used to reconstruct the oral cavity and a biphase appliance was used to temporarily fixate the mandible.

take nutrition orally after no longer than a 1-month period of adjustment to their disability. Unfortunately, a significant number of patients must undergo resection of structures other than the tongue to achieve adequate control of their cancer.

Patients with resections of the tongue, neck, floor of the mouth, and mandible (Figure 4.3) have different degrees of dysphagia impairment: of the masticatory process, bolus control, anteroposterior propulsion, and difficulty with airway protection. Reconstruction of the structures in the mandibular region can create scar tissue contractures and temporomandibular joint pain interfering with normal mastication. Not only is it difficult to place food

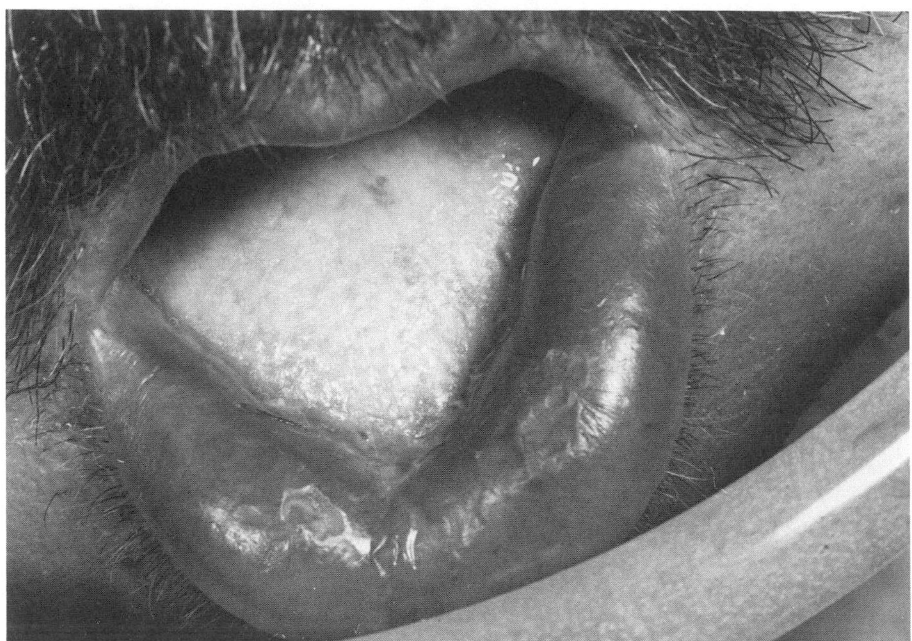

Figure 4.4 Floor of the mouth of the patient in Figure 4.3. Absence of a mobile tongue and a lower immobile lip made anterior/posterior propulsion difficult.

because of limited excursion, but subsequent swallows may also be poorly timed because of abnormal occlusal relationships (Figure 4.4). These poor mandibular/maxillary contacts make biting and chewing more of an effort and tend to interfere with bolus formation. McConnell and Logemann (1990) found that in glossectomized patients with T2 and T3 lesions, the type of surgical reconstruction that produced the most favorable swallowing outcomes were those that had either primary closure, skin grafts, or postsurgical defects that were allowed to granulate. Poorer outcomes were associated with larger lesions that required myocutaneous flaps to close the surgical defect.

Oropharyngeal Lesions

Oropharyngeal lesions may include anterior tongue resections, as well as resections of the soft palate, retromolar trigone, tonsils, base of tongue, and superior and lateral pharynx. In general, patients with oropharyngeal resections may experience nasal regurgitation, decreased bolus transit, aspiration, and pharyngoesophageal segment dysfunction.

Patients who undergo glossectomy that includes the base of the tongue are susceptible to persistent dysphagia, although the majority can successfully eat orally. Combining dynamic radiography and manometry (manofluorography),

McConnell (1988) demonstrated that patients with tongue base lesions lose not only the proplusive tongue-driving force of the oral stage of swallow but also have an increased resistance to bolus flow in the pharynx because the force generated is unable to produce sufficient negative pressure in the pharyngoesophageal segment. Eighty percent of patients with tongue base lesions and adequate reconstructions will have favorable swallowing outcomes, although some will need laryngeal suspension, laryngoplasty, or both if total oral alimentation is a goal (McConnell and Mendelsohn 1987). Donaldson et al. (1968) reported that 8 of 14 patients with total glossectomy had no dysphagia, while the remaining six had to rely on tube feedings. One of the six eventually had to undergo elective total laryngectomy to control the dysphagia. Myers (1972) reported a higher swallowing success rate in a series of 14 patients after glossectomy, all but one of whom were able to take nutrition orally. Summers (1974) noted that the majority of patients with glossectomy do well following surgery because they are able to protect their airway with an intact laryngeal sphincter.

Summers (1974) found that patients with composite resections required weeks or months to relearn swallowing and usually had a much more pronounced degree of frustration with eating than those who had only glossectomy. Conley (1960) supported this observation by noting that patients who had a hemiglossectomy with dissection of the floor of the mouth, adjacent mandible, and ipsilateral neck did recover the ability to swallow but with some aspiration, coughing, and anxiety associated with swallowing attempts.

Patients who undergo glossectomy and bony palate resections lose the ability to generate the adequate force necessary to propel a bolus into the pharynx. Aspiration can occur because of loss of bolus control and nasal regurgitation. Lack of tongue strength and mobility results in an inability to generate the pressure required to move the bolus from the mouth to the pharynx (McConnell and Mendelsohn 1987). This may result in premature leakage of contents into the pharynx, with subsequent aspiration or nasal regurgitation. For those with bony palate deficits, a palatal stent may be placed at the time of surgery. However, it may not allow for complete occlusion between the oral and nasal cavity because air pressure may be lost along the lateral sulcus. For this reason, patients may complain of dysphagia, although it is transitory and they learn to compensate. Dietary modifications such as pureed food textures with thin liquids and head posturing techniques generally facilitate swallow.

Ablative surgery on the oropharynx usually includes combined resection of the soft palate and tonsillar pillars. This type of resection may interfere with transportation of bolus material through the pharynx because normal sensory input is interrupted as a result of reconstructive efforts using tissue flaps that contain no sensory innervation. These tissue flaps also interfere with swallowing since they act passively rather than actively, resulting in the loss of the normal propulsive action supplied by the pharyngeal constrictor musculature. If the flaps are bulky, they may interfere mechanically with the passage of a bolus.

Patients who must undergo glossectomy and submental resections may lose tongue propulsion and lip sensation. The protective tilting action of the larynx provided by the hypomandibular constrictors is also sacrificed. This loss can result in significant aspiration. Conley (1960) reported that patients who had undergone total glossectomy with bilateral dissections of cervical lymph nodes swallowed poorly, but if both superior laryngeal nerves (SLNs), the hyoid, and the epiglottis were intact, they could swallow a liquid diet without aspiration.

Partial Laryngectomy

Partial laryngectomy is a general category of surgical resection of the pharyngeal and laryngeal region that seeks to control a malignancy while preserving vocal function and deglutition. These procedures are principally hemilaryngectomy and supraglottic laryngectomy.

Hemilaryngectomy

Definitions of hemilaryngectomy vary because some are complete and others are partial. Leonard et al. (1972) defined it as unilateral excision of the vocal fold plus extension to the anterior commissure, vocal processes, or both. Weaver and Fleming's (1978) definition includes unilateral resection of the vocal fold, vestibular fold, ventricle, and SLN with preservation of the epiglottis. The present discussion uses the latter definition. The typical resection that comprises a hemilaryngectomy is illustrated in Figure 4.5.

Weaver and Fleming (1978) studied a group of 11 patients undergoing hemilaryngectomy at periods of 6 weeks and 6 months postresection. The results showed that 7 of 11 had no swallowing difficulty with solids or liquids at either evaluation. Two patients had initial problems that resolved at 6 months, one failed to swallow adequately after 6 months, and one had recurrence of disease. The only patient who did not recover swallow had preoperative irradiation, neck dissection, and a postoperative fistula.

Leonard et al. (1972) found similarly encouraging results. Of the 75 patients with excised unilateral lesions that had not extended significantly, aspiration was not a problem except in those who were already debilitated and also had poor pulmonary function. None of the 75 had an immobile vocal fold before surgery. The authors implied that this may have contributed significantly to their good results.

The results reported by Schoenrock and associates (1972) were less encouraging. After unilaterally severing and elevating the infrahyoid muscles to form a perichondrial muscle pedicle flap, the thyroid ala, arytenoid cartilage, and vestibular and vocal folds were removed. In addition, the ipsilateral SLN was sectioned and the piriform sinus obliterated. Seven of the 11 patients who were studied 2 months postoperatively aspirated thin barium; one aspirated thick barium. Of the seven patients, only three subjectively complained of aspiration. Schoenrock's group (1972) attributed their findings to the fact that the larynx did not rise evenly on the excised side. If the excised vocal fold is not reconstructed at the same level as the intact one, aspiration will result. The unevenness will result in tilting the larynx, directing the barium to the resected

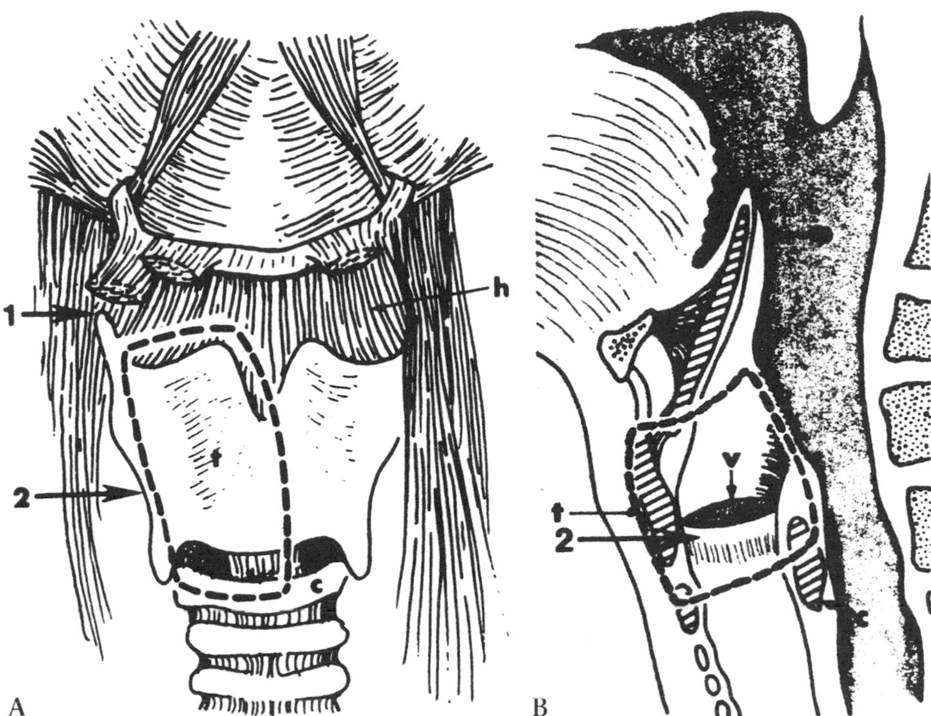

Figure 4.5 Frontal (A) and lateral (B) schematic views of structures excised during vertical hemilaryngectomy (enclosed within dashed lines). (1) Level of the superior cornua of the thyroid cartilage; (2) Level of the glottis; t = thyroid cartilage; c = cricoid cartilage; h = thyrohyoid membrane; e = epiglottis; v = laryngeal ventricle. (Reprinted with permission from DJ Disantis, DM Balfe, R Hayden, et al. The neck after vertical hemilaryngectomy: computed tomography. Radiology 1984;151:683.)

side, with eventual spilling into the trachea. Cineradiography showed seven patients' larynges failed to meet the base of the tongue on the excised side during swallow, thus offering limited protection against penetration into the trachea. In addition, normal sequential pharyngeal constriction was absent on the involved side, further contributing to aspiration. These authors noted that all seven patients had incompetent glottal chinks. Four of the seven could not achieve enough movement to get closure and three had good movement, but the functioning true vocal fold met the excised mucosal surface at a different level. Interestingly, even though aspiration in some of these patients was not subjectively apparent, it was demonstrated by chest radiography. This finding seemed to suggest that patients may be asymptomatic for a long period of time and then develop pulmonary complications, including minimal basilar pneumonia, pulmonary fibrosis, multiple lobe aspiration, aspiration pneumonia, and lung abscess.

Because there are alternatives to a complete hemilaryngectomy, such as laryngofissure and frontal lateral partial laryngectomy, fewer total hemilaryngectomies are being performed.

Supraglottic Laryngectomy

Supraglottic laryngectomy has several definitions. Weaver and Fleming (1978) defined it as a resection that "typically includes both false cords, both aryepiglottic folds, and one or both superior laryngeal nerves." Summers (1974) defined the resection as a "block resection of the vallecula, epiglottis, hyoid bone, aryepiglottic folds, ventricular bands, upper third of the thyroid cartilage, and thyrohyoid membrane." Flores and coworkers (1982) agreed with Summers and included the pre-epiglottic space. They pointed out that some supraglottic resections extend to include the resection of one arytenoid cartilage, the piriform sinus (partial laryngopharyngectomy), the base of the tongue, or a combination of these. The careful reader will note the potential differences in data interpretation relative to supraglottic resections as different criteria for patient selection may bias the results. For the purposes of this discussion, a supraglottic laryngectomy includes resection of both vestibular and aryepiglottic folds and one or both SLNs (Figure 4.6) (Weaver and Fleming 1978).

Most investigators agree that supraglottic resections are not without dysphagic complications, especially in the immediate (2- to 4-week) postoperative period. The incidence of postoperative aspiration in supraglottic resections can be as high as 50% (McConnell and Logemann 1990), with a 6% incidence of aspiration pneumonia (Freeman et al. 1979). An early study reported a 19% incidence of postoperative mortality secondary to supraglottic laryngectomy (Murray 1976). The eventual severity and duration of dysphagia beyond this period appears to be highly variable, however, partly because not all supraglottic resections remove identical structures, some patients develop postsurgical complications, and some receive either preoperative or postoperative irradiation. While a small majority eventually do swallow with minimal aspiration, resections that compromise the arytenoid cartilages and extend into the piriform sinus and tongue base create significant and sometimes persisting dysphagia (Conley 1960; Staple and Ogura 1966; Litton and Leonard 1969; Summers 1974; Weaver and Fleming 1978; Flores et al. 1982). The loss of the tongue base apparently impairs glottic protection as the larynx is elevated; the loss of arytenoid cartilage mass also results in impairment of the glottis at the laryngeal level. However, in a retrospective review of the respiratory and deglutition outcomes in 46 patients who had supraglottic laryngectomy resections that extended beyond the traditional limits and patients that did not, there were no significant differences (Beckhardt et al. 1994). The poorest outcomes in this series of patients were associated with a poor forced expiratory volume in 1 second to forced vital capacity ratio (FEV_1/FVC) on pulmonary function tests (Beckhardt et al. 1994).

Sacrificing one SLN during supraglottic resection does not significantly interfere with swallowing, although bilateral excision carries a negative prognosis for pharyngeal deglutition (Shedd 1976; Weaver and Fleming 1978). Bocca et

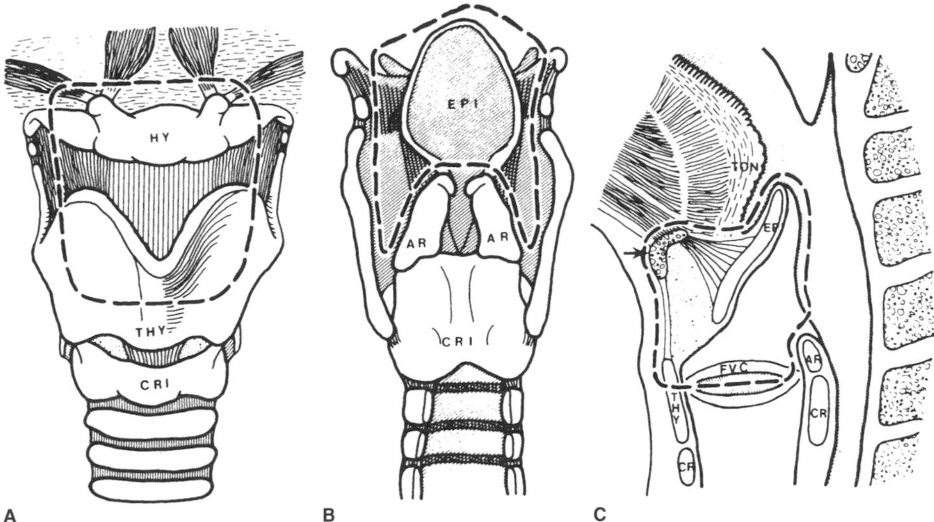

Figure 4.6 Subtotal supraglottic laryngectomy: surgical procedure. Line drawing of the larynx. Dashed lines indicate the margin of resection. A. View from the front; the surgeon resects portions of the hyoid bone (HY), thyrohyoid, and thyroid cartilage (THY) (CRI = cricoid cartilage). B. View from the rear; the resection includes the epiglottis (EPI), aryepiglottic folds, and portions of the piriform sinuses. The arytenoid cartilages (AR) are spared in routine operations; in extended procedures, a portion of one arytenoid may be shaved. C. View from the side; the resection extends into the vallecula and tongue base and removes the hyoid bone (arrow), pre-epiglottic fat, and false vocal cord (FVC). (Reprinted with permission from Springer-Verlag from DM Balfe. Dysphagia after laryngeal surgery. Dysphagia 1990;5:20.)

al. (1968) and Flores et al. (1982) did not find that bilateral excision of the SLN influenced the severity or duration of dysphagia. In fact, the latter group reported that immediate success at deglutition (as a proportional percentage) was higher with bilateral SLN resections, although this was not statistically significant. They pointed out that this variable "probably should not be considered separately since preservation of one superior laryngeal nerve is related to the preservation of the hyoid bone." Their patients with hyoid resections had a better prognosis for swallowing.

Weaver and Fleming (1978) measured swallowing competence of 23 patients after unilateral and bilateral supraglottic resections at 6 weeks and 6 months postsurgery. All 23 patients had swallowing difficulty with both liquids and solids. After 6 months, 16 patients still had dysphagia that ranged from mild to persistent. The most severely affected patients also had had resections of the tongue base. Not one of the four who underwent bilateral supraglottic resections regained their normal swallow, although three were able to maintain their weight with acceptable levels of aspiration (e.g., no pulmonary complications). The patient who had persistent aspiration had both SLNs severed and also had postoperative irradiation.

Staple and Ogura (1966) followed 36 patients with supraglottic laryngectomy who had excision of the epiglottis, both aryepiglottic folds and the pre-epiglottic space, vestibular folds, upper one-third of the thyroid cartilage on the affected side, and a smaller segment on the unaffected side. Eighteen of the 36 patients had initial periods of barium aspiration but regained their swallowing function so that oral nutrition could be maintained. Five patients evidenced persistent dysphagia but swallowed with minimal difficulty after 1–2 years. This improvement led the authors to remark on the potential adaptability of the surgically interrupted swallowing mechanism. Because half of this group did experience some mild aspiration, a follow-up study (Staple et al. 1967) was done to assess the long-term effects on the lungs of mild aspiration. Chest films were taken at 4 months and an average of 2.5 years after surgery. At 4 months, 14 of the 27 patients reviewed had pneumonia. At 2 years, 13 of the 39 patients studied had pneumonia. The authors concluded that although patients who aspirated during these measurements had a poor prognosis for recovery of deglutition, the outcome was, in most cases, not fatal.

Flores and coworkers (1982) studied the particular factors that might correlate with success in oral deglutition in 46 patients after supraglottic laryngeal surgery. Most of the 46 patients received high-dose preoperative irradiation. All underwent a typical (Weaver and Fleming 1978) procedure. Some had additional resections, including the arytenoid cartilage, piriform sinus, and tongue base. Twenty-eight patients were able to rely solely on oral intake within 5 days after removal of the nasogastric tube. Nine experienced delayed recovery but could rely solely on oral intake after 4 weeks to 5 months. Nine patients failed to swallow. Neither age nor preservation of the superior larynx or hyoid seemed to be important factors in predicting recovery. Of the 15 patients in whom one arytenoid cartilage was sacrificed, a higher proportion (47%), compared to 20% of the entire sample, failed to swallow than when both were preserved. Partial laryngopharyngectomy carried a negative prognosis for swallowing, although the most successful outcome in this group was in the only patient with preserved arytenoid cartilage function.

Logemann and Bytell (1979) studied eight patients with supraglottic laryngectomy with resections ranging from 10% to 50% of the tongue base. Fifty percent of the patients aspirated, with test materials falling diffusely into the pharynx in 75–92% of the patients. Laryngeal constriction was limited in one-half of the patients. This group also had some slowing of oral and pharyngeal transit times when compared with healthy individuals.

In a mixed group of 16 patients with partial laryngectomy, 12 were swallowing without difficulty in a mean of 37 days (Schima et al. 1994). The four patients who did not improve had similar bolus transit times to the group who did swallow well but did not have adequate laryngeal closure or normal (shorter) cricopharyngeal sphincter opening times.

Of 24 patients undergoing traditional and more extensive supraglottic resections, 16 aspirated thick barium paste, although in none was swallow incapacitated (Litton and Leonard 1969). Cineradiography revealed that 13 of the 16 had barium trapped over the laryngeal inlet and could not clear it on repeated attempts. All 16 who aspirated had pharyngeal involvement in addition to the supraglottic resection. Six also underwent tongue resections. The eight who did not aspirate all evidenced elevation of the laryngeal remnant, and none had a resection that involved the pharyngeal wall.

Bocca's group (1968) reported on 223 cases of classic supraglottic resection. No patient received irradiation and only six experienced dysphagia incident to poor arytenoid cartilage movement. In the majority of cases, dysphagia subsided within 3 weeks. Of 192 patients who received irradiation only for treatment of supraglottic lesions, none experienced significant dysphagia as a result of this treatment (Fayos 1975).

Epiglottic reconstruction after supraglottic laryngectomy for the prevention of dysphagia has been successfully performed. Calcaterra (1985) demonstrated reconstruction of a neoglottis from an epiglottis that was microscopically free of tumor. The neoglottis functionally projects over one-half of the laryngeal inlet and diverts food to the piriform fossae. Calcaterra (1985) studied 14 patients over a 3-year period who underwent reconstruction of a neoglottis at the time of supraglottic laryngectomy. Of these 14 patients, most were able to swallow on their first attempt without significant aspiration, and none exceeded 3 days of intravenous or nasogastric tube feeds. Additionally, there were no instances of airway obstruction that required long-term tracheostomy.

Numerous conclusions become apparent when assessing the potential effects on deglutition after supraglottic laryngectomy. First, patients who undergo the classic resection without bilateral denervation of the SLN experience mild and transitory dysphagia (Staple and Ogura 1966; Bocca et al. 1968; Weaver and Fleming 1978). If the resection extends into the piriform sinus, pharynx, or the tongue base, approximately one-half of patients have moderate to severe dysphagia but may be able to tolerate limited oral feedings (Staple and Ogura 1966; Litton and Leonard 1969; Logemann and Bytell 1979).

Second, patients who do best after supraglottic resections have the following characteristics: a mobile tongue base (Staple and Ogura 1966; Shedd 1976; Weaver and Fleming 1978; Sessions et al. 1979), a larynx that rises far enough to meet the tongue base (Bocca et al. 1968; Litton and Leonard 1969), a resected hyoid bone (Flores et al. 1982), and a glottis that allows for bilateral approximation of the vocal folds (Staple and Ogura 1966; Summers 1974; Sessions et al. 1979; Flores et al. 1982). Support for myotomy (surgical relaxation of the cricopharyngeal muscle) at the time of surgery as a procedure to prevent aspiration is provided by Staple and Ogura (1976), rejected by Weaver and Fleming (1978), and is thought to be useful when the hyoid or arytenoid cartilage must be sacrificed (Bocca et al. 1967). Myotomy produces more immediate successful swallowing but is not effective postoperatively in assisting patients who do not swallow well after supraglottic resection (Flores et al. 1982). Summers (1974)

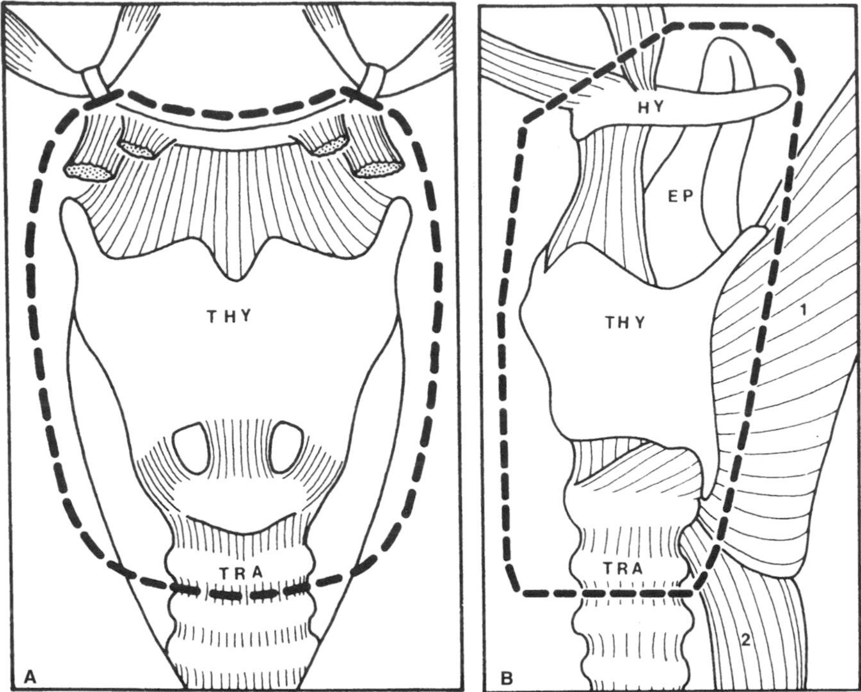

Figure 4.7 Line drawings of the surgical procedure of total laryngectomy. A. Frontal view: the surgeon removes the hyoid bone, thyroid cartilage (THY), cricoid cartilage, and often the first tracheal ring (TRA). B. Lateral view: the posterior margin of the resection severs the connections of the inferior constrictor (1) and cricopharyngeal (2) muscles. (HY = hyoid bone; EP = epiglottis; THY = thyroid cartilage; TRA = trachea.) (Reprinted with permission from Springer-Verlag from DM Balfe. Dysphagia after laryngeal surgery. Dysphagia 1990;5:20.)

felt the myotomy should be considered in patients expected to have significant postoperative sialorrhea.

Laryngectomy

Even though the alimentary and respiratory tracts are separated surgically (Figure 4.7), patients undergoing total laryngectomy are still at risk for dysphagic complications, especially in the acute stages of recovery. The reported incidence of dysphagia ranges from 10% to 58% (Balfe et al. 1982; Nayar et al. 1984). As might be expected, most of these focus on the physiologic changes the surgery might produce on the cricopharyngeal muscle. Early reports (Schobinger 1958) concluded that postoperative dysphagia was the result of the cricopharyngeal muscle in spasm. More recent investigations have shown that the cricopharyngeal muscle fails to perform, but not necessarily in a spasmodic fashion.

Using manometrics, Hanks and colleagues (1981) concluded that after laryngectomy, the cricopharyngeal muscle was not spastic, but weaker. Summers (1974) pointed out that in the absence of stricture at this level, the cricopharyngeal muscle performs in an uncoordinated manner because of detached inferior constrictor muscles. Summers (1974) and Kirchner and colleagues (1963) are in agreement that the changes in cricopharyngeal muscle function create a pharyngeal pseudodiverticulum that, in turn, may become the source of regurgitation. Such pseudodiverticula are found at the base of the tongue and in the posterior pharyngeal wall.

Following laryngectomy, the percentage of patients with postsurgical chronic dysphagia is poorly documented. In one study, five of ten patients developed dysphagia (Duranceau et al. 1976). Based on manometrics, all ten were found to have marked derangements in the upper esophageal sphincter.

Balfe et al. (1982) performed barium esophagrams on 45 total laryngectomy patients whose follow-up ranged from 6 months to 17 years. Forty of these patients had pharyngeal symptoms and 26 complained of dysphagia. Of the 40 patients with pharyngeal symptoms, the final diagnosis included recurrent neoplasm (15 patients), benign stricture (14 patients), fistula (13 patients), cricopharyngeal muscle dysfunction (12 patients), second primary tumor in the esophagus (2 patients), and abscess (1 patient). Seventeen patients had more than one abnormality. Neither the effect of irradiation on swallow nor to what extent dysphagia interfered with oral intake was described in this study.

Kirchner and Scatliff (1962) used cineradiography to examine 43 laryngectomized patients for dysphagia at different periods of time postsurgery. Of the 26 patients examined immediately postoperatively, 12 had dysphagia. Eight of the 12 had fistulas and four did not. Even though the majority of the 43 could eventually take nutrition orally, some had anterior pouch formation with regurgitation, constant accumulation of food and mucus, and complaints of a foreign-body sensation.

In a follow-up study, Kirchner and coworkers (1963) examined 35 patients with laryngectomy. They found that dysphagia was caused by a pharyngeal pseudodiverticulum resulting from separation of the pharyngeal suture line at its junction with the tongue base or by uncoordinated contraction of the detached pharyngeal muscles in the absence of stricture.

McConnell et al. (1986) used manofluorography to study 14 total laryngectomy patients to analyze the pharyngeal phase of swallow with respect to tongue propulsion, laryngeal movement, and constrictor contraction. Subjects were divided into two groups: nine without tongue impairment and five with tongue impairment. They found that the major functional change in the pharynx after total laryngectomy was increased pharyngeal resistance. Those without tongue impairment could compensate by using increased lingual propulsion to overcome increased pharyngeal resistance, whereas those with tongue impairment could not. This tongue weakness resulted in increased pharyngeal transit times for the latter group. Factors that may account for pharyngeal resistance include tongue impairment, anterior pouches, pseudoepiglottis, and pharyngeal or sphincter dismotility. While all of the patients with tongue impairment complained of difficulty swallowing, its effect on weight, diet selection, and nutrition was not documented.

There is some evidence to suggest that a higher percentage of the laryngectomized patients who also receive irradiation experience dysphagia. Three of the five patients examined by Duranceau and colleagues (1976) had postoperative dysphagia. Hanks et al. (1981) studied ten patients who were dysphagic after laryngectomy, seven of whom had received irradiation. This finding led the authors to conclude that although dysphagia following total laryngectomy was not common, irradiation may adversely influence upper esophageal motility.

Our own experience and that of Weaver and Fleming (1978) suggest that a large majority of those undergoing laryngectomy who have no medical complications swallow a soft diet after 14 days and that irradiation retards this recovery in a small number of patients. Most complain that they are unable to easily swallow tough meats and larger-sized boluses. Forty-seven of 59 laryngectomized patients reported postoperative dysphagia, but all were taking their nutrition orally after discharge from the hospital (Volin 1980). Only one patient had persistent dysphagia. There was no significant correlation between preoperative and/or postoperative irradiation and dysphagia.

Jung and Adams (1980) did a retrospective review of 226 laryngectomized patients. Of this group 36 (16%) patients experienced dysphagia: 16 had benign pharyngeal stricture, 14 had an obstructive stricture that was due to recurrence of cancer, four had malignant esophageal cancer, and two had benign lower esophageal stricture. The majority had preoperative irradiation. Most of those who experienced dysphagia had laryngopharyngectomy. The authors suggested that the complaint of persistent dysphagia may be a sign of early recurrence, especially if the postpharyngeal space is wider than normal or if patients have benign strictures.

Tracheoesophageal Puncture

The creation of a tracheoesophageal fistula during or after primary laryngectomy has been described as an alternate method for achieving communication (Singer and Blom 1980; Hamaker et al. 1985; Juarbe et al. 1986; Stiernberg et al. 1987; Maniglia et al. 1989). A tracheoesophageal fistula allows the patient to shunt pulmonary air from the trachea into the pharyngoesophageal segment, which acts as a vibrating source for the production of voice. In the usual circumstance a prosthetic valve is placed into the puncture site to facilitate speaking and prevent aspiration.

Numerous surgical interventions for the production of alaryngeal speech have been described. None is without complications. Conley et al. (1958), Asai (1972), Taub and Spiro (1972), Staffieri (1973), Singer and Blom (1980), Panje (1981), Wetmore et al. (1981), Li (1985), Andrews et al. (1987), and Saito et al.

(1989) have reported complications that may affect swallow, such as aspiration or leakage of saliva and food; aspiration of the voice prosthesis; stenosis of the hypopharynx, tracheostoma, or esophagus; stoma and fistula infection; development of a secondary fistula; pharyngoesophageal spasm; and migration or progressive fistula enlargement.

After the creation of a tracheoesophageal fistula, a stent or voice prosthesis may be in place at the tracheoesophageal site when oral feedings are begun. During these initial trial feedings, one should suspect leakage around the prosthesis if the patient coughs during swallow. Aspiration or leakage may also occur through the voice prosthesis. Inspection for dislodgement, improper fit, or faulty functioning of the voice prosthesis should follow. A modified barium swallowing study performed with the stent or voice prosthesis in place is often helpful to determine the site and amount of aspiration or leakage when clinical information is not available.

Irradiation and Deglutition

It is not infrequent for patients who undergo conservative surgical resections for carcinoma also to receive either preoperative or postoperative irradiation that produces many potential side effects that may further compromise swallowing, including oral and pharyngeal inflammation with subsequent pain in the soft tissues and bone, a drying effect on the mucosal tissues, diminished volume and thicker consistency of saliva, changes in taste sensation, and loss of appetite. Not all patients experience these symptoms, but when they do, the severity and duration of effects on deglutition are highly variable (Dreizen et al. 1977b).

Loss of Saliva Flow

If sufficient amounts of irradiation are directed toward the salivary glands, patients experience a marked reduction of salivary flow. These changes tend to be permanent and irreversible (Frank et al. 1953; Dreizen et al. 1977a). Of 42 patients with oral cancers who received 260 rads per day, 5 days per week, salivary flow rates after mastication dropped to 57% after the first week, to 76% after 6 weeks, and to 95% 3 years after irradiation (Dreizen et al. 1977a).

Hansen et al. (1970) studied the subjective complaints of 80 patients receiving irradiation for oral lesions. Seventy-eight percent experienced xerostomia during the second week of treatment. This complaint ranked first in a list of six. After 6 weeks of treatment the same individuals were troubled by xerostomia, and after 3 months of treatment it continued to be their major complaint.

When the salivary glands can no longer produce a normal mixture of serous and mucous saliva, deglutition is affected in two ways besides xerostomia: increased dental caries resulting from loss of the natural defense against decay and accumulation of stringy mucus that has lost its lubricating abilities (Carl 1980).

Dental caries create pain during mastication if left untreated (Dreizen et al. 1977a; Weaver and Fleming 1978). Decay can begin on any tooth and progresses rapidly toward destruction of the dental crown (Figure 4.8) (Dreizen et al.

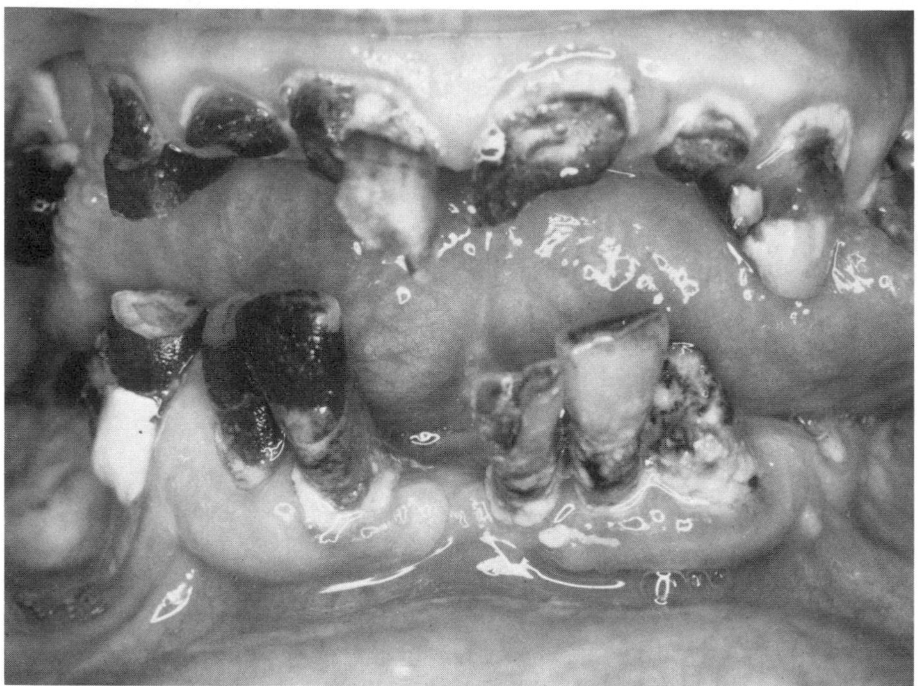

Figure 4.8 Xerostomia-related dental decay 2 years after radiotherapy in a patient with cancer of the tongue. (Reprinted with permission from S Dreizen, TE Daly, JB Drane, et al. Oral complications of cancer radiotherapy. Postgrad Med 1977;61:85.)

1977b). Accumulation of thick mucus can in itself mechanically interfere with swallowing (Figure 4.9). Hansen and colleagues (1970) found that an accumulation of stringy mucus was the second most common complaint (59%) after 2 and 6 weeks of irradiation. Patients reported that they were most uncomfortable when the dryness and thick mucus were at their highest point on the twelfth day of radiotherapy. These thick secretions also interfere with denture retention, tissue tolerance to the denture, and taste (Summers 1974).

Kuten and associates (1986) examined the effects of field arrangement, number of salivary glands irradiated, clinical manifestations such as dryness of the mouth, taste impairment, dysphagia, salivary secretion, and composition, and oral yeast flora on 32 patients treated with external irradiation to the head and neck. The patients received either primary or postoperative radiation therapy and were divided into four groups based on the volume of area irradiated. After 1,000–2,000 cGy, 29 of the 30 patients developed a variety of oral symptoms, with each patient experiencing at least one symptom, including xerostomia (81%), taste impairment (62%), dysphagia (59%), soreness (37%), and increase in salivary viscosity (16%). Twenty-two percent of the patients who reported xerostomia were experiencing this symptom before radiotherapy. The

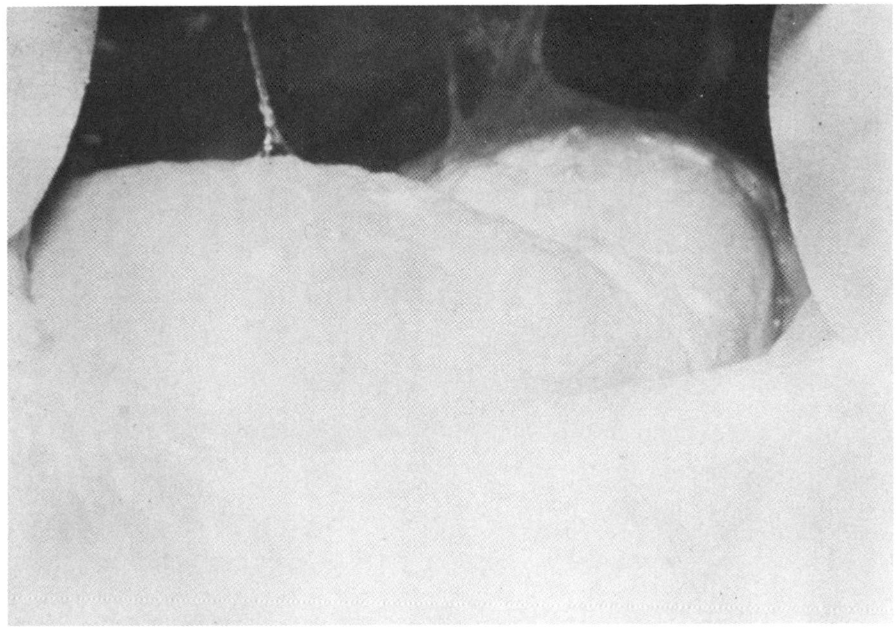

Figure 4.9 Patient with thick mucous secretions secondary to radiotherapy after resection of cancer of the tongue.

examiners concluded that at least 50% of the parotid gland must be spared from the field of radiation to prevent severe dryness. The severity of oral symptoms was shown to increase as salivary gland involvement in the radiated field was extended. Decrease in salivary secretions was accompanied by an increase in salivary sodium concentration and oral yeast flora.

Mucositis

Irradiation can produce significant inflammatory changes in the mucous lining, resulting in tenderness and burning not unlike a severe sore throat. A more marked form of these complaints may surface as mucositis (Figure 4.10). When the pain spreads to the pharyngeal mucosa, swallowing can be difficult. This discomfort is antagonized by coarse and highly seasoned foods. Hansen's group (1970) found that 33% of the patients in their study complained that inflamed mucosa impeded swallowing. Three months after irradiation, patients no longer had this complaint. In their study of 32 patients who received primary or postoperative head and neck irradiation, Kuten and associates (1986) found clinical manifestations of mucositis 3 weeks after the initiation of full-course radiation therapy. Patients had dry oral mucosa (53%), erythema of the mucosal surface (45%), and mucosal plaque formation (64%). They concluded that dysphagia was secondary to not only dryness caused by decreased salivary secretion

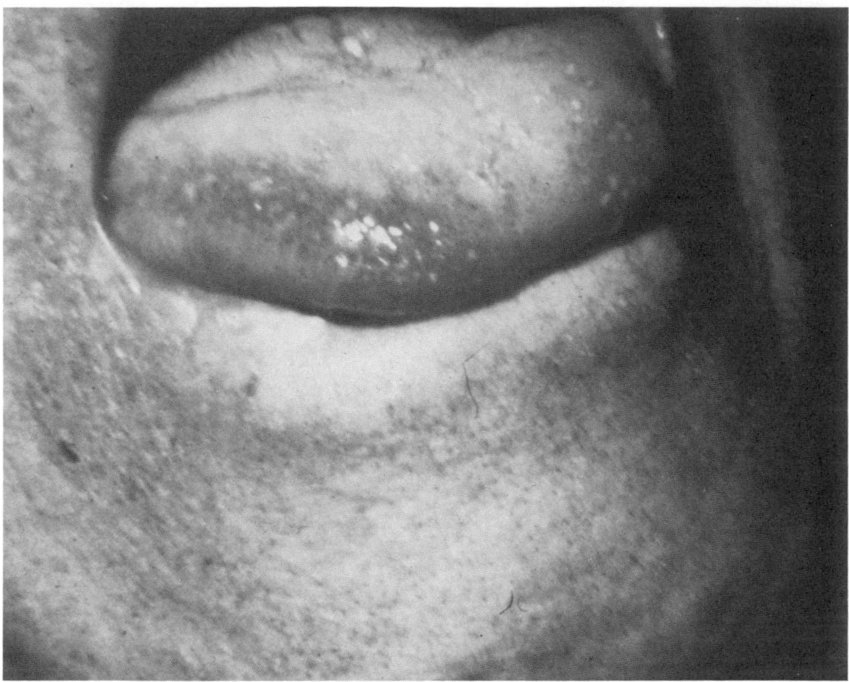

Figure 4.10 Early radiation mucositis of the tongue in a patient treated for cancer of the floor of the mouth. (Reprinted with permission from S Dreizen, TE Daly, JB Drane, et al. Oral complications of cancer radiotherapy. Postgrad Med 1977;61:85)

but also, to a greater degree, factors such as radiation damage to mucosal surfaces, edema, and infection. Dreizen et al. (1977b) reported that mucositis gradually improved spontaneously 3 weeks after termination of radiotherapy. Oral mucositis may also result from the use of chemotherapeutic agents such as doxorubicin (Adriamycin), methotrexate, and cyclophosphamide (Carl 1980).

Osteoradionecrosis

Osteoradionecrosis can result from oral mucosal destruction at the primary site of irradiation. Developing fibrosis and reduction of blood supply result in the formation of necrotic ulcers that, left untreated, can invade bony structures through infectious processes. Ulcers can develop 2–3 months after radiotherapy or any time thereafter (Dreizen et al. 1977b). The resultant pain can impair oral feeding actions and swallowing to a point at which patients are not able to take nutrition orally. Patients are most vulnerable to osteoradionecrosis of the jaw during the 2 years following irradiation (Dreizen et al. 1977b). Spongy bones are more susceptible to osteoradionecrosis than flat bones. As a result, the mandible and zygomatic bones are more often affected than the maxilla. A clinical example is presented in Figure 4.11.

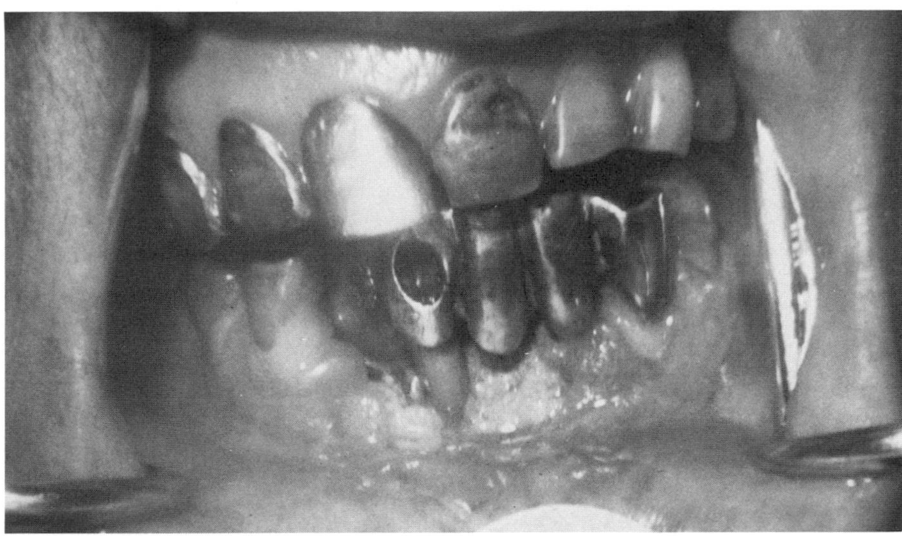

Figure 4.11 Osteoradionecrosis of the mandibular alveolar bone in a patient treated for cancer of the tongue. (Reprinted with permission from S Dreizen, TE Daly, JB Drane, et al. Oral complications of cancer radiotherapy. Postgrad Med 1977;61:85.)

Trismus

Patients who have mastication difficulty in the form of tonic spasms during or following irradiation may be suffering from trismus. Trismus is believed to occur secondary to fibrosis of the muscles of mastication (Parsons 1984). Radiation-induced trismus occurs most often after irradiation of the nasopharynx, tonsil, retromolar trigone, or paranasal sinuses. Patients who have received both surgery and irradiation are at greater risk of developing trismus than those patients who are treated with either modality alone (Parsons 1984). If severe trismus develops, dental extraction may become necessary for feeding. In addition, jaw excursions may be painful and limited. Temporomandibular joint exercises should begin after surgery and continue during and after radiotherapy to prevent the development of trismus. The success of therapeutic exercise methods depends on the severity of the fibrosis and patient compliance (Barrett et al. 1988).

Loss of Taste and Appetite

Patients often experience weight loss during radiation therapy as a result of a decreased ability to taste, chew, smell, and swallow. All of these factors contribute to a reduction in appetite. Hansen and associates (1970) reported that 53% of the patients in their study experienced loss of appetite during and shortly after irradiation. Twenty-two percent said that this was due to a loss of taste; the remaining 78% felt it was related to feelings of nausea and a general dissatisfaction with their diet. Acuity of taste is recovered rapidly at first and then more slowly. A tumor that is necrotic or infected may also predispose the patient to nausea and vomiting. Patients generally recover taste acuity 20–60 days after radiotherapy, and it fully returns after 120 days (Dreizen et al. 1977b). Others have reported specific losses of sweet, salt, and bitter tastes (Conger 1973; DeWys and Walters 1975). Sour and bitter tastes are suppressed more than sweet and salty tastes; however, most patients complain that all food has lost its flavor (Jepson 1985). Aversions to meat and vegetable proteins have also been noted (Fleming et al. 1982). Such aversions can lead to loss of appetite, disinterest in food, and, eventually, to poor nutrition. Severe loss of proteins, calories, vitamins, and minerals can lead to a nutritional deficiency type of stomatitis.

CERVICAL SPINE DISEASE

Osteophytic changes in the cervical spine that put undue mechanical pressure on the proximal pharynx or esophagus must be considered in the differential diagnosis of mechanical dysphagia.

Although pressure on the pharynx from the cervical spine is rare (Umerah et al. 1981), some investigators feel that it may just be overlooked as a potential cause and therefore is not as rare as once believed (Lambert et al. 1981). Radiographically, cervical osteophytes appear as bony projections from one or more of the cervical vertebrae, with displacement of the posterior pharyngeal or common esophageal wall. Typically, it is found in elderly patients with cervical spondylosis (Umerah et al. 1981) and usually is seen at the level of C4–C7 (Lambert et al. 1981). Patients complain of pain at the cricopharyngeal level, probably caused by the pressure of food on the osteophytes (Umerah et al. 1981). All patients complain that solids are harder to swallow than liquids (Lambert et al. 1981). In addition to dysphagia, other symptoms, such as cough, stridor, hoarseness, and other laryngeal or pharyngeal disorders, may be present (Girgis et al. 1982). A review of the history of spinal diseases and dysphagia is provided by Gamache and Voorhies (1980).

NASOENTERIC TUBES

Acutely ill patients may be placed on either enteral or parenteral nutrition as a primary means of nutritional support or as a supplement in patients with inadequate oral intake. Nasoenteric tubes may complicate oral feedings because of mechanical interference and by their association with an increased incidence of aspiration pneumonia.

We have clinically observed that large-bore nasogastric feeding tubes are more likely to interfere with the smooth passage of semisolid and solid bolus textures. Bolus residual may remain in the hypopharynx or be directed toward the airway. Consequently, in those patients who require supplemental nasoenteric feeding tubes it is preferable to have a small-bore feeding tube in place during dysphagia evaluations and when oral feedings are begun.

Enteral support using a nasogastric tube may lead to aspiration resulting from hypersalivation, depressed cough reflex, laryngopharyngeal injuries, gastroesophageal reflux, and dislodgement of the tube into the esophagus or trachea (Noone and Graham 1973; Alessi and Berci 1986). Risk factors predisposing a patient with nasoenteral feedings to aspiration pneumonia include reduced level of consciousness (less than alert and oriented) with consequent compromise in glottic closure and cough reflex, dysphagia from neurologic or esophageal mechanisms, vomiting, ileus or gastric dilation, and failure to maintain elevation of the head (Awe et al. 1966; Cameron and Zuidema 1972; Bartlett and Gorbach 1975; Torosean and Rombeau 1976; Metheny et al. 1986).

In a study conducted by Sitzmann (1990), 90 patients who had been admitted to Johns Hopkins Hospital with a primary complaint of dysphagia were reviewed. Patients were divided into two groups based on the etiology of dysphagia: neurogenic (43 patients) and mechanical (47 patients). All patients were placed on enteral (63%) or parenteral (37%) nutrition because of marked malnutrition. Patients with nasoenteric tubes had a 40% complication rate (aspiration or endotracheal placement of the tube), resulting in a 30% mortality. This mortality was significantly higher than that seen with other treatment modalities, such as jejunostomy tube feedings and total parenteral nutrition. Both nasoenteric and gastrostomy tube feedings were associated with an increased risk of aspiration pneumonia. Sitzmann concluded that patients admitted to a hospital with the primary complaint of dysphagia that has led to severe malnutrition should not be placed on nasoenteric or gastrostomy feeding tubes until the dysphagia has resolved. It was also suggested that hospitalized dysphagic patients should be evaluated by cineradiography to rule out reflux or aspiration before oral or nasoenteric feedings are begun.

TRACHEOSTOMA TUBES

Tracheostoma tubes create a mechanical interference to swallowing by restricting normal laryngeal elevation. Loss of elevation compromises glottal protection and invites aspiration. Butcher (1982) reported that tracheostoma tubes increased the chances of aspiration by fixing the larynx anteriorly and preventing its axial rotation. Arms et al. (1974) demonstrated that one is at a greater risk for aspiration if a tracheostoma tube is in place.

Bonanno (1971) attempted to investigate the theory that tracheostoma tubes could contribute to dysphagia. He studied 43 patients who underwent elective or semi-elective tracheostomy for general surgery. All were considered to be poor pulmonary risks for general anesthesia. None had head or neck cancer. Previous medical health was not reported. Three of the 43 patients had postoperative dysphagia because, Bonanno felt, the tracheostoma tube appeared to be anchoring the trachea to the pretracheal strap muscles and the skin of the neck, thus limiting anterior elevation and rotation. Lack of this movement interfered with relaxation of the cricopharyngeal muscle.

Stauffer et al. (1981) prospectively studied the complications and consequences of endotracheal intubation and tracheotomy in 150 critically ill patients. Of the 150 patients, 97 received only endotracheal intubation, 46 received tracheotomies following endotracheal intubation, and seven received only tracheotomy. Of the 53 patients who received a tracheotomy, 51 were standard tracheotomies and two were cricothyroidotomies. The 8% incidence of aspiration was similar for patients who received endotracheal intubation or tracheotomy. Two follow-up visits after extubation were conducted on the patients in this study to assess late complications. In the first follow-up visit, 47 patients were evaluated. The incidence of dysphagic complaints was not reported. During a second follow-up visit of 21 patients, dysphagia was reported by 38% of patients with tracheotomy and 8% of patients with endotracheal intubation.

It has been our experience that the incidence of dysphagia is greater in patients who have tracheostomy combined with surgical resection of the head and neck. In these cases, patients already have compromised deglutition, and the tracheostoma tube serves as an additional barrier to normal laryngeal elevation.

Patients who have cuffed tracheostoma tubes that are overinflated are at risk for esophageal obstruction from the pressure on the tracheoesophageal wall. The obstruction keeps nutrition from entering the esophagus easily, creating spillover and possible aspiration.

An additional complication is that the presence of the tube prevents expiratory air from being shunted superiorly, resulting in a decrease of expired air needed to clear the larynx after swallowing (Weaver and Fleming 1982). This reduction of the ability to clear the airway because of mechanical interference may impede rehabilitation (see Chapter 11).

SUMMARY

Mechanical swallowing dysfunction is usually the result of the oral or pharyngeal structures or both being surgically removed or altered. This impairs the displacement of food in the mouth and the bolus in the pharynx. Even though some patients have adequate sensory and motor components for postoperative oral and pharyngeal feeding, most have significant dysphagia. Additionally, the majority have adequate cortical skills needed for the rehabilitation of feeding.

The dysphagia liability is increased by radiotherapy, chemotherapy, or both. A careful evaluation of the pathology as discussed should assist the clinician in working out the diagnostic dilemmas that these patients often present. Treatment suggestions are provided in detail in Chapter 11.

REFERENCES

Alessi DM, Berci G. Aspiration and nasogastric intubation. Otolaryngol Head Neck Surg 1986;94:486.

Andrews JC, Mickel RA, Hanson DG, et al. Major complications following tracheoesophageal puncture for voice rehabilitation. Laryngoscope 1987;97:562.

Arms RA, Dines DE, Tinstman TC. Aspiration pneumonia. Chest 1974;65:136.

Asai R. Laryngoplasty after total laryngectomy. Arch Otolaryngol Head Neck Surg 1972;95:114.
Awe W, Fletcher W, Jacobs S. The pathophysiology of aspiration pneumonia. Surgery 1966;60:232.
Baker BM, Fraser AM, Baker CD. Long-term postoperative dysphagia in oral/pharyngeal surgery patients: subjects' perceptions versus videofluoroscopic observations. Dysphagia 1991;6:11.
Balfe DM, Koehler RE, Setzen M, et al. Barium examination of the esophagus after total laryngectomy. Radiology 1982;143:501.
Barrett NVJ, Martin JW, Jacob RF, et al. Physical therapy techniques in the treatment of the head and neck patient. J Prosthet Dent 1988;59:343.
Bartlett JG, Gorbach SL. The triple threat of aspiration pneumonia. Chest 1975;68:560.
Beckhardt RN, Murray JE, Ford CN, et al. Factors influencing functional outcome in supraglottic laryngectomy. Head Neck 1994;16:232.
Blomquist IK, Bayer AS. Life-threatening deep facial space infections of the head and neck. Infect Dis Clin North Am 1988;2:237.
Bocca E, Pignataro O, Mosciaro O. Supraglottic surgery of the larynx. Ann Otol Rhinol Laryngol 1968;77:1005.
Bonanno PC. Swallowing dysfunction after tracheostomy. Ann Surg 1971;174:29.
Butcher BR. Treatment of chronic aspiration as a complication of cerebrovascular accident. Laryngoscope 1982;92:681.
Calcaterra TC. Epiglottic reconstruction after supraglottic laryngectomy. Laryngoscope 1985;95:786.
Cameron JL, Zuidema GD. Aspiration pneumonia: magnitude and frequency of the problem. JAMA 1972;219:1194.
Carl W. Dental management of head and neck cancer patients. J Surg Oncol 1980;15:265.
Cohen EL. Epiglottitis in the adult. Postgrad Med 1984;75:309.
Conger AD. Loss and recovery of taste acuity in patients irradiated to the oral cavity. Radiat Res 1973;53:338.
Conley JJ. Swallowing dysfunctions associated with radical surgery of the head and neck. Arch Surg 1960;80:602.
Conley JJ, DeAmesti F, Pierce MK. A new surgical technique for the vocal rehabilitation of the laryngectomized patient. Ann Otol Rhinol Laryngol 1958;67:655.
Coyle JL, Wood JL, Robbins JA, et al. Changes in swallow duration and bolus velocity in head and neck cancer patients treated with radiotherapy. Presented at the meeting of the Dysphagia Research Society, McLean, Virginia, 1995.
DeWeese DD, Saunders WH. Textbook of Otolaryngology. St. Louis: Mosby, 1973.
DeWys WD, Walters K. Abnormalities of taste sensation in cancer patients. Cancer 1975;36:1888.
Doberneck R, Antoine A. Deglutition after resection of oral, laryngeal and pharyngeal cancers. Surgery 1974;75:87.
Donaldson RC, Skelly M, Paletta FX. Total glossectomy for cancer. Am J Surg 1986;116:585.
Dreizen S, Brown LR, Daly TE, et al. Prevention of xerostomia-related dental caries in irradiated cancer patients. J Dent Res 1977a;56:99.
Dreizen S, Daly TE, Drane JB, et al. Oral complications of cancer radiotherapy. Postgrad Med 1977b;61:85.
Duranceau A, Jamieson G, Hurwitz A, et al. Alteration in esophageal motility after laryngectomy. Am J Surg 1976;131:30.
Fayos JV. Carcinoma of the endolarynx: results of irradiation. Cancer 1975;35:1525.
Fleming SM, Weaver AW. Clinical management of dysphagia in head and neck cancer patients. Dysarthria Dysphonia Dysphagia 1982;1:80.
Flores TC, Wood BG, Koegel L Jr, et al. Factors in successful deglutition following supraglottic laryngeal surgery. Ann Otol Rhinol Laryngol 1982;91:579.

Frazell EL, Lucas JC. Cancer of the tongue: report of the management of 1,554 patients. Cancer 1962;15:1085.
Freeman RB, Marks JE, Ogura JH. Voice preservation in treatment of carcinoma of the pyriform sinus. Laryngoscope 1979;11:1855.
Fujiu M, Logemann JA, Pauloski BR. Increased postoperative posterior pharyngeal wall movement in patients with anterior oral cancer: preliminary findings and possible implications for treatment. Am J Speech Lang Pathol 1995;4:24.
Gamache FW, Voorhies RM. Hypertrophic cervical osteophytes causing dysphagia. J Neurosurg 1980;53:338.
Girgis IH, Guirguis NN, Mourice M. Laryngeal and pharyngeal disorders in vertebral ankylosing hyperostosis. J Laryngol Otol 1982;96:659.
Greenspan D, Greenspan JS. The oral features of HIV infection. Gastroenterol Clin North Am 1988;17:535.
Groher ME, Enderle EE. Mechanical dysphagia secondary to macroglossia: a case report. Department of Veterans Affairs Medical Center, New York, 1988.
Hamaker RC, Singer MI, Blom ED, et al. Primary voice restoration at laryngectomy. Arch Otolaryngol Head Neck Surg 1985;111:182.
Hamlet S, Jones L, Patterson R, et al. Swallowing recovery following anterior tongue and floor of mouth surgery. Head Neck 1991;13:334.
Hanks JB, Fisher ST, Myers WC, et al. Effect of total laryngectomy on esophageal motility. Ann Otol Rhinol Laryngol 1981;90:331.
Hansen D, Meyer E, Werner H. Function disorders of the oral cavity as a side effect of radiotherapy. Z Laryngol Rhinol Otol 1970;49:534.
Hawkins DB, Miller AH, Sachs GB, et al. Acute epiglottitis in adults. Laryngoscope 1973;83:1211.
Hirano M, Kuriowa Y, Tanaka S. Dysphagia following various degree of surgical resection for oral cancer. Ann Otol Rhinol Laryngol 1992;101:138.
Jepson J. Nutrition in patients irradiated for head and neck cancer. Nutri Supp Serv 1985;5:27.
Juarbe C, Shemen L, Eberle R, et al. Primary tracheoesophageal puncture for voice restoration. Am J Surg 1986;152:464.
Jung TT, Adams GL. Dysphagia in laryngectomized patients. Otolaryngol Head Neck Surg 1980;88:25.
Kander PL, Richards SH. Acute epiglottitis in adults. J Laryngol Otol 1977;91:295.
Kerr DA, Ash MM. Oral Pathology. Philadelphia: Lea & Febiger, 1978.
Keyes KS. Oral Mucosal Diseases. In MM Paparella, DA Shumrick (eds), Otolaryngology: Head and Neck. Philadelphia: Saunders, 1980;2136.
Kirchner JA, Scatliff JH. Disabilities resulting from healed salivary fistula. Arch Otolaryngol Head Neck Surg 1962;75:46.
Kirchner JA, Scatliff JH, Dey FL, et al. The pharynx after laryngectomy. Laryngoscope 1963;73:18.
Knuff TE, Benjamine SB, Castell DO. Pharyngoesophageal (Zenker's) diverticulum: a reappraisal. Gastroenterology 1982;82:734.
Kothary PM, DeSouza LJ. Swallowing without tongue. Bombay Hosp J 1973;15:58.
Kuten A, Ben-Aryeh H, Berdicevsky I, et al. Oral side effects of head and neck rotation: correlation between clinical manifestations and laboratory data. Int J Radiat Oncol Biol Phys 1986;12:401.
Lambert JR, Tepperman PS, Jimenez J, et al. Cervical spine disease and dysphagia. Am J Gastroenterol 1981;76:35.
LaVelle CLB, Proctor DB. Clinical Pathology of the Oral Mucosa. Hagerstown, MD: Harper & Row, 1978.
Lazarus CL. Effects of radiation therapy and voluntary maneuvers on swallowing function in head and neck cancer patients. Clin Comm Disord 1993;4:11.

Leonard JR, Holt GP, Maran AG. Treatment of vocal cord carcinoma by vertical hemilaryngectomy. Ann Otol Rhinol Laryngol 1972;81:469.

Li SL. Functional tracheoesophageal shunt for vocal rehabilitation after laryngectomy. Laryngoscope 1985;95:1267.

Litton WB, Leonard JR. Aspiration after partial laryngectomy: cineradiographic studies. Laryngoscope 1969;75:887.

Logemann JA, Bytell DE. Swallowing disorders in three types of head and neck surgical patients. Cancer 1979;44:1095.

Maniglia AJ, Lundy DS, Casiano RC, et al. Speech restoration and complications of primary versus secondary tracheoesophageal puncture following total laryngectomy. Laryngoscope 1989;99:489.

Mayosmith MF, Hirsch PJ, Wodzinski SF, et al. Acute epiglottitis in adults. N Engl J Med 1986;314:1133.

McConnell FMS. Analysis of pressure generation and bolus transit during pharyngeal swallowing. Laryngoscope 1988;98:71.

McConnell FMS, Logemann JA. Diagnosis and Treatment of Swallowing Disorders. In CW Cummings (ed), Otolaryngology, Head and Neck Surgery (Update II). St. Louis: Mosby, 1990;57.

McConnell FMS, Mendelsohn MS. The effects of surgery on pharyngeal deglutition. Dysphagia 1987;1:145.

McConnell FMS, Mendelsohn MS, Logemann JA. Examination of swallow after total laryngectomy using manofluorography. Head Neck Surg 1986;9:3.

Metheny NA, Eisenberg P, Spies M. Aspiration pneumonia in patients fed through nasoenteral tubes. Heart Lung 1986;15:256.

Murray GM. Pulmonary complications following supraglottic laryngectomy. Clin Otolaryngol 1976;1:241.

Myers EN. The role of total glossectomy in the management of cancer of the oral cavity. Otolaryngol Clin North Am 1972;5:343.

Nayar RC, Sharma VP, Arora MML. A study of the pharynx after laryngectomy. J Laryngol Otol 1984;98:807.

Noone RB, Graham WP. Nutritional care after head and neck surgery. Postgrad Med 1973;53:80.

Panje WR. Prosthetic voice rehabilitation following laryngectomy. Ann Otol Rhinol Laryngol 1981;90:116.

Parsons JT. The Effect of Radiation on Normal Tissues of the Head and Neck. In RR Million, NJ Cassisi (eds), Management of Head and Neck Cancer. Philadelphia: Lippincott, 1984;173.

Patterson HC, Kelly LH, Strome RR. Ludwig's angina: an update. Laryngoscope 1982;92:370.

Pauloski BR, Logemann JA, Rademanker AL, et al. Speech and swallowing function after oral and oropharyngeal resections: one year follow-up. Head Neck 1994;16:313.

Raufman JP. Odynophagia/dysphagia in AIDS. Gastroenterol Clin North Am 1988;17:599.

Saito H, Yoshida S, Saito T, et al. Simple mucodermal tracheoesophageal shunt method for voice restoration. Arch Otolaryngol Head Neck Surg 1989;115:494.

Sarant G. Acute epiglottitis in adults. Ann Emerg Med 1981;10:58.

Schabel SI, Katzberg RW, Burgener FA. Acute inflammation of epiglottis and supraglottic structures in adults. Radiology 1977;122:601.

Schima W, Denk DM, Schober E, et al. Swallowing function after laryngeal resections: videofluoroscopic assessment of prognostic factors. Presented at the meeting of the Dysphagia Research Society, McLean, Virginia, 1994.

Schobinger R. Spasm of cricopharyngeus muscle as a cause of dysphagia after total laryngectomy. Arch Otolaryngol 1958;67:271.

Schoenrock LD, King AY, Everts EC, et al. Hemilaryngectomy: deglutition evaluation and rehabilitation. Trans Am Acad Ophthalmol Otolaryngol 1972;76:752.

Schumaker HM, Doris PE, Birnbaum G. Radiographic parameters in adult epiglottitis. Ann Emerg Med 1984;13:588.

Sessions DG, Zill R, Schwartz SL. Deglutition after conservation surgery for cancer of the larynx and hypopharynx. Otolaryngol Head Neck Surg 1979;87:779.

Shedd DP. Rehabilitation problems of head and neck cancer patients. J Surg Oncol 1976;8:11.

Singer MI, Blom ED. An endoscopic technique for restoration of voice after total laryngectomy. Ann Otol Rhinol Laryngol 1980;89:529.

Sitzmann JV. Nutritional support of the dysphagic patient: methods, risks, and complications of therapy. JPEN J Parenter Enteral Nutr 1990;14:60.

Staffieri M. Laringectomia totale con ricostruzione di "glottide fonataria." Nuovo Arch Ital Otol 1973;1:181.

Staple TW, Ogura JH. Cineradiography of the swallowing mechanism following supraglottic subtotal laryngectomy. Radiology 1966;87:226.

Staple TW, Ragsdale EF, Ogura JH. The chest roentgenogram following supra-glottic laryngectomy. AJR Am J Roentgenol 1967;100:583.

Stauffer JL, Olson DE, Petty TL. Complications and consequences of endotracheal intubation and tracheotomy. Am J Med 1981;70:65.

Stiernberg CM, Bailey BJ, Calhoun KH, et al. Primary tracheoesophageal fistula procedure for voice restoration: the University of Texas Medical Branch experience. Laryngoscope 1987;97:820.

Summers GW. Physiologic problems following ablative surgery of the head and neck. Otolaryngol Clin North Am 1974;7:217.

Taub S, Spiro RH. Vocal rehabilitation of laryngectomees. Am J Surg 1972;124:87.

Torosean M, Rombeau J. Feeding by tube enterostomy. Surg Gynecol Obstet 1976;143:273.

Umerah BC, Mukherjee BK, Ibekur O. Cervical sypondylosis and dysphagia. J Laryngol Otol 1981;95:1179.

Volin RA. Predicting failure to speak after laryngectomy. Laryngoscope 1980;90:1727.

Weaver AW, Fleming SM. Partial laryngectomy: analysis of associated swallowing disorders. Am J Surg 1978;136:486.

Weber RS, Ohlms L, Bowman J. Functional results after total or near total glossectomy with laryngeal preservation. Arch Otolaryngol Head Neck Surg 1991;117:512.

Wetmore SJ, Johns ME, Baker SR. The Blom-Singer voice restoration procedure. Arch Otolaryngol 1981;107:674.

Williams AC, Guralnick WC. The diagnosis and treatment of Ludwig's angina: report of twenty cases. N Engl J Med 1943;228:443.

5

Esophageal Dysphagia

William J. Ravich

A large number of subspecialties are involved in evaluating and caring for patients with swallowing disorders. Most subspecialists have a limited understanding of the knowledge and technical expertise of other fields. The following chapter offers a gastroenterologist's perspective on dysphagia of presumed and documented esophageal origin, written for clinicians from other subspecialties who want to acquire a working familiarity with esophageal causes of swallowing problems and their management.

MECHANISMS OF ESOPHAGEAL DYSPHAGIA

The esophagus is a distensible tube, about 20 cm long, connecting the pharynx and stomach. It is separated from the pharynx by the upper esophageal sphincter (UES) and from the stomach by the lower esophageal sphincter (LES). Under resting conditions, the esophageal lumen is collapsed, a potential space that can distend easily to accommodate swallowed air, liquids, or solids. The act of swallowing initiates pharyngeal peristalsis as well as relaxation of both the upper and lower esophageal sphincters. The pharyngeal peristaltic contractile wave is propagated through the UES and continues down the length of the esophagus, pushing the swallowed bolus into the stomach (Figure 5.1).

Esophageal dysphagia can be caused by motor or structural abnormalities (Table 5.1). Structural mechanisms include luminal stenosis and, less often, luminal deformity. Motor disorders include abnormalities of esophageal peristalsis and of LES function.

STRUCTURAL DISORDERS

Esophageal Stenosis

Esophageal stenosis (narrowing) is conceptually the easiest mechanism of dysphagia to understand. When the lumen narrows, solid food may be too large to pass through it. Esophageal stenosis typically causes dysphagia for solid food. In addition, the nature of the solid material ingested is important for symptom production. Dysphagia is more likely when solids are tough or fibrous. Softer, more easily chewed foods are much less likely to cause difficulty. An exception to this tough food–soft food dichotomy is that many patients also experience particular trouble with soft, absorbent foods such as bread or pasta,

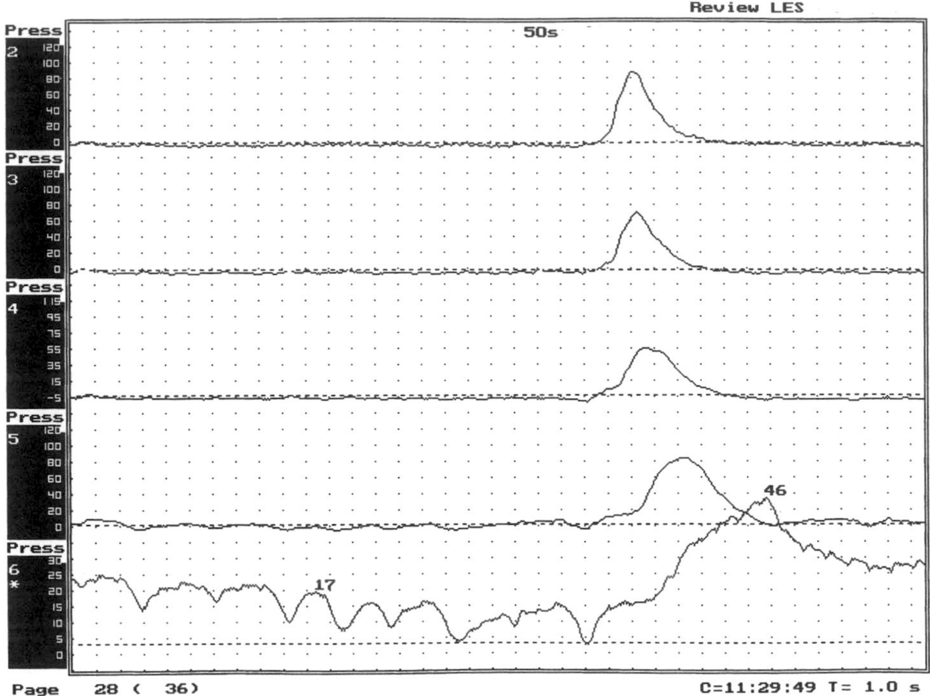

Figure 5.1 Normal esophageal peristalsis. In the manometric study shown here, the bottom sensor is within the LES segment, while the upper four pressure sensors are positioned at 2-cm intervals above the LES (distance of distal sensor from nares and timing of swallow indicated by number and letter at the top). Peristalsis proceeds in an orderly fashion down the length of the esophagus. The LES relaxes to intragastric pressure and remains open until the peristaltic wave passes through it, allowing the swallowed bolus to pass unimpeded into the stomach. The broken line represents the intragastric baseline pressure. Swallowing initiates esophageal peristalsis, as well as LES relaxation. (Vertical scale, 1 increment = 20 mm Hg; horizontal scale, 1 increment = 1 second.)

which swell when mixed with saliva during mastication. Once bolus impaction occurs, the patient may have difficulty with liquids as well, obscuring the characteristic solids-only nature of esophageal stenosis. However, a careful history usually reveals that liquid dysphagia begins with ingestion of solids.

Physicians often rely too much on on the patient's sensation of where food is sticking. The common wisdom that patients "accurately localize symptoms to the site of obstruction" is often inaccurate. In fact, approximately one-third of patients with obstructing lesions of the distal esophagus point to the neck as the site of obstruction (Edwards 1974). Conversely, one-third of patients with dysphagia localized to the pharynx have an isolated abnormality of the esophagus (Jones 1985).

Table 5.1 Mechanisms of Dysphagia

Structural abnormalities
Luminal stenosis
Luminal deformity
Motor dysfunction
Abnormalities of peristalsis
Abnormalities of sphincter function

It is surprising how well some patients do despite dramatic stenosis. It is often stated, based on radiographic observations in patients with Schatzki's rings (Schatzki 1963), that patients with luminal diameters of greater than 18 to 20 mm are never symptomatic, whereas those with diameters less than 10–12 mm are always symptomatic. Between these extremes, symptoms vary both in frequency and severity, depending on the presence of associated motor dysfunction and the choice and preparation of food. The treatment of a stenosis is to open or remove the narrowed segment, depending on the specific cause.

Common intrinsic structural abnormalities that narrow the esophagus include mucosal rings, benign strictures, and malignant tumors.

Rings and Webs

The esophagus may be narrowed by a band of tissue composed of mucosa and submucosa. By tradition, this type of lesion is called a ring when located at the esophagogastric junction and a web when located elsewhere in the esophagus or hypopharynx.

Although classically described in patients with iron-deficiency anemia (sideropenic dysphagia), the vast majority of esophageal webs now seen are not associated with iron deficiency. Webs of the pharyngoesophageal segment or cervical esophagus are frequently asymmetric, most often impinging on the esophageal lumen from the anterior wall (Figure 5.2A).

The most common bandlike constriction of the esophagus is the Schatzki's ring. This lesion is typically symmetric and located at the esophagogastric junction (Figure 5.2B). Asymptomatic Schatzki's rings are detected in about 10% of the population (Goyal et al. 1971). The ring is always noted in the presence of a hiatal hernia. However, most hiatal hernias are not associated with Schatzki's ring. The etiology of a Schatzki's ring is unknown. Since they are rarely seen in childhood and generally present in middle age, it is unlikely that a Schatzki's ring represents a congenital abnormality.

Webs and rings typically produce dysphagia for solids only. Patients often report that symptoms are intermittent and less likely if they select their food wisely and chew carefully. Conversely, symptoms are more likely if the patient eats out or carries on a conversation while eating, situations where the choice of food is

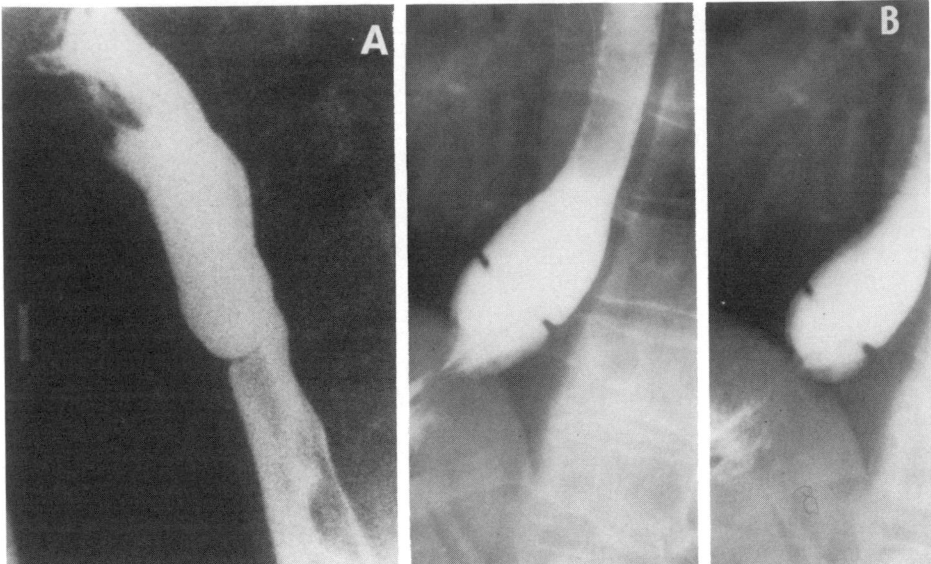

Figure 5.2 Webs and rings. Thin, band-like, stenotic lesions are generally referred to as rings when located at or near the esophagogastric junction, and webs when located elsewhere in the esophagus. A. A web located at the pharyngoesophageal segment. B. Schatzki's ring located at the esophagogastric junction. (Courtesy of Bronwyn Jones, MD.)

more restricted and proper preparation of food before swallowing more difficult. The patient often must end the episode by inducing regurgitation. Once the food is dislodged, the patient can often return to the meal without further difficulty.

The extent to which attention to the mechanics of cutting and chewing controls symptoms is limited. When the lumen is severely compromised, the patient may find it impossible to maintain the level of attention required to remain symptom-free without avoiding solids entirely. The patient may describe symptoms without any apparent progression in frequency or severity, going back for many years. Progression, when it does occur, usually is slow.

Radiographically, these lesions appear as thin (2–4 mm) bands that form shelf-like constrictions anywhere along the esophagus. Although radiologists occasionally refer to thicker lesions as webs or rings, these are probably short strictures or muscular contractions.

Treatment of webs or rings involves dilatation or rupture of the ring by any one of a variety of esophageal dilator systems. The ring is thin, nonfibrotic, and easy to dilate. Complete, or nearly complete, symptomatic relief can be anticipated. Failure to respond is unusual. Dilatation may provide permanent relief, although a large proportion of patients (perhaps a majority) need periodic redilatation at variable intervals (Groskreutz and Kim 1990).

Table 5.2 Differential Diagnosis of Esophagitis

Gastroesophageal reflux
Infections (*Candida*, viral)
Trauma (prolonged nasogastric intubation)
Acute chemical ingestion (lye, industrial acids)
Drug-induced esophagitis (tetracycline, iron, potassium, quinidine, nonsteroidal anti-inflammatory drugs)
Radiation
Skin conditions (pemphigus, cicatricial pemphigoid, epidermolysis bullosa dystrophica, lichen planus, toxic epidermal necrolysis, Stevens-Johnson syndrome)
Others (Crohn's disease, Behçet's syndrome)

Benign Stricture

Strictures are rarely seen in children, although congenital strictures do occur. The vast majority of benign esophageal strictures are acquired in adulthood as a consequence of esophagitis. In a circular structure like the esophagus, edema due to ongoing inflammation and fibrosis as part of the healing process occurs at the expense of luminal diameter.

As with webs and rings, dysphagia is generally for solids only. However, dysphagia is progressive, with episodes becoming more frequent and severe over a period of months or years. As luminal narrowing increases, the patient reports trouble with food that previously caused no difficulty. Occasionally, stenosis can become so severe that even thick liquids cause dysphagia. Even then, however, dysphagia is virtually always greater for solids than liquids.

Because benign strictures are most often a sequelae of reflux-induced esophagitis, patients usually describe a history of heartburn or chest pain and may report the frequent use of antacids or other ulcer medications. In some patients the esophagus appears to be relatively insensitive to acid exposure. These individuals never experience significant reflux symptoms despite severe esophagitis and progression to stricture formation. While most benign esophageal strictures are a result of reflux esophagitis, any cause of esophagitis can cause stricture formation (Table 5.2).

Radiographically, a benign stricture is seen as a narrowed segment of esophageal lumen that may range from a centimeter to many centimeters long (Figure 5.3). The stricture usually is smooth and gradually tapering, with a symmetric lumen that follows the anticipated path of the normal esophagus. Ongoing inflammation may produce an eroded appearance along its course.

Proper management requires both treatment of the underlying inflammation and dilatation of the stricture. Treatment of the cause of esophagitis requires accurate diagnosis. While reflux is the most common cause of esophagitis, other possibilities must be considered, especially in patients with atypical histories, an unusual distribution of inflammation, or failure to respond to reflux treatment.

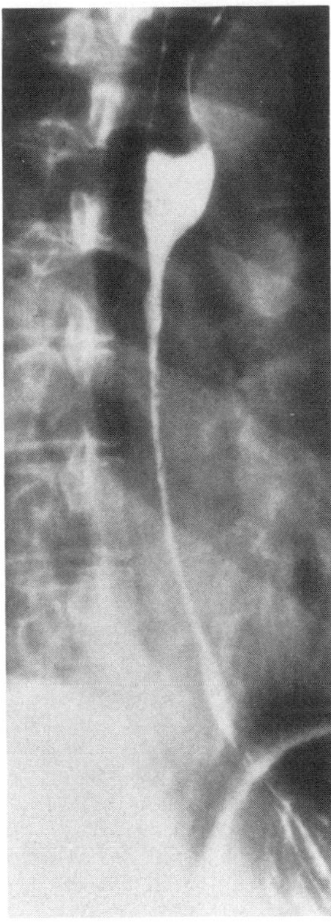

Figure 5.3 Benign stricture. This stricture is long and symmetric, with a lumen that tapers gradually. The lumen follows the anticipated line of the normal esophagus. The barium within the narrowed lumen has a somewhat irregular appearance due to the presence of erosions. (Courtesy of Bronwyn Jones, MD.)

Dilatation can often be performed using the same techniques available for a Schatzki's ring. However, the stricture may be relatively unyielding and require stiffer dilator systems. Effective dilatation usually improves symptoms, although edema from inflammation may result in less complete symptomatic relief than with a Schatzki's ring and in relatively rapid restenosis. Frequent dilatations are more often required in benign strictures than with Schatzki's rings. Even when ongoing inflammation completely ceases, periodic dilatation may be necessary, especially during the first year after initial treatment, when maturation of the fibrotic reaction continues at the expense of luminal diameter.

Malignant Stricture

Although benign tumors may arise from the esophagus, the vast majority of clinically significant tumors of the esophagus are malignant. In the past, most esophageal malignancies were squamous cell carcinomas, although recent studies suggest a dramatic increase in adenocarcinoma of the distal esophagus. Most esophageal adenocarcinomas appear to arise from Barrett's esophagus, a prema-

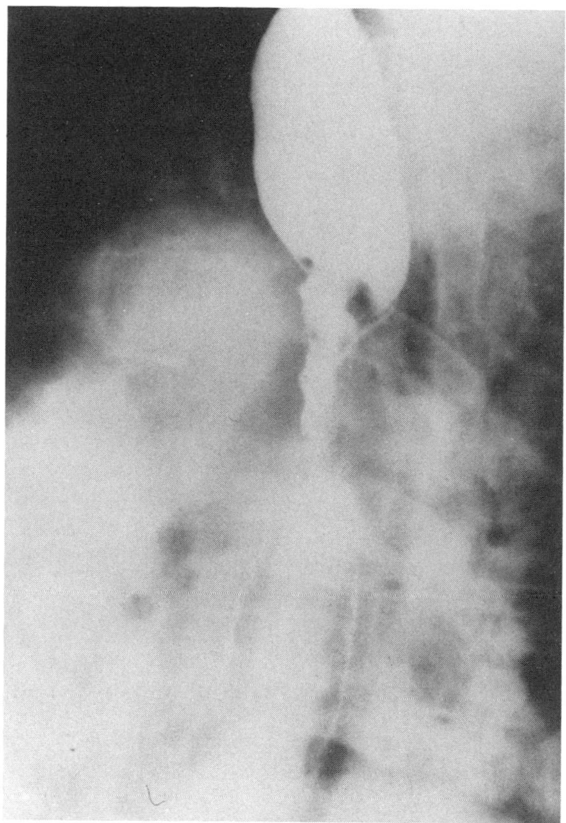

Figure 5.4 Malignant stricture. The stricture is circumferential. Characteristics distinguishing it from a benign stricture include the sharp, shelf-like proximal margin and the more irregular configuration of the stenotic segment. Unlike some malignant strictures, this stricture follows the anticipated path of the esophageal lumen. Compare the appearance to the benign stricture shown in Figure 5.3. (Courtesy of Bronwyn Jones, MD.)

lignant condition in which columnar cells replace the usual squamous epithelium covering the lower end of the esophagus as a result of severe gastroesophageal reflux.

As with other types of stenotic lesions, dysphagia is initially for solids only. However, it usually progresses rapidly, with dysphagia for soft foods and even liquids developing within a few months of the onset of symptoms.

Radiographically, esophageal malignancies appear as strictures of variable length. By the time of presentation, the cancer is usually many centimeters long and involves the entire circumference of the esophageal lumen, producing a stricture. The typical malignant stricture is characterized by its shelflike proximal margins and irregular channel, which may diverge substantially from the anticipated course of the esophageal lumen (Figure 5.4). However, not all esophageal cancers are obviously malignant on barium radiography, and occasional malignant-looking strictures may be benign (Ravich et al. 1986). For this reason, endoscopy with tissue sampling by biopsy, cytologic brushing, or both is essential to distinguish between benign and malignant strictures.

Curative treatment is primarily surgical, although apparent cures by radiotherapy have been reported. Unfortunately, by the time symptoms develop, the cancer is usually far advanced and incurable. The overall 5-year survival rate for esophageal cancer is only about 5%. Even among those in whom resection for apparent cure is possible, the 5-year survival rate is only about 15% (Earlam and Cunha-Melo 1980). Recent studies suggested that the 5-year survival rate could be doubled with a combination of preoperative radiotherapy and chemotherapy (Forastiere et al. 1993). Surprisingly, almost 25% of patients had no evidence of cancer by gross or histologic examination; among these patients, survival was improved fourfold over rates reported for surgery alone and twofold over those with evidence of residual tumor at surgical resection.

For patients in whom curative resection is not possible, palliative resection is often still feasible and provides good symptomatic relief. In the past, a high perioperative mortality rate of about 29%, in combination with the infrequency of cure, made surgery unattractive (Parker and Moertel 1978). However, with better nutrition provided by preoperative and perioperative hyperalimentation, the risk of palliative surgery has declined (Kinoshita et al. 1978).

Alternative approaches include dilatation, tumor ablation (thermal treatment to destroy tumor obstructing the esophagus) by means of laser or bipolar electrocautery, or stent placement. Each of these approaches is directed at opening the esophageal lumen to permit eating, in recognition that the major cause of early death in patients with esophageal cancer is malnutrition and aspiration pneumonia.

Dilatation generally provides limited and short-lived relief but is useful in preparing for other forms of therapy. The choice between other modalities depends on specific features of the tumor and local technical expertise and resources. Endoscopic laser therapy and bipolar electrocautery can be used to destroy tumor tissue that blocks the esophageal lumen. This may provide a number of months of relief, allowing continuing oral intake. Should obstruction recur, treatment can be repeated.

An esophageal stent is a tube with a large channel, which can be placed through the strictured segment to maintain luminal patency. The stent permits ingestion of a modified diet, concentrating on soft, easily chewed foods and purees. Since the development of thermal methods of treatment, the use of stents for palliation has decreased dramatically. However, they continue to be useful in certain situations, especially in the presence of a tracheoesophageal fistula that often complicates the natural history or treatment of esophageal cancer. In this situation, a properly placed stent can maintain the esophageal lumen while covering the opening to the airway. The recent introduction of expandable metal stents has made insertion easier and provides a larger internal luminal diameter, allowing patients to eat a less restrictive diet.

Although endoscopic treatment with laser, bipolar electrocautery, or stent placement may be highly successful in reestablishing luminal patency, a substantial proportion of patients with esophageal cancer have poor appetites and are unable to gain weight. The early use of endoscopically placed or fluoroscopically guided gastrostomies should be considered in patients who fail to eat once the lumen is reestablished or who are scheduled to undergo chemotherapy or radiotherapy, treatments that may produce or exacerbate anorexia.

Luminal Deformity

Extrinsic Compression

Some degree of luminal deformity due to extrinsic compression by normal mediastinal structures (i.e., the aortic knob, the left mainstem bronchus, and the left atrium of the heart) is normally seen on barium studies and rarely, if ever, causes symptoms. More pronounced compression can occur with mediastinal pathology such as aortic aneurysm, cardiomegaly, congenital abnormalities of the large mediastinal arteries (e.g., aberrant subclavian artery), enlarged mediastinal lymph nodes, and lung cancer. The elasticity of the contralateral wall tends to minimize symptoms until compression is far advanced. By the same token, dilatation is usually ineffective because the force of dilatation is absorbed by the elastic, uninvolved wall. Effective treatment, when necessary, would require shrinking or removing the mass-producing compression. Unfortunately, this is often not practical in patients in whom compression produces significant symptoms.

Esophageal Diverticulum

Compared with diverticula of the hypopharynx, esophageal diverticula are rare and most often asymptomatic, even when they reach relatively large size. When symptoms do occur, they include dysphagia for liquids and solids, regurgitation of previously swallowed food back to the mouth, or both. Regurgitation without dysphagia is not uncommon.

Most often, esophageal diverticula are a consequence of downstream obstruction, either motor or structural in origin (pulsion diverticulum) (Figure 5.5). Increased pressure in the esophagus results in bulging at a point of relative weakness. Less commonly, diverticula can result from periesophageal inflammation, which causes traction on the esophageal wall (traction diverticulum). Although most traction diverticula occur in the midesophagus, most midesophageal diverticula, like their distal esophageal counterparts, are pulsion in origin.

Treatment of pulsion-type diverticula is only necessary if the diverticulum is symptomatic. Because of the frequent causative role of motor or structural disorders, it is important to look for these abnormalities. It may be difficult to distinguish between the underlying obstructive disorder and the diverticulum as a cause of symptoms. It is appropriate to attempt to treat the underlying cause of increased pressure with dilatation in the case of structural obstruction or with drugs for dysmotility. In some patients, symptoms initially thought to be a consequence of the diverticulum improve significantly or resolve entirely with such conservative therapy.

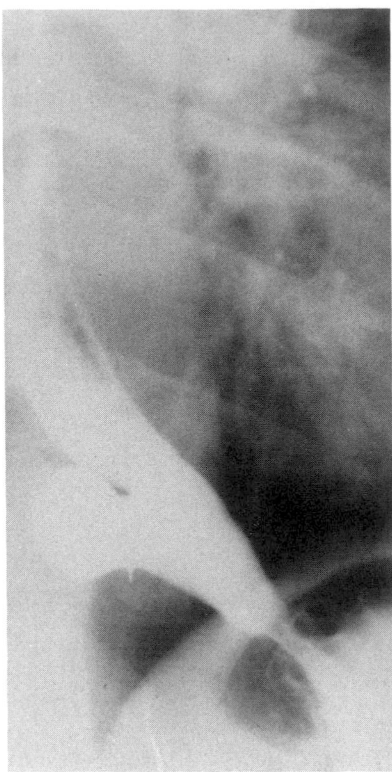

Figure 5.5 Esophageal diverticulum. A pulsion-type diverticulum located in the distal esophagus. Notice the narrowed appearance of the esophagogastric junction, suggesting the presence of a stricture. In most cases, esophageal diverticula are presumed to be caused by increased luminal pressure, secondary to motor or structural obstruction distally. (Courtesy of Bronwyn Jones, MD.)

Should medical management fail, surgical removal of the diverticulum is required. Surgery limited to diverticulectomy, however, is associated with a high incidence of early anastomotic leakage or late recurrence, probably because it fails to deal with the underlying cause of increased intraesophageal pressure and creates an area of relative wall weakness. Therefore, diverticulectomy should be combined with treatment of the underlying disorder, whether that be motor (with a surgical myotomy) or structural (with dilatation).

ESOPHAGEAL DYSMOTILITY

Classification of Esophageal Motility Disorders

An orderly, progressive peristaltic wave is not uniformly present after every swallow, even in individuals without dysphagia. The dividing line between normal and pathologic degrees of dysmotility is poorly defined.

In one study of 95 healthy adults (Richter et al. 1987), 5-ml wet swallow induced double-peaked contractions in 14.3 ± 22.4% of swallows, nonperistaltic contractions in 6.0 ± 10.3% of swallows, and nonpropagated contractions in 5.2 ± 1.5% of swallows. Interestingly, the frequency of simultaneous contractions was 0.8–2.7%, substantially lower than previously reported. The incidence of abnormal contractions changes with bolus type (it is increased with dry swallows), although not with age.

There have been a variety of schemes for the classification of esophageal dysmotility. In abnormalities of esophageal peristalsis, contraction amplitude may be too high or low, contraction duration prolonged, or the orderly progression of the contractile wave down the length of the esophagus uncoordinated. In abnormalities of LES function, the pressure may be too high or low, and relaxation may be incomplete. Finally, the esophageal body and LES can misbehave separately or together. The individual characteristics of commonly described motility disorders are not necessarily unique. In many ways, the separation between entities is somewhat arbitrary.

Disorders of Esophageal Peristalsis

Motor dysfunction of the body of the esophagus may cause symptoms of dysphagia, chest pain, or regurgitation. Dysphagia is usually for liquids as well as solids, although not necessarily in equal measure. Chest pain may mimic that of cardiac disease and cause considerable concern on the part of both patient and physician. Although pain initiated or exacerbated by swallowing would strongly implicate the esophagus as the site of origin, a clear relationship to eating is often absent. Similarly, the presence of other symptoms implicating the swallowing mechanism would support the possibility that the esophagus is the cause of chest pain. However, cardiac disease is sufficiently common, especially in an older age group, that a cardiology evaluation may be justified.

Diffuse Esophageal Spasm

Esophageal spasm is a graphic term with an imprecise meaning. The diagnosis of esophageal spasm is used quite freely among physicians, including gastroenterologists. All too often, esophageal spasm is diagnosed on the basis of minor degrees of dysmotility seen radiographically or manometrically, or even on the basis of consistent symptoms in the absence of radiographic or manometric confirmation. Esophageal spasm constitutes the end of a spectrum of nonspecific esophageal dysmotility. At one end of the range are the abnormal contractions seen occasionally in normal individuals; at the other are repeated high-amplitude, prolonged, simultaneous, or multiphasic contractions, or some combination of these, in the absence of any normal peristaltic activity (Figures 5.6 and 5.7). While few would argue against calling the latter "spasm," there is little agreement on where less severe abnormalities of esophageal peristalsis end and spasm begins.

An interesting feature of these criteria is the inclusion of high LES pressures and incomplete relaxations as an associated finding. LES dysfunction in

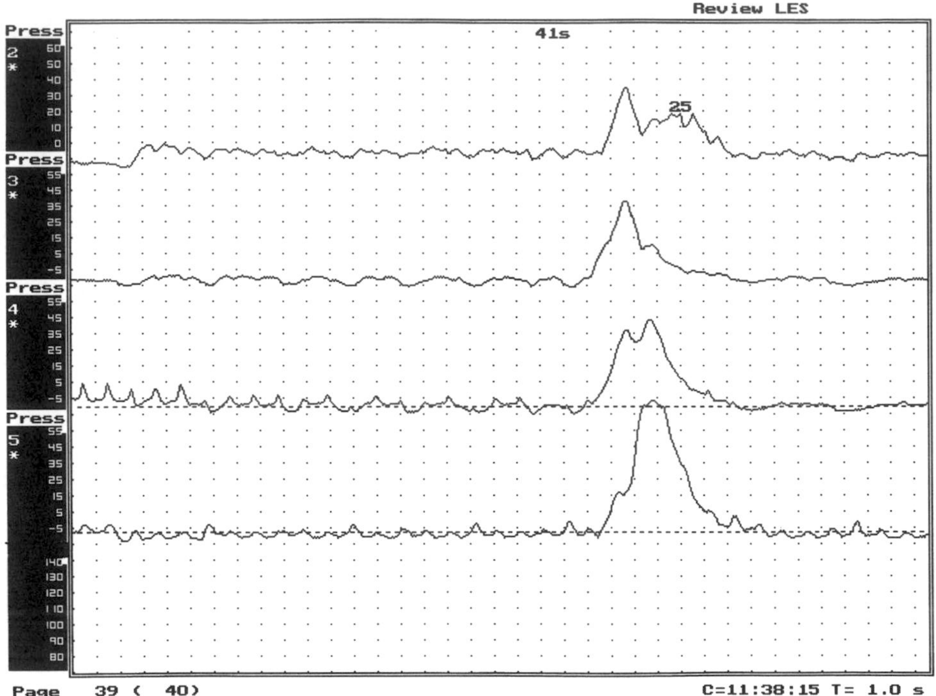

Figure 5.6 Manometric appearance of esophageal spasm. The manometric findings in esophageal dysmotility are characterized by various combinations of simultaneous, multiphasic, high-amplitude, and prolonged contractions. The more severe forms are designated diffuse esophageal spasm, although the boundaries between this diagnosis and lesser degrees of dysmotility are not well-established. In addition, occasional abnormal contractions may be seen in normal individuals. In the manometric study shown, the four tracings are from pressure sensors spaced at 2-cm intervals in the distal esophagus (distance of distal sensor from nares and timing of swallow indicated by number and letter at the top). The initial upstroke in all leads are simultaneous. In addition, each demonstrates a secondary upstroke that also begins simultaneously. The amplitude and duration of contractions are within normal limits. The broken lines represent intraesophageal resting pressure. (Vertical axis scale, 1 increment = 10 mm Hg; horizontal scale, 1 increment = 1 second.)

diffuse esophageal spasm is well recognized, with failure of complete relaxation noted in one-third of patients (DiMarino and Cohen 1974). The presence of LES dysfunction in diffuse esophageal spasm and of spastic contractions in a variant of achalasia ("vigorous achalasia") obscures the distinction between the two (see section on Achalasia).

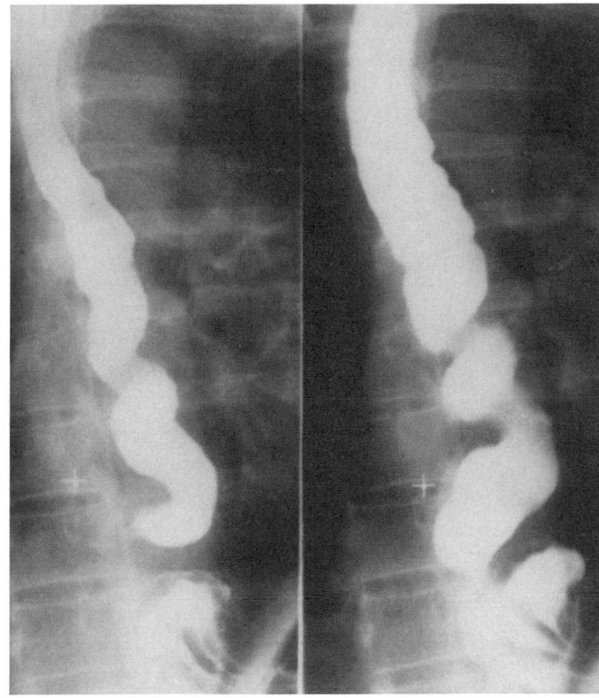

Figure 5.7 Radiographic appearance of esophageal dysmotility. A variety of patterns of abnormal peristalsis may be seen on barium radiography. In spot film, the silhouette of the barium column in the upper portion of the esophagus has a serrated appearance, whereas in the lower portion there is a "corkscrew" configuration. In addition, there is a hiatal hernia. (Courtesy of Bronwyn Jones, MD.)

Nutcracker Esophagus

In 1977, Brand et al. described a group of patients with chest pain or dysphagia, occurring in association with manometric findings of high amplitude, but with normally progressive peristaltic waves. This syndrome, often called the "nutcracker esophagus," is considered by some authorities to be the most commonly detected disorder of esophageal motility.

A number of questions surround the manometric pattern of the nutcracker esophagus. First, the criteria for diagnosis has changed over time. Originally described as a mean pressure of more than 120 mm Hg, recent studies of normal individuals indicate that this value is too low, especially for the older population. Castell (1987) has suggested that, to avoid overdiagnosis, the term *nutcracker esophagus* should be restricted to patients with mean pressures greater than 180 mm Hg.

Second, the pressures measured during serial motility studies performed in the same individual may change substantially, resulting in the manometric interpretations changing from abnormal (i.e., nutcracker) to normal on different recordings in the same patient (Dalton et al. 1988). Interestingly, the pressures tend to be highest at the initial recording, suggesting that anxiety associated with the procedure may play a role in this manometric pattern.

Third, it is not clear why nutcracker esophagus produces symptoms. Barium esophagram studies demonstrate normal stripping function. While increased pressure could conceivably cause discomfort, most patients with high-amplitude contractions during motility do not have pain at the time of the examination, and it is often difficult to appreciate differences between contraction amplitude and appearance during spontaneous episodes of pain that are witnessed manometrically. It is possible that the nutcracker esophagus represents a marker of patients with intermittent diffuse esophageal spasm.

Nonspecific Esophageal Motility Disorders

Disagreement about the criteria for esophageal spasm aside, a large number of patients referred to the esophageal function laboratory have abnormalities of esophageal motility in which the degree and type of motility abnormalities detected are not sufficient to be labeled esophageal spasm or nutcracker esophagus. Such lesser patterns of dysmotility are called "nonspecific esophageal motor disorders." Their clinical significance remains unclear. On one hand, it is difficult to ignore the potential significance of disordered peristalsis in patients with dysphagia. On the other, similar degrees of abnormality are so common in normal volunteers that their mere presence cannot be considered proof of causality.

Treatment of Disorders of Esophageal Motility

The medical therapy for esophageal dysmotility is often of limited benefit. A variety of smooth-muscle-relaxant drugs (nitrates, hydralazine, calcium channel blockers) have been used in an attempt to decrease esophageal contractile amplitude and repetitive contractions. Although some patients respond dramatically, many do not. Controlled clinical trials have thus far failed to demonstrate a convincing beneficial effect of these drugs on symptoms (Davis et al. 1987). Clinical experience suggests that the symptomatic response is quite variable and often incomplete, that side effects related to the hypotensive effects of the drugs severely limit the use of these medications, and that patients who fail to respond to the first drug used usually fail to respond to subsequently prescribed drugs.

The most common mistake in the treatment of esophageal dysmotility is to assume that the patient has a primary disorder of esophageal motility. Esophageal dysmotility is like anemia, a laboratory finding that requires further evaluation. Like anemia, there is a differential diagnosis of esophageal dysmotility. The most common cause of dysmotility is esophageal irritation, most commonly by gastroesophageal reflux. Disordered esophageal peristalsis also may result from esophageal obstruction, ganglion degeneration (i.e., vigorous achalasia), autonomic neuropathies (e.g., due to diabetes or alcohol abuse), or collagen vascular diseases (especially scleroderma and mixed connective tissue disease). Only patients with esophageal dysmotility in the absence of an underlying etiology are considered to have a primary (or idiopathic) esophageal dysmotility.

Reflux-induced dysmotility is probably the most common cause of esophageal dysmotility and is more easily treated than idiopathic dysmotility. As heartburn is not always present, reflux should be considered in any patient with symptoms of esophageal spasm. Ironically, the drugs used to treat idiopathic dysmotility may make reflux worse by further impairing LES pressure. Esophageal stenosis, another cause of esophageal dysmotility, may be missed occasionally by barium studies and endoscopy. Dilatation should be considered if there is any question of a structural obstruction.

Primary esophageal dysmotility accounts for only a minority of these patients. Whether idiopathic esophageal dysmotility is a single disorder or a number of disorders awaiting differentiation remains to be seen. Recent studies suggest that esophageal distention may be a cause of symptoms commonly attributed to spasm (Barish et al. 1986). The possibility that the pain of esophageal spasm derives from acute esophageal dilatation proximal to an area of spasm, rather than from the muscular contraction per se, must be considered.

ABNORMALITIES OF LOWER ESOPHAGEAL SPHINCTER FUNCTION

Achalasia

Achalasia is a condition in which a nonrelaxing or incompletely relaxing LES prevents the passage of swallowed material into the stomach. Patients usually present with dysphagia for both liquids and solids. Regurgitation is common, characteristically resulting in regurgitation of recognizable food hours after it was eaten. Late regurgitation of undigested food is a feature seen in only a few cases of dysphagia, primarily achalasia and hypopharyngeal (Zenker's) or esophageal diverticulum. During barium swallow, with the patient in the upright position, the esophagus is generally dilated and a column of barium of variable height is maintained above a tight esophagogastric junction (Figure 5.8). The possibility that this appearance could represent a tight esophageal stricture is ruled out at endoscopy when the endoscope passes into the stomach with mild to moderate resistance.

Although the impairment of LES response to swallow is key to the functional obstruction to the flow of food into the stomach, the motor abnormalities of achalasia include the complete loss of progressive peristalsis (Figure 5.9). In the more common variant of achalasia ("classic achalasia"), low-amplitude, aperistaltic contractions in the body of the esophagus are combined with a high or high-normal, nonrelaxing sphincter. The simultaneous low-amplitude increases in pressure with swallow are often attributed to pharyngeal pressure, transmitted into the dilated esophagus, rather than to true esophageal contractile activity.

In recent years, the presence of a variant of achalasia, called *vigorous achalasia*, has been recognized. In this condition, the typical LES findings of achalasia are associated with higher-amplitude, prolonged, multiphasic contractions, indicating that intrinsic esophageal motor response to swallowing, however deranged, is still present.

It also has been assumed that the complete absence of progressive peristalsis and the failure of LES relaxation represented the sine qua non of achalasia; a consequence of degeneration of the ganglion cells of the myenteric plexus. However, there have been reports of return of peristalsis after successful treatment. It has

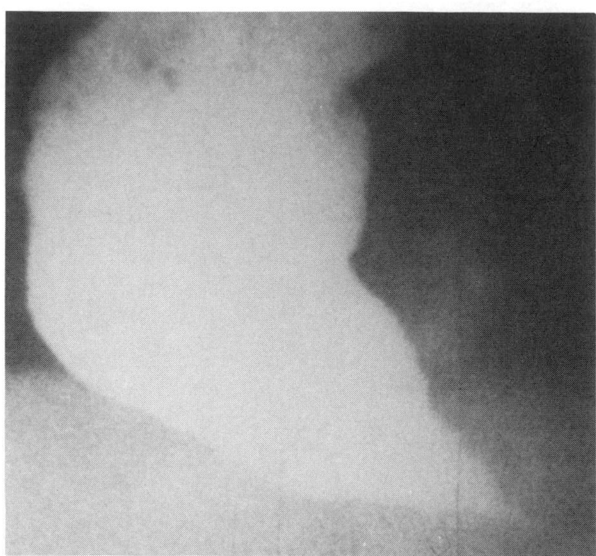

Figure 5.8 Radiographic appearance of achalasia. A barium esophagram with the patient in an upright position demonstrates the typical features of achalasia: a dilated esophagus and a smooth, tapering narrowing at the esophagogastric junction (the "parrot-beaked deformity"), holding up a column of barium mixed with retained food. In more extreme cases, the esophagus may take on a tortuous appearance (the "sigmoid esophagus"). (Courtesy of Bronwyn Jones, MD.)

been suggested that the absence of progressive peristalsis is an artifact of the recording systems used, and that progressive peristalsis could be present, but unrecognized, until esophageal dilatation reverses after therapy (Vantrappen and Hellemans 1980). However, cine or video recordings of barium esophagrams do not support this suggestion. Regardless, the return of peristalsis after treatment must be relatively rare and may represent an early stage of disease.

More recently, complete relaxation of the LES has been described (Katz et al. 1986). Although conceptually earth-shaking from the esophagologist's perspective, the pattern of relaxation appears distinctly different from normal. It would appear to correspond to the limited degree of opening of the esophagogastric junction commonly noted on barium studies and does not require a complete reassessment of the manometric definition of achalasia.

The manometric features of achalasia are nearly, but not absolutely, pathognomonic. These include a lower esophageal sphincter with a high or high-normal resting pressure that fails to relax appropriately with swallow. In addition, there is a complete loss of progressive peristalsis. Occasional patients with identical manometric findings secondary to tumor infiltration of the esophagogastric junction have been described, a condition labeled *secondary achalasia* or *pseudoachalasia* (Kahrilas et al. 1987). This condition also has been described in a few nonmalignant conditions. Features that should raise suspicion of secondary achalasia include older age of onset, shorter duration of symptoms, modest dilatation of the esophagus, and rapid and profound weight loss.

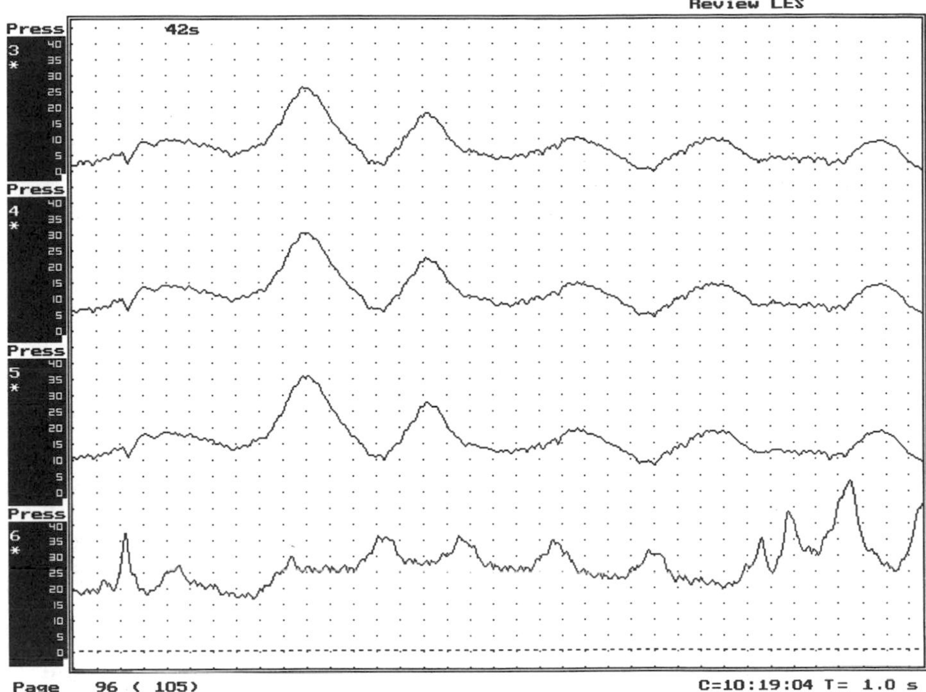

Figure 5.9 Manometric findings in achalasia. The LES, examined in the bottom pressure channel, fails to relax to intragastric resting pressure (represented by the broken line) with swallow (distance of distal sensor from nares and timing of swallow indicated by number and letter at the top). In addition, the contraction in the other three pressure recordings, from sensors located at 2-cm intervals within the distal esophagus, are low amplitude and simultaneous. A second simultaneous wave detected by these sensors represents a secondary contraction, while fluctuation later in the tracing is probably due to the effect of respiration. (Vertical scale, 1 increment = 5 mm Hg; horizontal scale, 1 increment = 1 second.)

Compared with other primary esophageal motor disorders, we usually are able to diagnose achalasia with confidence and treat it with success. Although achalasia involves motor abnormalities of both the esophageal body and LES, it is the LES dysfunction that is largely responsible for obstruction with resultant symptoms. Most patients are sufficiently symptomatic at presentation to warrant therapy. The major absolute indication for treatment is nighttime regurgitation, which puts the patient at risk for aspiration during sleep. Treatment also would be warranted if the obstruction is severe, nutrition is impaired, or the esophagus progressively dilates over time.

Until recently, there have been three treatment choices: smooth muscle relaxant drugs, pneumostatic dilatation, and surgery. All aim at decreasing LES pressure, thereby diminishing the resistance to the flow of food and liquid. None have a clinically significant effect on abnormal motor function in the esophageal body.

For many years it was said that there is no drug therapy for achalasia. However, calcium channel blockers and long-acting nitrites do lower LES pressure significantly and have been used for achalasia. Because esophageal transit, and therefore drug absorption, are problematic in achalasia, a sublingual route of administration is preferred. Although early reports suggested that most patients respond to calcium channel blockers, clinical experience has been less impressive. A recent double-blind, placebo-controlled trial (Traube et al. 1989), showed symptomatic improvement, but this improvement was rarely complete. Objective improvement in esophageal emptying could not be confirmed.

Sooner or later, most patients require more definitive therapy. The choice between pneumostatic dilatation or surgery is most often dictated by local tradition. Few centers have extensive experience with both techniques as primary therapy. Either the initial therapy is pneumostatic dilatation, with the relatively few refractory patients proceeding to surgery, or myotomy, with the extremely-poor-risk patients sent for dilatation. Either way, the cards are stacked against the second choice. In a number of series, pneumostatic dilatation, using a number of different dilator types and techniques, provided good to excellent results in 60–94% of patients, whereas myotomy produced good to excellent long-term responses in 70–100% (Vantrappen and Janssens 1983).

Both pneumostatic dilatation and surgery have their advantages and limitations. Dilatation is less demanding technically, can be performed as an outpatient procedure, and costs less. The major risk is perforation, occurring in 1–4% of patients, depending on the series. Surgery costs more and requires greater skill and a prolonged recovery period. Mortality has been reported in 0–2%. A variable, but often high, incidence of clinically significant postoperative reflux-induced esophagitis and strictures has led to a lively argument in the surgical literature about technique, with a strong tendency among gastroenterologists to favor dilatation as an initial approach.

Recently the endoscopic injection of a potent neurotoxin (botulinum toxin, [BOTOX]) directly into the sphincter segment has been used successfully in achalasia. A placebo-controlled study has demonstrated a symptomatic response similar to that found with pneumostatic dilatation (Pasricha 1995). This approach is technically simple and the risks appear to be confined to those associated with endoscopy alone. The effect of a successful injection lasts on average for 1–4 years; those who respond initially often respond to repeated injection. The role of botulinum toxin in the long-term management is still undetermined.

Isolated Abnormalities of Lower Esophageal Sphincter

LES dysfunction is not limited to patients with achalasia. As previously mentioned, incomplete relaxation of the LES occurs in perhaps one-third of patients with other evidence of severe esophageal dysmotility. In addition, occasional patients referred for esophageal manometry have isolated abnormalities of LES function, either a hypertensive LES pressure or incomplete relaxation in response to swallow. Few of these patients have any radiographically detectable impairment of function. They may represent a preclinical stage in the evolution of achalasia, abnormalities related to esophageal spasm during periods of otherwise normal peristaltic activity, or a secondary reaction to intragastric phenomenon in which the LES reaction is directed at preventing gastroesophageal reflux. In most patients, the explanation and clinical significance of isolated abnormalities of LES function cannot be determined.

MOTOR WEAKNESS

Intermittent impairment of contraction amplitude or peristalsis is relatively common. Radiologists frequently mislabel weakness as spasm when they see the escape of barium above the peristaltic wave. The distinction is important, as medication directed toward esophageal spasm, which generally decreases contractile amplitude, would be inappropriate if the problem actually is weakness. In practice, the esophagus can empty by gravity, and many patients with esophageal paresis are asymptomatic. Although some medications can increase esophageal contractility, their effect in patients with severe paresis usually is limited.

Severe esophageal weakness is relatively rare. It is most characteristically found in patients with collagen vascular disease, such as scleroderma and mixed connective tissue disease. The esophagus is the second most common organ involved in scleroderma (D'Angelo et al. 1969). Esophageal involvement varies from mild to nonspecific to the complete absence of a contractile response to swallow; a condition referred to as "the sclerodermatous esophagus." Many of these patients have low LES pressure on manometry. The resulting severe gastroesophageal reflux with poor esophageal clearance makes them particularly susceptible to esophageal inflammation and strictures.

GASTROESOPHAGEAL REFLUX DISEASE

Despite its name, heartburn (or the sensation of burning in the chest) is generally of esophageal origin. Heartburn is the archetypic symptom of gastroesophageal reflux, although it may occasionally represent a nonspecific response to other types of esophageal dysmotility. Patients with gastroesophageal reflux often complain of regurgitation of sour or bitter material with or without food.

Dysphagia associated with gastroesophageal reflux may be due to a variety of mechanisms. Gastroesophageal reflux, with or without esophagitis, is a common cause of esophageal dysmotility. It also can produce esophageal paresis. Finally, chronic inflammation of any type can cause strictures.

Our understanding of the pathophysiology of gastroesophageal reflux has progressed substantially over the past decade, but still remains incomplete. The major components of the "antireflux barrier" are the LES acting in combination with the anatomic configuration of the esophagogastric junction. Reflux is most likely to occur when the pressure in the LES is low and when the esophagogastric junction is pulled up into the chest creating a hiatal hernia.

Other factors, however, play variable roles in different individuals. It now appears that the ability of the sphincter to prevent reflux is not simply a matter of the pressure of the sphincter measured during standard esophageal manometry. The sphincter pressure is dynamic, changing throughout the day under the influence of neural, hormonal, and mechanical influences. Additional factors that may either produce or exacerbate the severity of reflux include the neutralizing capacity of saliva, the ability of esophageal motility to clear refluxed material, and the efficiency of gastric emptying, which decreases pressure against the antireflux barrier.

All reflux is not pathologic. Gastroesophageal reflux is a common physiologic event. Many apparently normal individuals describe heartburn on a regular basis. A study of apparently healthy hospital employees indicates that approximately 33%, 14%, and 7% complained of heartburn on a monthly, weekly, and daily basis, respectively (Nebel et al. 1976). It would appear that reflux is a feature of normal life and does not necessarily reflect a pathologic condition.

Continuous pH monitoring has demonstrated that the vast majority of normal individuals experience gastroesophageal reflux on a daily basis (DeMeester and Johnson 1976). Most reflux episodes in normal individuals are of short duration, occur during the day, and do not provoke any symptoms.

Continuous pH monitoring permits the objective evaluation for reflux under near-physiologic conditions. The patient performs the activities of normal daily living, including eating, working, and sleeping. Continuous pH monitoring provides quantitative information on both the presence and severity of acid reflux. The incidence and duration of reflux events can be calculated and analyzed for the entire recording period and for segments of particular interest. The severity of reflux detected by pH monitoring correlates fairly well with the probability of esophageal inflammation and Barrett's esophagus (Iascone et al. 1983). Continuous pH monitoring is currently considered the best single test for the diagnosis of gastroesophageal reflux, with a sensitivity and specificity of approximately 90% (Richter and Castell 1983).

Barium studies, although important in evaluating patients with dysphagia, confirm the presence of reflux in only the minority of patients with symptomatic reflux disease.

Esophagitis refers to inflammation of the lining of the esophagus. Esophagitis may vary in severity from microscopic inflammation, to mucosal edema, to frank erosions or ulcerations. Although the most common cause of esophagitis is gastroesophageal reflux disease, most patients with gastroesophageal reflux disease do not have esophagitis (Behar et al. 1976).

Treatment is directed at enhancing the strength of the antireflux barrier, improving esophageal clearance and gastric emptying, and decreasing the noxiousness of gastric contents. Antireflux therapy has three components: alteration in lifestyle, drugs, and surgery.

For many patients, reflux is provoked by dietary indiscretion and physical activity. Decreasing or eliminating foods that decrease LES pressure (e.g., fat, chocolate) or stimulate gastric acid production (e.g., coffee, tea) is important, especially in patients who ingest large amounts or note the association of symptoms with their ingestion. In some patients with reflux, dietary modification is enough to control symptoms. Smoking also impairs esophageal function and should be eliminated. In addition, patients are instructed to elevate the head of the bed on 6-inch blocks and avoid lying down within 2 hours of eating. These measures allow gravity to assist in reflux prevention and enhance esophageal clearance.

Self-medication with antacids is common in patients with heartburn. Unfortunately, antacids alone are rarely sufficient to control esophagitis. Antacids are primarily used for symptomatic relief in patients with intermittent, infrequent heartburn. Most patients with severe symptoms or esophagitis require more potent acid-lowering agents, most often one of the available histamine antagonists, the H_2-blockers (i.e., cimetidine, ranitidine, nizatidine, famotidine), in combination with lifestyle changes.

Although prokinetic drugs (e.g., bethanechol, metoclopramide, cisapride) have potentially beneficial effects on upper gastrointestinal motor function, they have generally been disappointing when used as single agents. The use of metoclopramide has been further limited by the frequent occurrence of neuropsychiatric side effects, including agitation, insomnia, and lethargy. Prokinetic agents are occasionally used as adjunctive agents, in combination with H_2-blockers in patients with more severe disease. Cisapride, a recently approved prokinetic agent, appears to be at least as effective as metoclopramide without the risk of neuropsychiatric side effects.

The vast majority of patients can be controlled by the measures mentioned previously. Surgical intervention has generally been reserved for the occasional patient who has been refractory to medical management. A number of operations have been described, most involving reestablishing the intra-abdominal location of the esophagogastric junction (hiatal hernia repair) in combination with wrapping a portion of the stomach around part or the whole circumference of the lower esophagus (fundoplication). Laparoscopic approaches to antireflux surgery have been developed and appear to be as effective as traditional surgical approaches with a more rapid recovery. Surgery is effective in controlling reflux in approximately 80–90% of patients in whom it is used.

The introduction of a more potent class of acid-reducing drugs, the proton pump blockers, has demonstrated that acid plays a critical role in producing symptoms even in the occasional patient who fails to respond clinically to H_2-blocker therapy. However, omeprazole and lansoprazole, the two available agents within this class of drugs, are only approved for short-duration (2 months) treatment of gastroesophageal reflux because of concerns about the carcinogenic potential of long-term, profound acid suppression. However, no cases of cancer in humans have been reported and the risk of developing cancer as a result of long-term use of proton pump blockers appears to be low. It seems likely that proton pump blockers will be used as an alternative to surgery in patients with refractory reflux disease who are poor surgical risks.

REFERENCES

Barish CF, Castell DO, Richter JE. Graded esophageal balloon distention: a new provocative test for non-cardiac chest pain. Dig Dis Sci 1986;31:1292.

Behar J, Biancani P, Sheahan DG. Evaluation of esophageal tests in the diagnosis of reflux esophagitis. Gastroenterology 1976;71:9.

Brand DL, Martin D, Pope CE. Esophageal manometrics in patients with anginal type chest pain. Am J Dig Dis 1977;23:300.

Castell DO. The Nutcracker Esophagus and Other Primary Esophageal Motility Disorders. In DO Castell, JE Richter, CB Dalton (eds), Esophageal Motility Testing. New York: Elsevier, 1987;130.

Dalton CB, Castell DO, Richter JE. The changing faces of the nutcracker esophagus. Am J Gastroenterol 1988;83:623.

D'Angelo WA, Fries JF, Masi AT, et al. Pathologic observations in systemic sclerosis (scleroderma): a study of 58 autopsy cases and 58 matched controls. Am J Med 1969;46:428.

Davis HA, Lewis MJ, Rhodes J, et al. Trial of nifedipine for prevention of esophageal spasm. Digestion 1987;36:81.

DeMeester TR, Johnson LF. Patterns of gastroesophageal reflux in health and disease. Ann Surg 1976;184:45.

DiMarino AT, Cohen S. Characteristics of lower esophageal sphincter function in symptomatic diffuse esophageal spasm. Gastroenterology 1974;66:1.

Earlam R, Cunha-Melo JR. Oesophageal squamous cell carcinoma: a critical review of surgery. Br J Surg 1980;67:381.

Edwards DAW. Diagnostic Procedures: History and Symptoms of Esophageal Disease. In G Vantrappen, J Hellemans, (eds), Diseases of the Esophagus. New York: Springer-Verlag, 1974;103.

Forastiere AA, Orringer MB, Perez-Tamayo C, et al. Preoperative chemoradiation followed by transhiatal esophagectomy for carcinoma of the esophagus. J Clin Oncology 1993;11:1118.

Goyal RK, Bauer JL, Spiro HM. The nature and location of the lower esophageal ring. N Engl J Med 1971;284:1175.

Groskreutz JL, Kim CH. Schatzki's ring: long-term results following dilatation. Gastrointestinal Endos 1990;36:479.

Iascone C, DeMeester TR, Little AG, et al. Barrett's esophagus: functional assessment, proposed pathogenesis, and surgical therapy. Arch Surg 1983;118:543.

Jones B, Ravich WJ, Kramer SS, et al. Pharyngoesophageal interrelationships: observations and working concepts. Gastrointest Radiol 1985;10:225.

Kahrilas PJ, Kishk SM, Helm JF, et al. Comparison of pseudoachalasia and achalasia. Am J Med 1987;82:439.

Katz PO, Richter JE, Cowan R, et al. Apparent complete lower esophageal sphincter relaxation in achalasia. Gastroenterology 1986;90:978.

Kinoshita Y, Endo M, Nakayama K, et al. Evaluation of ten-year survival after operation for upper- and midthoracic esophageal cancer. Intern Adv Surg Oncol 1978;1:173.

Nebel OT, Fornes MF, Castell DO. Symptomatic gastroesophageal reflux: incidence and precipitating factors. Am J Dig Dis 1976;21:953.

Parker EF, Moertel CF. Is there a role for surgery in esophageal carcinoma? Am J Dig Dis 1978;23:730.

Pasricha PJ, Ravich WJ, Hendrix TR, et al. Intrasphincteric botulinum toxin for the treatment of achalasia. N Engl J Med 1995;332:774.

Ravich WJ, Kashima H, Donner MW. Drug-induced esophagitis simulating esophageal cancer. Dysphagia 1986;1:13.

Richter JE, Castell DO. Gastroesophageal Reflux Disease: Pathogenesis, Diagnosis, and Therapy. In DO Castell, LF Johnson (eds), Esophageal Function in Health and Disease. New York: Elsevier, 1983;151.

Richter JE, Wu WC, Johns DN, et al. Esophageal manometry in 95 healthy adult volunteers: variability of pressure with age and frequency of "abnormal" contractions. Dig Dis Sci 1987;32:583.

Schatzki R. The lower esophageal ring: long term follow-up of symptomatic and asymptomatic rings. Am J Roentgenol Rad Ther Nuclear Med 1963;90:805.

Traube M, Dubovik S, Lange RC, et al. The role of nifedipine therapy in achalasia: results of a randomized, double-blind, placebo-controlled study. Am J Gastroenterol 1989;84:1259.

Vantrappen G, Hellemans J. Treatment of achalasia and related motility disorders. Gastroenterology 1980;79:14.

Vantrappen G, Janssens J. To dilate or to operate? That is the question. Gut 1983; 24:1013.

6

Development and Impairments of Feeding in Infancy and Childhood

James F. Bosma

Feeding is central within the living experience of the young infant, and it continues to be a major element of experience in the older infant and child. The young infant's manner of arousal toward feeding and competence in suckle feeding reflect his or her general health and neurologic status. Conversely, many forms of neurologic impairment and some forms of systemic illness are associated with dysphagia; failure to thrive is common, and frank malnutrition may occur rapidly in young infants. These conditions may be associated with an increase in impairment, including dysphagia. When dysphagia and other conditions have this reciprocal influence, the detection, evaluation, and therapy of dysphagia are strategic. This review is concerned particularly with evaluating the performances of suckle feeding and the later acquisition of voluntary oral manipulation and swallow of particulate foods in normal and neurologically impaired individuals. The review incompletely refers to the several recent volumes concerned with dysphagia in the pediatric population (Wolf and Glass 1992; Arvedson and Brodsky 1993; Tuchman and Walter 1994; Rosenthal et al. 1995). These volumes record the remarkable advances in observation, insight, and care that have accompanied the rapid evolution of this clinical field.

SUCKLE FEEDING

Our reference for description of suckle feeding is the normal young term-born infant who has had several successful bottle feedings by a single care person; breast feeding is separately considered. Suckle feeding, in this circumstance, is a mature neurologic performance (Peiper 1963; Blass and Teicher 1980; Bosma 1986a; Selley et al. 1990a). It is consistent in its relation to arousal and in its initiating responses and sequences. It is consistent and efficient in actions of suckle, swallow, and adapted adjacent respirations. The efficiency of formula intake in relation to time varies between normal newborn infants, without relation to weight or incidental actions of the mother or care giver (Rybski and Gisel 1984; Rybski et al. 1984).

This quality of performance is appropriate to stable coordination patterns of suckle and pharyngeal swallow in the bulbar area neural networks. The infant is expected to rouse stably, with increasing readiness of rooting in response to oral area touching and to promptly begin suckling on a nipple or equivalent object. The suckle action, perceived by the examiner's finger or imaged by videosonography or videoradiography, is a coordination of the tongue, the hyoid and mandibular muscles, and the lower lip. Videosonography in horizontal plane, with the ultrasound probe on the cheek (Figure 6.1), demonstrates a posteriorward moving peristaltic wave. Each wave consists of a downward displacement followed by an upward displacement, such that suction and nipple compression succeed each other (Bosma et al. 1990). According to Rudolph (1994), "depression of the tongue and mandible generates suction up to 150 mm Hg in the oral cavity." The peristaltic wave conveys the expressed bolus of formula toward the pharynx. Sonography, in transverse projection with the probe under the chin (Figure 6.2), demonstrates that these vertical motions occur differentially in the medial portion of the tongue, into which the genioglossus muscle is inserted. An understanding of anatomy allows us to infer that the peristaltic motions of the medial portion of the tongue are accomplished by reciprocal coordination of the genioglossus and the transverse intrinsic lingual muscles, which relate the medial portion of the tongue and the adjacent lateral portion into which the styloglossus and hyoglossus muscles insert. These intrinsic motions of the tongue, which immediately begin the milking actions of suction and nipple compression, are central within the more general concerted motions of the tongue, lower lip, mandible, and hyoid. This composite of structures, the *suckle motor organ*, is moved alternately upward and backward in relation to the palate and then downward and forward, and these gross actions are coordinated with those of pharyngeal swallow.

Videoradiography in lateral projection (Figure 6.3) demonstrates the conveyance of the suckled bolus from the nipple through the faucial isthmus (between the pharyngeal palate and tongue), through the pharynx, and into the esophagus. If suckle and swallow occur in simple one-to-one sequence, milk filling of the oral accumulation area alternates rhythmically with pharyngeal swallow. If two or more suckles precede a swallow, a bolus is accumulated adjacent to the junction of the oral, or bony, and pharyngeal, or muscular, palate and also in the valleculae, between the tongue, epiglottis, and pharyngeal palate and palatopharyngeal folds. These two accumulation sites are separate, as the faucial isthmus is closed after each conveyance of bolus.

The pharynx is moved extensively during a swallow. Videoradiography in lateral and in posteroanterior projection demonstrates a peristaltic wave descending in the constrictor wall. The constriction begins at the level of cervical vertebra 1 and the oral, or bony, palate. At the beginning of swallow the palatopharyngeal isthmus is closed by combined action of the constrictor and palatine muscles. The descent of the peristaltic wave is demonstrated prominently in the constrictor wall. In some instances, a lucency is seen advancing ahead of the bolus through the lower portion of the pharynx and the pharyngoesophageal segment, indicating relaxation of the constrictor muscle. Simultaneously, the hyoid bone moves upward and forward, and the tongue, having conveyed the bolus into the pharynx, is pressed posteriorward. The

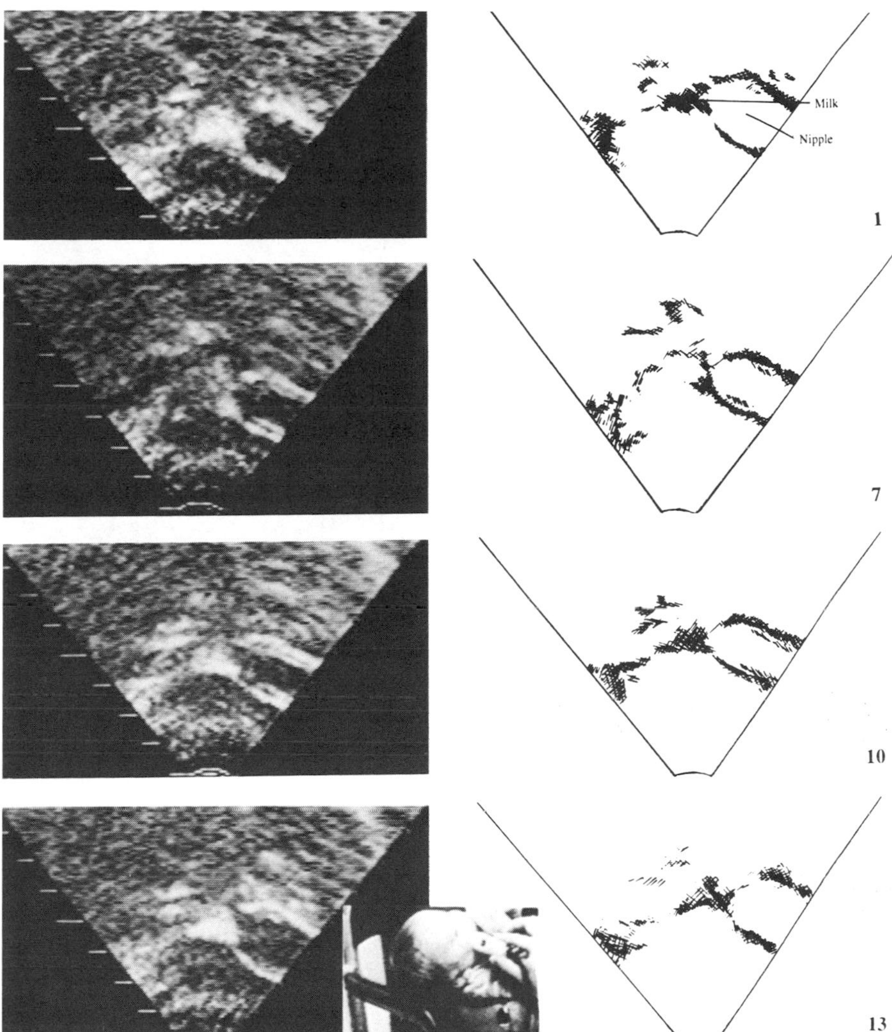

Figure 6.1 Ultrasound demonstration of tongue motions during suckle feeding. Imaging is in the transverse plane with probe held on the cheek; the video inset, expanded, shows the position of the probe. Selected video frames at 30 per second and derived tracings: frame 01, tip of the nipple is in reference contour; frame 07, tip of the nipple is compressed and the tongue dorsum is slightly separated from the tip of the nipple; frame 10, tip of the nipple is compressed and milk is expressed; frame 13, tip of the nipple is reopened nearly to reference contour.

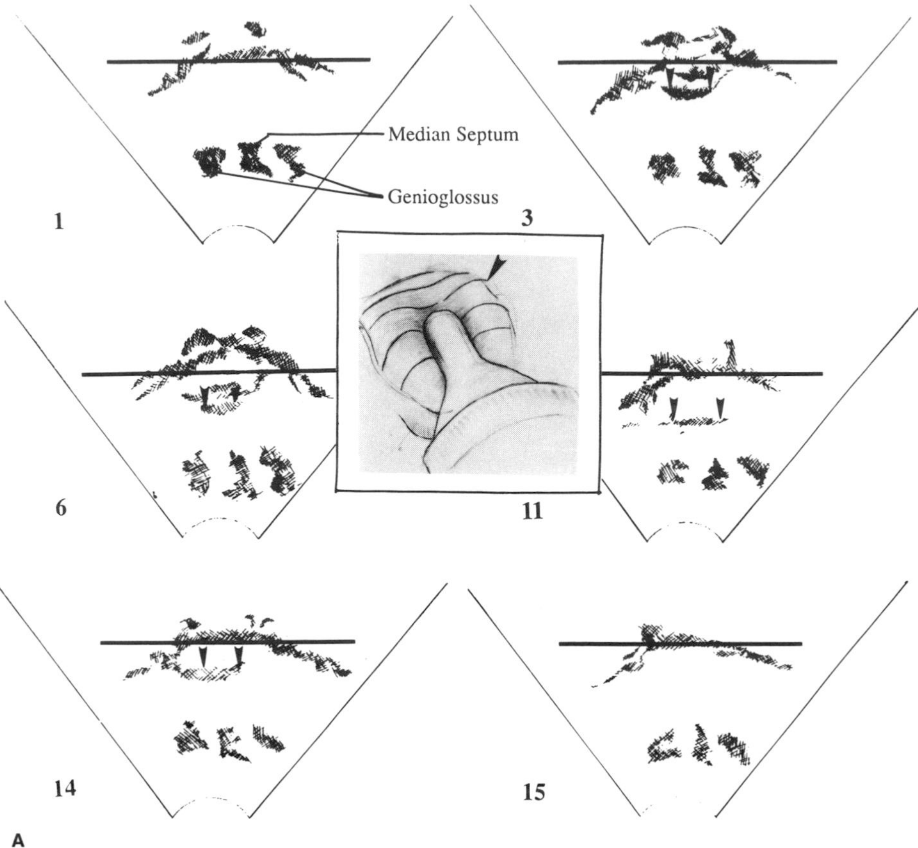

Figure 6.2 A. Ultrasound demonstration of tongue motions during suckle feeding. Imaging is in the coronal plane (arrow), with the probe in the submental area. The frames illustrate motions of the medial portion of the tongue, into which the genioglossus muscle is inserted, in relation to the lateral portions, into which the styloglossus and hyoglossus muscles are inserted. The arrows point to the superior margin of the medial portion. Frame 1: The superior margin of medial portion and of lateral portions are aligned. Frame 3: The margin of the medial portion is displaced inferiorly; milk is visible superior to the margin. Frames 6 and 11: The margin of the medial portion is displaced further inferiorly and milk is seen superior to the margin. Frames 14 and 15: Progressive return of the superior margin of the medial portion to alignment with the lateral portion. B. Sections of the infant tongue distinguishing its medial and lateral portions. The sections are approximately sagittal in the plane of the lingual artery. The right genioglossus is shown extending fan-like into the tongue from its attachment on the gonial process of the mandible. A portion of the genioglossus, which is extended toward the lingual artery, is in the pattern of gross bundles. Distally, the muscle is divided into small fascicles, similar in diameter to intrinsic lingual muscles. (From JF Bosma. Anatomy of the Infant Head. © 1986. The Johns Hopkins University Press.)

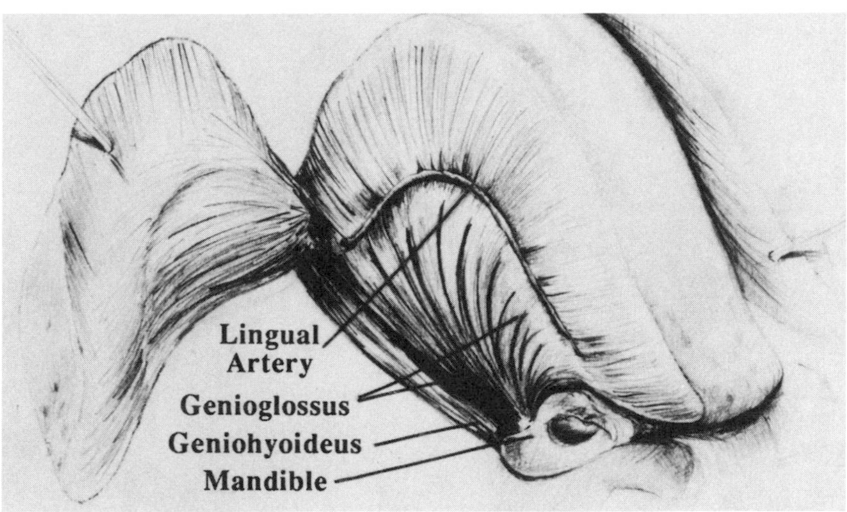

B

tongue thus participates in initiating pharyngeal swallow. The larynx is raised, along with the hyoid, and is also undergoing closure. The pharyngoesophageal segment is stably closed except during swallow or retrograde transit by belching, regurgitation, or vomiting. It is opened during swallow by a combination of the inhibition that precedes the activation wave of peristalsis and of upward and forward displacement of the cricoid cartilage, on which the cricopharyngeus muscle and the suspensory ligament of the esophagus are attached.

During a rhythmic suckle-feeding run, the pharyngeal swallow is coordinated in remarkable duplication. Exceptionally, during the initial swallow of a run, or during an isolated swallow, a small portion of the barium bolus may briefly penetrate into the laryngeal vestibule and be promptly and fully extruded again into the pharynx within 30–90 milliseconds (one to three video frames).

The centers of respiration control and feeding are developing simultaneously in the brain stem. The coordination of individual pharyngeal swallows is consistently capable of superseding and displacing respiration (Doty 1968; Wilson et al. 1981; Miller 1982; Sessle and Henry 1989).

The alternation of pharyngeal actions in swallow and respiration are well shown in lateral-projection videoradiography, as the pharynx reopens after completion of swallow. During dyspnea, as in crying, the pharyngeal participation in inspiration is conspicuous, as it is enlarged transversely, with forward displacement of the tongue and hyoid, and is also enlarged vertically, with descent of the hyoid, larynx, and hypopharynx in relation to the basicranium and the midfacial skeleton. The inspiratory expansion of the pharynx is also well shown in the posteroanterior projection as a transverse expansion of the oropharynx and laryngopharynx. The expansion demonstrates the available mobility and also

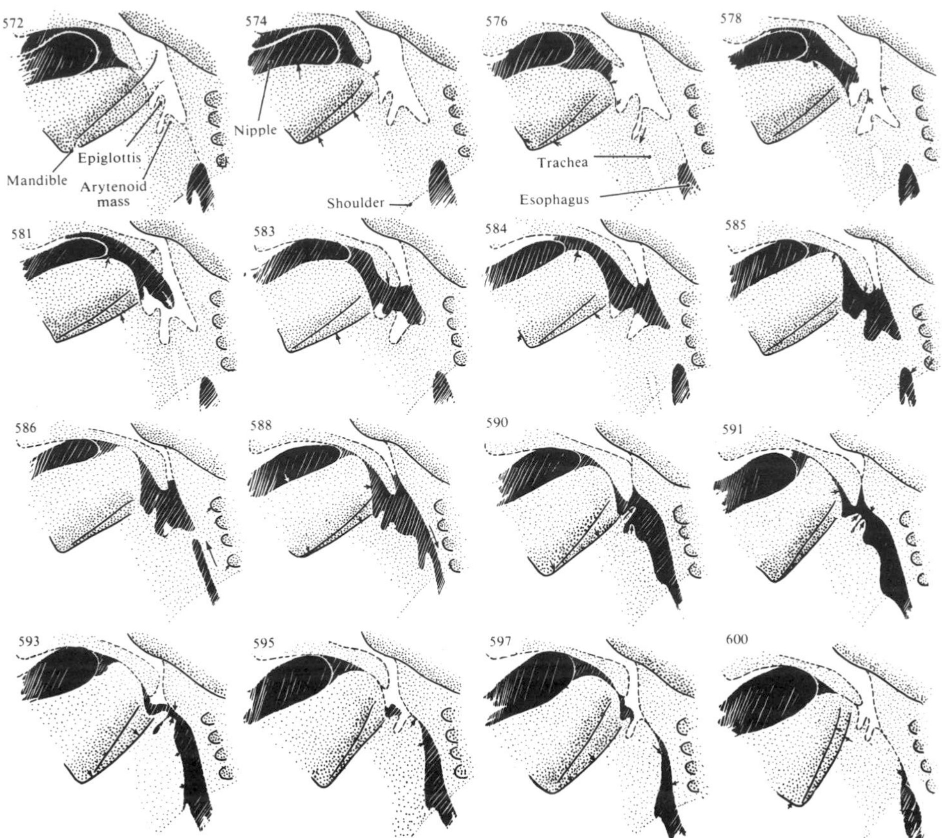

Figure 6.3 Cineradiographic frame tracings of established suckle feeding of a barium mixture at 50 frames per second. In frame 572, the undistorted nipple is within the mouth surrounded by barium. The barium bolus is retained in the primary oral accumulation area by apposition between the velum and tongue. The pharynx is open in respiration. In frames 574–584, the mandible and tongue are elevated and the nipple is compressed. Coincidentally, the increased mass of the free bolus penetrates the junction of the mouth and pharynx and fills the oropharynx. The reciprocal phase of the suckle performance is shown in frames 585–600, in which the mandible and tongue body are displaced inferiorward, allowing the nipple to resume its original contours; the velum and tongue are approximated, separating the oral and pharyngeal cavities. The pharyngeal stage of swallow occurs with elevation of the palate and anterior motion of the posterior pharyngeal wall, which is representative of general convergence of the posterior and lateral constrictor walls of the pharynx. The pharyngoesophageal segment is open in frames 588–593. (Reprinted from FL Vice, JM Heinz, G Giuriatti, et al. Cervical auscultation of suckle feeding in newborn infants. Dev Med Child Neurol 1990;32:766.)

the resources of dilating muscles of the pharyngeal area. During expiration, the pharynx is constricted in each of these planes. The constriction is generalized and simultaneous; thus, it differs from the constriction of peristalsis and affords an additional criterion of pharyngeal-area motor resources. Radiography in lateral projection during effortful expiratory constriction demonstrates near-complete closure of the airway in the larynx and pharynx. The expiration may be valved at the glottis for phonation, grunt, or cough.

During rhythmic suckle feeding, respiration is incorporated into the rhythmic sequence, so that pairs of expiration and inspiration (less commonly, the sequence is of inspiration and expiration) are interposed between swallows (Wilson et al. 1981; Daniels et al. 1990; Bamford 1991). This incorporation may be delayed during a run, so that respiration is omitted between the first swallows. In some premature infants, and in occasional term or neurologically impaired infants, this feeding apnea may continue during the duration of the run, causing hypercapnia, hypoxia, and secondary bradycardia.

Increasingly, clinicians use cervical auscultation, via stethoscope or a microphone over the larynx, to evaluate feeding, particularly the competence of pharyngeal swallow and the previously noted interactions of swallow and respiration (Logan and Bosma 1967). Cervical auscultation is used in physiologic studies of swallow and respiration (Selley et al. 1990a). It demonstrates bolus transit sounds and also abrupt discrete actions of the larynx and pharynx preceding and succeeding the bolus transit sounds (Vice et al. 1995) (Figure 6.4). The initial and final discrete sounds may be remarkably consistent in form in successive swallows (Figures 6.5 and 6.6). In pharyngeally dysphagic infants and children, cervical auscultation may demonstrate the occasion or absence of pharyngeal swallow and also possible bubbling sounds, wheezes, or stridor, which may indicate the presence of unswallowed bolus or secretions in the airway.

The esophagus differs from the pharynx in structure, innervation, and pattern of performance in feeding. As stable suckle feeding is developing, esophageal peristalsis is also evident. Single boluses delivered from the pharynx are peristaltically conveyed, after a brief pause, down the length of the esophagus and through the esophagogastric junction (Gryboski et al. 1963; Gryboski 1965; Gryboski 1975; Boix-Ochoa and Canals 1976; Herbst 1989; Milla 1991). Each pharyngeal swallow briefly inhibits esophageal peristalsis so that, during a suckle-feeding run, the boluses of successive swallows may accumulate in the esophagus. Transit of the accumulated milk into the stomach may be irregular, with little distinct peristalsis until the suckle-feeding run is completed. Neural control of the esophagus and the esophagogastric junction is incomplete in the infant and young child, permitting reflux of gastric contents into the esophagus (Gryboski 1975; Grand et al. 1976).

Neural control of the pharyngoesophageal segment is stable. Per manometry, the resting pressure in the pharyngoesophageal segment is increased by acidification within the esophagus, simulating reflux (Sondheimer 1983). The extent of increase in resting pressure is the same in infants known to reflux frequently and in normal infants. Neural control of the esophagogastric junction is also

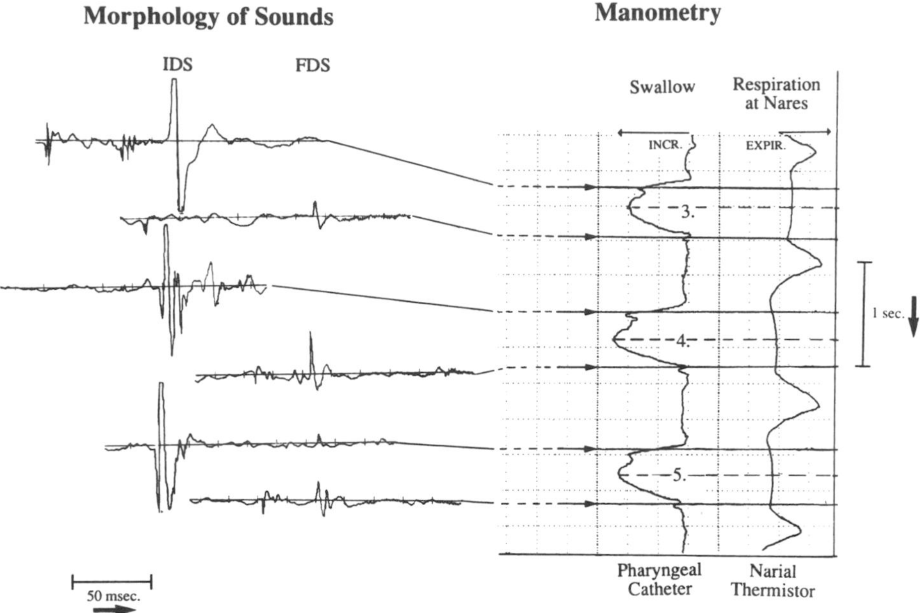

Figure 6.4 Correlation of cervical sounds with pharyngeal swallows and respiration at nares. Swallows 3–5 of a rhythmic suckle feeding run. Normal term-born infant. The initial discrete sounds (IDS) and final discrete sounds (FDS) occur, respectively, early and late in relation to the pharyngeal swallow, as indicated by manometry at the pharynx. (From FL Vice, JM Heinz, G Giurriatti, et al. Cervical auscultation of suckle feeding in newborn infants. Dev Med Child Neurol 1990;32:766.)

mature. Manometric pressure in the lower esophageal sphincter in postterm infants and in children is comparable to that in adults (Moroz and Beiko 1981). The sphincter pressure is lower in preterm infants and increases with gestational age (Newell et al. 1988).

CAUSES AND MECHANISMS OF SUCKLE-FEEDING IMPAIRMENTS

The infant who transiently fails to initiate suckle feeding or who suckles or swallows poorly may be demonstrating current problems of feeding readiness or illness or injury. The clinician is more concerned about an infant who continues in feeding failure. The causes and mechanisms of continuing feeding failure probably lie in the developmental history of the mouth and pharynx and in the representations, or patterning, of feeding and other oral and pharyngeal functions in the brain. Abnormalities of the mouth and pharynx or of the bulbar

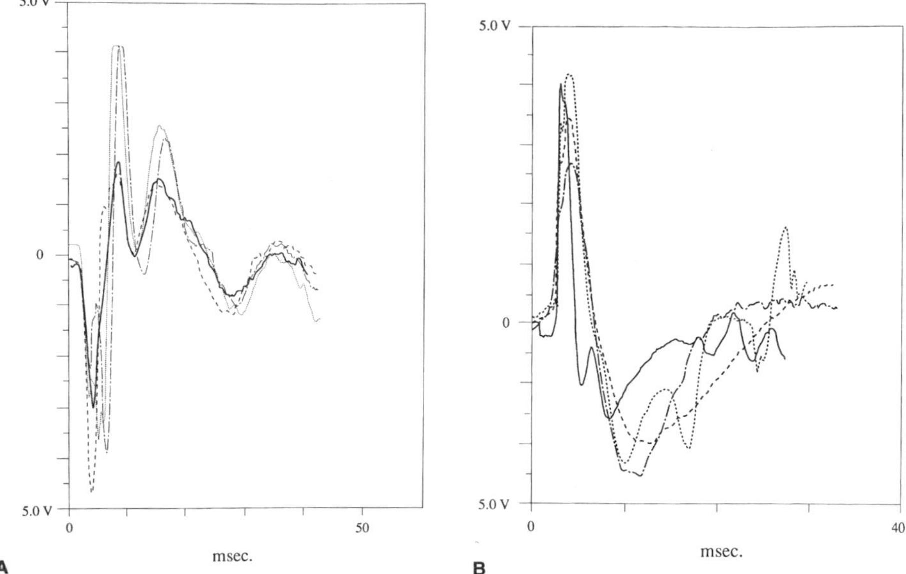

Figure 6.5 A. Morphologic details of initial discrete sounds (IDS) compared using overlays of these sounds of successive swallows during rhythmic suckle feeding. B. IDS of three successive swallows of another infant.

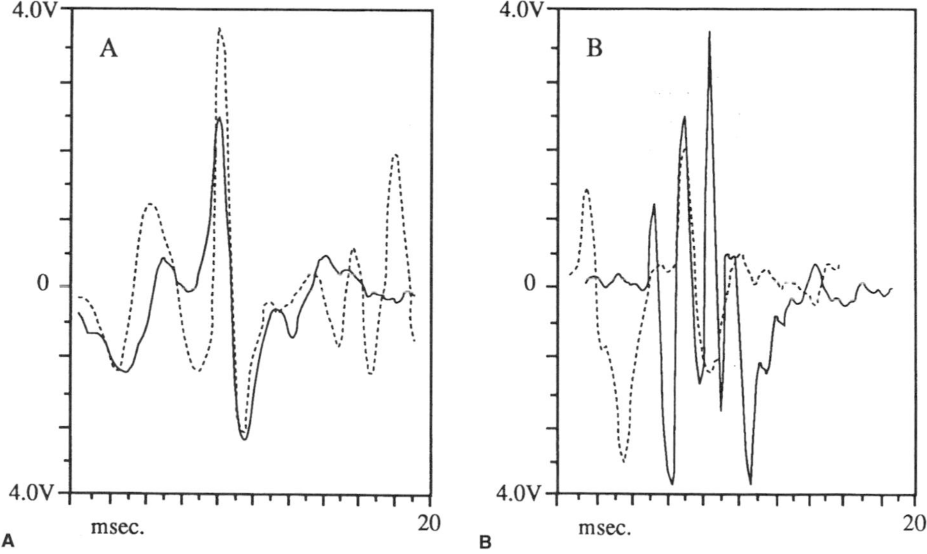

Figure 6.6 A. Morphologic details of final discrete sounds (FDS) of consecutive swallows. B. FDS of consecutive swallows of another infant.

portion of the brain may have occurred during initial development in the embryo or small fetus. The resulting gross abnormalities of the mouth and pharynx or the brain are readily discerned. The greater challenge is to distinguish impairments of the development shared between the oral and pharyngeal area and the bulbar portion of the brain, which occur later in development in the fetus and infant. This sharing is involved in the performance of suckle feeding, and also in participation of the pharynx and larynx in respiration and in the maintenance of the pharyngeal airway, which is the developmental prologue of postural control of the head and neck. The current concept of the development of this sharing is that it occurs by a reciprocating mechanism—i.e., sensory inputs from the mouth and pharynx during feeding stimulate the development of brain regions representing the various feeding movements, which then generate more refined movements. These, in turn, generate further performance-appropriate input. The system is thus reciprocating in both its peripheral and central aspects.

As clinicians gain experience with dysphagia in neurologically impaired infants and children, they are increasingly concerned with the development of the separate representations of these categorical functions in the medulla and at higher levels. It is necessary to view abnormalities in the development of feeding from this perspective, because we then may understand the influence of abnormal early feeding performance on the pattern of feeding of the neurologically impaired child. Abnormalities of early respiratory and positional performances also are cumulative in their effects on performance in each of these categories. These categorical functions combine in their influences on the developing structure and form of the muscles and skeleton in the mouth, pharynx, and larynx. Thus, we may understand the mechanisms by which the peripheral effector structures grow and develop into shapes that further handicap the feeding performance.

For purposes of this review, the causes and mechanisms of suckle-feeding impairments are classified into embryopathy of the oral and pharyngeal area, embryopathy of the brain and peripheral nerves, acquired neurologic impairments, acquired impairments of the mouth and pharynx, and iatrogenic mechanisms.

Embryopathy of the Oral and Pharyngeal Area

The embryogenesis of the pharyngeal and oral area is complex, because it is derived from convergence of the foregut with the branchial arches and with the cervical segmental muscles of the ventral median bar. The peripheral sensory and motor innervation is of corresponding diversity, as it includes the trigeminal, facial, glossopharyngeal, vagal, hypoglossal, and upper cervical nerves. The simplest impairments, in terms of detection and clinical management, are those of the tongue and palate. Infants who have hypoplasia of the tongue may achieve adequate suckle feeding by compensatory actions of the constrictor wall, pharyngeal palate, palatine folds, and hyoid suspensory muscles. The mandible and palate and other portions of the midfacial skeleton are adapted in shape so that they form functionally appropriate chambers about the hypoplastic tongue (Weinberg et al. 1969).

Analogously, an infant who has cleft palate but who has normal feeding incentive and normal sensory inputs and central representations of suckle and swallow, may demonstrate remarkable motor compensations for this anatomic defect by muscles of the pharyngeal palate, adjacent constrictor wall, and tongue (Bosma et al. 1966).

A lesser degree of pharyngeal palate hypoplasia may be evidenced by cleft of the uvula or by a palate that is visibly short or lax under fingertip palpation. The lesser mass of the hypoplastic palate may be more clearly evidenced by radiography in lateral projection than by inspection or palpation. An infant who has palate hypoplasia may have greater problems of pharyngeal dysphagia, including nasal regurgitation, than the infant with a cleft palate. The greater disability may be coincident with sensory impairment. The most extensive impairment associated with palatal hypoplasia or cleft is that described by Robin (1931), which includes retrusion and possible hypoplasia of the mandible and ptosis of the tongue, with secondary pharyngeal airway obstruction (Takagi et al. 1966; Bruston 1978; Rickham et al. 1978; Williams et al. 1981).

Embryopathy of the Medulla and Pons

The primary nuclei of the cranial nerves are distinguishable soon after the medullary portion of the brain stem achieves its basic form. The most common embryopathies are aplasia of motor nuclei and syringobulbia. Nuclear aplasia in the oral musculature is an infrequent but significant mechanism of suckle dysphagia, as part of the syndrome of aplasia. Aplasia in the hypoglossal or trigeminal motor innervation may cause impairment of the suckle actions. Aplasia in the facial innervation may cause general or discrete weakness in the orbicularis oris or in the fanlike arrangement of mimetic muscles, resulting in leakage at the labial seal about the nipple. Aplasia of vagal striated motor innervations may cause weakness of the pharyngeal or laryngeal muscles or both. Since nuclear aplasia, or agenesis, may be disseminated throughout the striated motor system (Warkany et al. 1981), evidence of the syndrome of localized muscle weakness, hypoplasia, or contracture may be sought in other motor innervations, such as the extraocular muscles (Möbius' syndrome), or muscles in the trunk or limbs (Evans 1954; Goldblatt and Williams 1986; Cohen and Thompson 1987).

Expansion of the central canal in the bulbar area, or syringobulbia, may expand in isolation or as part of a more general myelodysplasia (Swaiman 1989). It may be associated with hypoplasia of primary nuclei (Sieben et al. 1971) or with impairment of performance coordination or regulation. Respiratory impairment may result from bilateral adductor vocal fold paralysis (Holinger et al. 1978) or from impairment of central regulation of respiration (Ward et al. 1986; Hays et al. 1989). We have seen failure of elicitation of pharyngeal swallow in two infants who had Arnold-Chiari malformation of the brain stem in association with lumbar myelomeningocele. In each, pharyngeal participation in respiration and crying and in airway maintenance was normal. In one comparably impaired infant, without radiographic evidence of malformation in the brain stem, an occasional swallow could be elicited in association with intensive suckling; these occasional swallows were seen by videoradiography to be normal in pattern. These selective impairments in eliciting swallow may imply a discrete lesion in the vicinity of nucleus tractus solitarius and adjacent internuncial cells of the swallowing center. This clinical topic awaits detailed comparison of bulbar impairments with the elegant demonstration of the brain stem that is now available by magnetic resonance imaging (Packer et al. 1985).

Acquired Neurologic Impairment

Dysphagia in infants is most commonly caused by neurologic impairment acquired in fetal or early postnatal life. The impairment may result from various respiratory or vascular problems shared by mother and fetus late in pregnancy or during delivery. The infant's respiration and neurocirculation may be impaired in the immediate newborn period. In spite of currently available therapy for Rh incompatibility, encephalopathy of hyperbilirubinemia still occurs. In many instances, no specific etiology of the impairment is identified.

Genetics has an increasing role in diagnosing and evaluating infants who have impairments of the oral and pharyngeal area, whether those impairments are of somatic structure or form or function. During the postnatal period, certain metabolic problems are demonstrated that were held in abeyance during pregnancy. The fetus may have shared an endocrinopathy with the mother and manifest it when the symbiosis was interrupted. For example, a diabetic mother's infant with hyperplasia of islet cells may be transiently hypoglycemic in the newborn period. A fetus may be defended by the maternal organism from its own metabolic anomaly, such as phenylketonuria. Progressive disorders may be demonstrated in the first postnatal weeks or months, including leukodystrophy or mitochondrial myopathy, which are not clearly related to the maternal-fetal symbiosis. The heritable problems, such as transient hypoglycemia in the infant of a diabetic mother or an infant with phenylketonuria, impair feeding by a mechanism of general depression or possible seizure. Progressive encephalopathy or neuropathy may specifically impair the oral or pharyngeal feeding actions.

Acquired Impairments of the Oral and Pharyngeal Feeding Apparatus

Acquired impairments of the oral and pharyngeal feeding apparatus are common but are usually benign and transient. Suckle feeding is usually diminished but not interrupted by acute upper respiratory infections; the infant has more feeding difficulties from nasal obstruction by secretions than by impairment of suckle or swallow. Similarly, oral mucositis of monilia (thrush) usually causes little impairment of suckle. The oral or pharyngeal lesions of herpes simplex cause feeding-related pain. The infant with oral pain from infectious, mechanical, or thermal inflammation of the mouth may initiate suckle and promptly discontinue it with indications of distress.

Iatrogenic Mechanisms

Some feeding impairments are incidental sequelae of pediatric care. The most common and increasing in frequency are those of infants who survive preterm births and have been nourished parenterally or by enteric intubation for weeks or months. These infants have been deprived of oral feeding experience and perhaps of spontaneous or pacifier-elicited suckling. Suckling deprivation is increased if the infant was ventilated via an orotracheal tube for a long time. The repeated stress of intubation may cause an infant or child to become orally defensive (Wolf and Glass 1992; Rudolph 1994).

An analogous deprivation of oral feeding experience may occur during early postnatal surgery in or near the route of feeding, with the incidental effect of delaying the onset of oral feeding. The infant may have been adversely conditioned by pain or distress associated with feeding, unskillful feeding, or interruption of the feeding schedule (Illingsworth and Lister 1964; Illingsworth 1969; Dowling 1977; Kaslon and Ruben 1978; Beraitis et al. 1981; Geertsma et al. 1985). Rudolph (1994) points out possible specific food aversion following association of the food with an adverse experience. Comparable aversion may occur after cancer chemotherapy (Bernstein 1978) and also as part of certain metabolic abnormalities (Hyman et al. 1987).

When oral feeding is impaired, the clinician is concerned about both nutrition and the oral feeding experience. An infant who suckle feeds with variable competence, possibly as a function of the skill of different caregivers, may graduate subtly into malnutrition. Conversely, an infant who is overtly malnourished, perhaps admitted to a hospital from an environment of privation, may suckle avidly but repair malnutrition only slowly. Intubation feeding, by nasogastric or gastrostoma tube, is indicated in either circumstance, in an effort to prevent neurodevelopmental failure from malnutrition (Cravioto and Arrieta 1979; Klein 1980; Prensky 1989).

PATTERNS OF SUCKLE-FEEDING IMPAIRMENT

To evaluate suckle feeding, one must understand the actions and development of suckle and swallow and how feeding relates to the infant's current state. Observation of a possibly feeding-impaired infant may begin with the infant in reference state, calmly awake or in light sleep. Cervical auscultation demonstrates frequent pharyngeal swallows. Non-nutritive suckle motions are common, either spontaneously or as elicited by a touch on the lips.

Much can be learned by observation and cervical auscultation of the infant in usual feeding circumstances. But the clinician should also feed the infant. Suckle feeding may be generally impaired, as in the infant who fails to arouse toward feeding, or feeding components may be impaired—i.e., rooting and latching, suckle, pharyngeal swallow, or esophageal swallow. Clinicians are particularly concerned about an infant who fails to initiate rooting and latching during oral area stimulation, after the infant has been roused by gross movements of the limbs and trunk. The oral area stimulation should be in a sequence of touching or stroking from the cheeks to the lips and thence to the tongue and lingual chamber (Morris and Klein 1987; Morris 1989). If an attempt to elicit rooting by stroking the cheeks or the skin of the lips does not produce rooting, lip closure is evaluated by crosswise stroking of mucosa of the inner lip (the pars villosa) (Bosma 1986a). Lip response may be in a pattern of vertical closure, or pucker, or a pattern of eversion, or pout, appropriate to participation in suckle. The tongue and lingual cavity is usually stimulated with the gloved finger, with the ball of the finger tip downward against the tongue. The stimulus motion is anteroposterior in direction. The response is enclosure by the tongue and lower lip graduating into anteroposterior tongue motions and then into the entire suckle motions, single and then rhythmic, of the tongue, lower lip, hyoid, and mandible. These gestures of evaluation of oral area responses are also the gestures employed in therapeutic stimulation, before feeding time, of the infant who demonstrates delay, deficiency, or variability of the oral stage of suckle feeding (Mueller 1972; Wilson 1977; Morris and Klein 1987; Morris 1989).

An impaired infant's effectiveness at bottle feeding varies with current response state and effort availability of the infant, and also with the general competence and skill of the feeding person. The advantage of one or few feeding persons (preferably the mother) is apparent. In some instances, merely changing the nipple may result in notable increase in feeding competence (Rudolph 1994).

Failure to elicit suckle in an infant who otherwise rouses well to stimulation outside of the oral area is found occasionally in infants who have had adverse conditioning experiences. The infant's aversion may be indicated at any stage of graduation toward suckle feeding, such as a disturbance during preparation for feeding or a negative response to rooting stimulation or nipple insertion. Suckling or suckle feeding may be initiated and then interrupted after a few swallows, possibly with the mouth then lax about the nipple. Renewal of feeding, in this circumstance, is a nursing or mothering skill. Often, it is necessary to continue nutrition by an indwelling soft nasogastric tube, which does not apparently impede suckle feeding.

The clinician is particularly concerned about an infant who suckles well but is impaired in pharyngeal swallow. This, again, may result from somatic embryopathy of form, such as cleft or hypoplasia of the palate, cleft of the epiglottis or cricoid cartilage, or motor unit aplasia. The impairment may be of pharyngeal area sensory inputs, possibly combined with impairment in bulbar coordination of swallow, as in familial dysautonomia. Identifying the mechanism of selective pharyngeal dysphagia is aided by evaluating other pharyngeal and laryngeal performances, including participation in tidal respiration, cry, and airway maintenance. For those with competence of nonfeeding performances of the pharynx and larynx, and incompetence in the suckle stage of feeding, selective pharyngeal dysphagia must be attributed to a localized lesion in the representation of swallow in the medulla. This selective impairment may be persistent. Cervical auscultation at the larynx, by stethoscope or by microphone and speaker, is useful in detecting pharyngeal swallow impairment, because the sounds indicate the event of swallow and also, if swallow of pharyngeal content fails to occur or is impaired, the sounds may demonstrate bubbles of respiration mixed with fluid, or choke, clearing, cough, or stridor. Further evaluation of pharyngeal dysphagia requires a videoradiographic study (Kramer 1989; Sivit 1990; Benson and Lefton-Greif 1994; Marquis and Pressman 1995). Radiography may demonstrate that a marginally impaired swallow performs adequately if the formula is thickened, as by mixing with rice flour or with one of the recently available starch-based agents. Combining cervical auscultation with videoradiography, with the acoustic recording on a channel of the video film, gives the clinician an acoustic reference, which may subsequently be used in cervical auscultation by stethoscope in guiding the feeding care of the infant.

Suckle has been used to facilitate swallow in an infant who had this selective impairment. Milk was delivered by syringe at the side of the pacifier. In this procedure, stethoscope auscultation was used to detect the effectiveness of this facilitation. Milk delivery was discontinued when swallows failed to empty the pharynx and retained swallow residua were evident, by cervical auscultation, in the airway.

The normally feeding infant indicates satiation by attenuation of the suckle runs and increased frequency of feeding pauses. This attenuation can be distinguished from fatigue of the feeding effort, such as is found in myasthenia or myopathy or as in nonspecific fatigue of motor effort, as in some infants who have marginal cardiac or respiratory adequacy. The infant may actively grasp the nipple like a pacifier, with intermittent suckling, at the conclusion of feeding; this is noted particularly in breast feeding. At the conclusion of feeding, the young infant usually graduates into sleep.

Gastroesophageal reflux (GER) and esophagopharyngeal regurgitation are continuing concerns and possible problems in orally and pharyngeally impaired infants. GER is demonstrated frequently, by esophageal pH monitor, in neurologically impaired infants and children (Morris 1979; Sondheimer 1983; Catto-Smith et al. 1991). It is variously attributed to primary central impairment of vagal control (Vane et al. 1982), to increased intra-abdominal pressure associated with spastic disorder (Kasson et al. 1965), or to prolonged time in supine position (Guttman 1972).

GER may be associated with chronic respiratory disease (Boyle et al. 1985; Pack 1990; McColley and Carroll 1994). This coincidence has been the basis for antireflux surgery (Wilkinson et al. 1981). Recently, GER is increasingly treated with potent acid inhibitors and prokinetic agents such as cisipride (Tuchman 1994).

Exceptionally, the infant may cry for a long time at the end of feeding. This postprandial crying, designated "fussiness" or "colic," has been attributed to esophagopharyngeal regurgitation secondary to inadequate burping, to irritable bowel, or protein hypersensitivity (Illingsworth 1954; Wessel et al. 1954). Whether this prolonged crying is an individual difference in state regulation or a difference in parental tolerance may be difficult to discern (Taubman 1984). Whether an increase in carrying the infant during the day may have an effect on this problem is controversial (Barr et al. 1991).

ACQUISITION OF SUCKLE FEEDING IN THE PRETERM INFANT

The pharyngeal performances of swallowing secretions, participating in respiration, and maintaining an airway are adequate in small, viable, unimpaired preterm infants. The fetus has been swallowing since the twelfth week of gestation or earlier (Humphrey 1970). Fetuses near term are said to swallow 450 ml/day, a greater volume than in the first neonatal weeks (Golubeva et al. 1959). Prenatal ultrasound demonstrates frequent suckle actions.

Preterm infants have an oral and pharyngeal feeding experience that differs remarkably from that of a fetus in utero and of a term-born infant. Initial suckle, as early as 18–24 weeks gestation (Golubeva et al. 1959), is rapid, non-nutritive in pattern, and interspersed with nonspecific mouthing. Non-nutritive suckling concomitant with tube feeding is associated with increased oxygenation (Paludetto et al. 1986), earlier gastric emptying (Widstrom et al. 1988), and increased weight gain in preterm infants nourished by intubation (Measel and Anderson 1979; Field et al. 1982; Bernbaum et al. 1983). Field et al. (1982) also showed that non-nutritive suckling was associated with less restlessness and earlier achievement of bottle feeding. Non-nutritive suckling also increased polypeptide hormone release, with greater gastric secretion and earlier gastric emptying (Widstrom et al. 1988). In preterm infants without embryopathy of the oral and pharyngeal area or of the brain stem and without extensive acquired encephalopathy, this graduation toward mature suckle feeding progresses stably (Wolff 1968). The perioral elicitations of rooting are acquired later in development. Gryboski (1969) observed preterm infants sequentially from gestational week 32 and noted graduation of nonspecific mouthing into single or few nutrient suckles. At 35–36 weeks, suckling was in bursts or runs, interspersed with swallows. These observations are confirmed by Colley and Creamer (1958), Casaer et al. (1982), Daniels et al. (1986), and Herbst (1989). Recent studies in preterm infants by our group have demonstrated developmental progression in separate components of suckle feeding at a bottle: stabilization of individual suckle, swallow sequences, stabilization of suckling rhythm, and finally interposition of breaths between swallows in the suckle-feeding runs. Before these breath interpositions, the runs are partially or entirely apneic. The nurse or mother feeding the infant at this stage must be alert to the liability of apnea; this alertness is aided by cervical auscultation. Various sugars, particularly sucrose, elicit increase in suckling effort and duration of runs (Maller and Turner 1973; Steiner 1977; Ashmead et al. 1980).

Tone in the esophagus and the esophagogastric junction is low in the early preterm infant, but tone in the pharyngoesophageal segment is comparable to that at term (Milla 1991). Esophageal peristalsis becomes more consistent and of higher amplitude as the preterm infant approaches term (Sondheimer 1983; Herbst 1989; Milla 1991).

Orogastric or nasogastric intubation feeding continues during these early feeding efforts, with supplementation of the oral feeding or replacement if the oral feeding attempt was unsuccessful. Of these methods, orogastric intubation is associated with fewer adverse effects on lung function than nasogastric intubation in preterm infants smaller than 2,000 g. Awareness of the adverse effects of gavage feeding on compliance of the lung and chest wall and on increase in diaphragmatic work requirement incline the clinician toward oral feeding (Heldt 1988). The greatest risk to this progression toward oral feeding is that of interruption of feeding experience by reason of clinical exigencies, such as sepsis or other intercurrent illness. An ailing preterm infant may occasionally regress or actually lose recently acquired advances in feeding. Orotracheal intubation for respiratory support particularly impedes feeding-equivalent experience, as the tube fills and immobilizes the mouth, particularly if the tube is supplemented by stabilizing flanges that cover the lips and cheeks. As increasing numbers of small preterm infants survive, the incidence and duration of respiratory assistance are increasing (Hack et al. 1991). The provision of oral feeding experience merits the best available skills of the mother or other caregiver. If suckle-feeding experience is not currently available, periods of passive suckle-equivalent oral stimulation should be provided (Morris 1989).

BREAST FEEDING OF THE PRETERM AND THE FEEDING-IMPAIRED INFANT

In the Western world, breast feeding of preterm and feeding-impaired infants has been largely replaced by formula feeding by nipple or by intubation (Jelliffe and Jelliffe 1978). Artificial milk-consistency feeding has been highly successful in nutrition and in the nonmaternal care of infants. But these clinical advances have been detrimental to the mother-infant relationship. During gestation, the mother and infant are each prepared for suckle feeding. The mother has been furnished with a responsive lactation apparatus and with nipples that are well contoured for the infant's mouth and will be further adapted in form during each feeding (Erenberg et al. 1986). The mother is prepared in mind and spirit to provide the ambience that is so much a part of suckle feeding. The mother provides olfactory cues to which the infant is responsive (Steiner 1977; Sarnat 1978; Meier 1980; Schaal 1988; Sullivan et al. 1991). The mother also provides duplication of feeding circumstance. The milk is warm. Initially, post-delivery, it consists of colostrum. At each feeding, the infant's initial suckling usually obtains little milk, so that the dysphagia-liable infant's first swallows may be safer. Subsequently, the quantity of milk released varies with suckle effort and corresponding stimulation to lactation. Late in the feeding, and during the attenuation of effort at the end of feeding, the infant's swallows may be followed by phonation.

In Western hospitals, neonatal intensive care units customarily graduate a premature infant from nasogastric tube feeding of formula or expressed breast milk to bottle feeding, using a premie nipple, and thence possibly to breast feeding, if the mother has been able to maintain milk production by breast pumping. However, some studies have demonstrated that premature infants as young as 32 weeks' gestational age or less than 1,500 g can be graduated directly to breast feeding if feeding coordination has been achieved (Meier and Pugh 1985; Meier and Anderson 1987; McCoy et al. 1988; Blackman 1991), and if the hospital routines can be adapted to permit flexibility in the time and duration of breast feeding. Breast feeding was found to be associated with greater stability of PO_2 levels than was bottle feeding (Meier and Anderson 1987). We anticipate that breast feeding of premature infants may become common practice in neonatal intensive care units in which this effort is well sponsored. Some intensive care units encourage mothers to express milk for intubation or bottle feeding of medically problematic postterm infants, with or without feeding impairment (Wilks and Meier 1988). No studies of breast feeding of dysphagic infants have been reported. Such studies of dysphagic infants are needed, for these infants may be particularly in need of the resources and mechanisms of communication that breast feeding affords. In the face of these benefits of satisfaction and interpersonal exchange, it is important to recognize that the nutritional adequacy of breast feeding depends on the potential lactation efficiency of the mother and on the mother's lactation response state at the time of individual feeding. The preterm or dysphagic infant may fail to thrive with breast feeding, just as normal infants occasionally fail to thrive (Evans and Davies 1977).

This experience of preterm infant feeding in modern contemporary nurseries is in striking contrast with the care of premature and small-for-dates infants born at high altitudes in parts of the Andean mountains. As reported by Anderson et al. (1986) and Leeuw et al. (1991), these infants are swaddled and bound between the mothers' breasts, with ad libitum access to nipple feeding.

TRANSITIONAL FEEDING

The transitional feeding period is a time of graduation from exclusive suckle feeding of liquids to voluntary ingestion of physically varied foods. It is also a time when various neurologic impairments of feeding actions are demonstrated. To recognize these impairments one must be familiar with the patterns of normal post-suckle-feeding development.

The supplementation of suckle feeding by addition of discriminate oral awareness and voluntary oral feeding actions begins in the first postterm months. At term, the feeding-ready infant is fully preoccupied with the suckle-feeding performance. During established suckle feeding, the young infant may tolerate, and fail to respond to, other stimuli, including those of some painful clinical procedures. In some pharyngeally dysphagic infants, suckle feeding may continue in spite of nasal or laryngeal penetration of pharyngeal content.

Within a few weeks of term, volition and variation are added, usually near the completion of the suckle-feeding session. The infant interrupts feeding to give visual attention or to phonate with the nipple still in place.

The graduation of oral responses and actions has been comprehensively described (Mueller 1972; Wilson 1977; Morris 1982; Morris and Klein 1987; Gisel 1988a; Morris 1989; Gisel 1991; Stolovitz and Gisel 1991). Spoon feeding of pablum or similar puree-consistency foods at 4–6 months elicits mouth opening. The pablum is ingested by suckle actions. At this time, the infant's hand actions graduate from a finger or a fisted hand in the mouth to bringing manually manipulated objects into the mouth. This can include manual delivery of soft foods or of crisp but soluble crackers. Spoon feeding or independent hand feeding is graduated toward semiparticulate foods, such as small vegetal bits in a puree matrix.

Chewing

The acquisition of chewing and of biting skills are separate achievements. As noted above, the suckle-feeding performance is oriented on the median portion of the mouth. Material of fluid consistency does not usually penetrate into the lateral portion of the mouth adjacent to the molar alveolar ridges. The buccal recess of the infant (Figure 6.7) is minimal in area.

In young children, the oral manipulations of chewing differ qualitatively from the suckle-pattern manipulation of purees (Stolovitz and Gisel 1991). Chewing is a lateralized performance and is oriented about the molar area (Dubner et al. 1978; Luschei and Goldberg 1981). The tongue has a major role in the chewing performance (Gisel 1988a) (Figure 6.8). It shifts the oral content to the molar area and interacts with the buccal musculature to repeatedly place the food on the moving molar table. At the completion of mastication, the tongue transfers the food to the primary bolus accumulation area, adjacent to the junction of the bony and muscular portions of the palate. These various components of chewing are guided by subjective cues generated by voluntary manipulation of the food. Firm or "solid" foods are more effective than viscous or pureed foods in eliciting chewing (Gisel 1988b; Gisel 1991). In normal children between 6 months and 2 years, the increasing chewing efficiency to the endpoint of swallow has been calibrated with videophotographic observation using gelatin masses of differing sizes (Archambault et al. 1991). The initiation of swallow by conveyance of the bolus through the faucial isthmus is also voluntary. The young child may be seen to interrupt oral feeding and give attention to the swallow.

The mandibular motions of mastication are usually vertical in their early manifestation. The motions become principally transverse ("grinding") and increase in efficiency. During transitional feeding, the sided incidence changes. At 2 years, 60% of chewing is on the right side; at 4 years, 60% is on the left

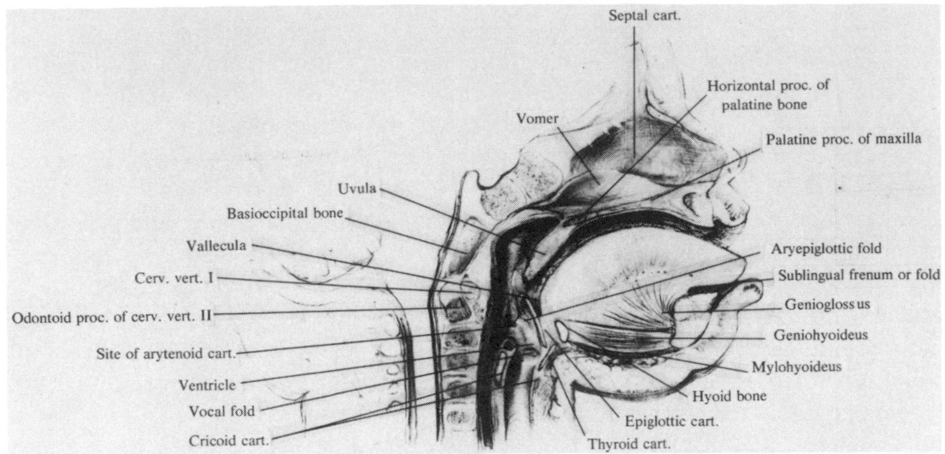

Figure 6.7 Midline section of oral and pharyngeal area in an infant. The tongue fills the lingual cavity, which is bounded in this demonstration by the oral palate, mandible, body of the hyoid bone, and mylohyoideus. The tongue is slightly separated from the oral and pharyngeal palate and is displaced anteriorly in this drawing. The pharynx is short in vertical dimension. The tip of the epiglottis approximates the uvula at the inferior end of the velum. The pharyngoesophageal segment is adjacent to the inferior margin of the cricoid cartilage; it is drawn in the open position. The infant's larynx differs notably from that of the adult. The arytenoid and corniculate cartilages are surrounded by a large mass of loose connective tissue, which diminishes the lumen of the laryngeal vestibule. The length of the vocal folds and of the ventricle is diminished in comparison with the internal diameters of the thyroid and cricoid cartilages.

(Gisel 1988a). The achievement of chewing is not dependent on eruption of molar teeth; the entire coordination of mastication is usually achieved before eruption of the molars begins, at 12 to 20 months (Gisel 1988b).

Evaluation of Chewing in Feeding-Impaired Children

Intraoral food manipulation is commonly impaired in young children who have disorders of oral area coordination. This manipulation in normal and in coordination-impaired children has been described in a standard manner (Gisel 1988a; Gisel and Patrick 1988). Evaluation of this manipulation requires patience. Bits of cracker or readily softened candy are placed in the mouth by the child or the clinician and "followed" by inspections during passive openings of the mouth. The test material may remain on the tongue during externally apparent chewing motions. The material may be extruded through the lips or held on the tongue dorsum until swallowed. The material may be displaced laterally and not be retrieved (this is termed "squirreling"). In some children who have oral dyspraxia, chewing may be elicited by the caregiver placing particulate

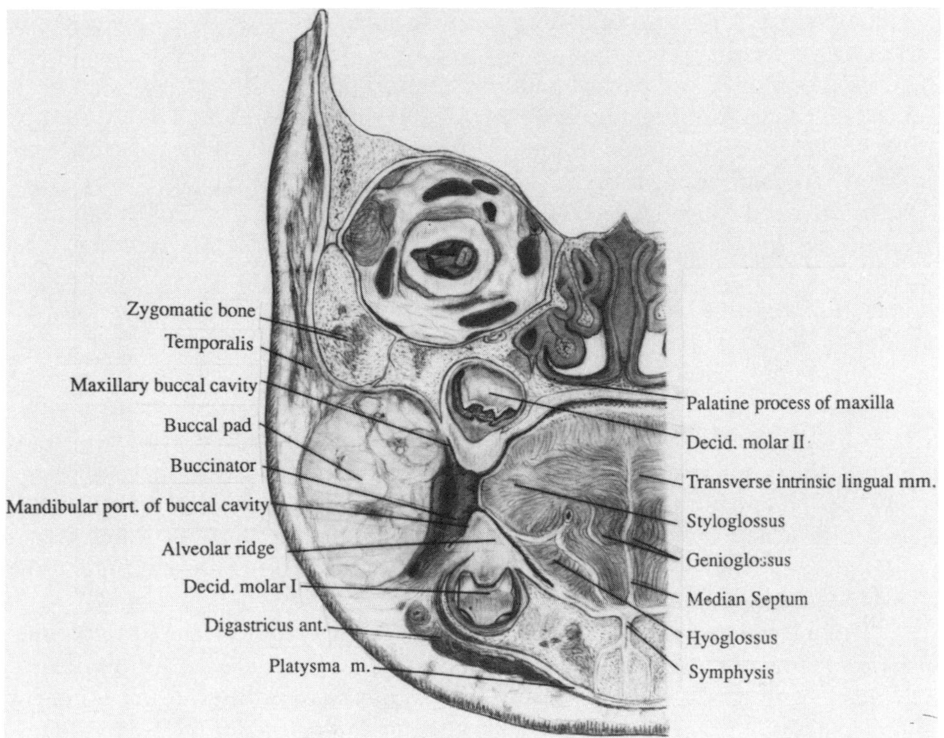

Figure 6.8 Coronal section of the facial area in an infant. A section through the body of the tongue, symphysis of the mandible, oral palate, central portion of the nasal chamber, and buccal pad. The tongue fills the oral cavity, which in this plane is bounded inferiorly by the mandible and the mandibular ridge and laterally by the buccal wall.

food on the molar table. At a lesser level of competence in such children, food placed on either molar table is moved by the tongue to its dorsum and there mashed by the tongue.

Infant-patterned suckle feeding is available in some orally dyskinetic children. They may retain rooting and latching responses. As part of their latching response, the head and neck are stabilized about a nipple equivalent. During videofluoroscopic study, barium-coated cracker bits deposited on the tongue of these children may be carried into the pharynx by suckle actions of the tongue and are swallowed.

Biting

Biting is separate from chewing in its coordination pattern and in the mechanism and schedule of its generation. Discrete voluntary biting can be readily distinguished from the sustained jaw closure that occurs in some forms of spastic dyskinesia. Biting on the nipple is first noted as a part of oral play at the end of suckle feeding. The infant of 6–12 months may bite objects that he or she brings to the mouth as a part of hand and mouth play. During transitional feeding the mouth may be voluntarily firmly closed by the jaw as well as by the lips during defensive resistance to feeding. During biting, the mandible is guided vertically in the midline toward such interincisor approximation as may be available in the child's arrangement of maxilla and mandible. The posteroanterior relation of the mandible and maxilla differs in biting and chewing. The mandible is commonly farther forward in biting than in chewing. The performance of biting is as liable to impairment as the performance of chewing in oral dyskinesia, but its impairment is less well defined.

These graduations of oral skills indicate increasing awareness of food and other possible ingesta and increasing attention to oral actions. Selection or rejection of foods, and participation in feeding, is discriminate and is initially varied, possibly changing with the caregiver or the circumstance. Studies by Davis (1939) of young children offered trays of varied foods demonstrated nutritionally irregular selection during each meal but a nutritionally balanced diet over a period of days. Much fluid intake during transitional feeding may continue to be by suckle feeding at the breast or by bottle.

These developmental generations of the feeding performance are uniquely individual (Bosma 1976). They depend on the individual's accumulation of experience with foods, feeding circumstances, and culture. But this development also depends on variations in innate elements, including the array of oral mucosal sensory receptors. The resultant feeding patterns, which are carried into childhood, are a product of feeding satisfaction and failure. The feeding distortions, disruptions, and experiences of distress and failure to which the neurologically impaired infant and child are liable are mechanisms that subsequently influence the individual's feeding patterns. In some circumstances, noted in the following section, the dysphagic child's feeding pattern may be determined extensively by experiences of failure.

If semiparticulate food or small food bits are delivered into the mouth of a child who has impairment of chew and bite, the food may be partially prepared for swallowing by tongue mashing.

To external observation, the motions of tongue mashing are similar to the early, vertical motions of chewing, but visualization of the oral cavity by passive opening of the mouth or by videoradiography in posteroanterior projection demonstrates that the food is not in the molar area. The tongue-mashed food, including particles, may be effectively swallowed. It is important to recognize, in this connection, that the feeding-related actions of the pharynx include more than swallowing accumulated secretions or a food bolus delivered from the mouth. The pharynx participates in more general performances of the upper portion of the alimentary tract, including gagging, vomiting, and rumination. The pharynx also participates with the larynx in the respiratory actions of coughing and choking and in the less effortful actions of clearing secretions or food residua in the trachea or the laryngeal vestibule.

Particularly during the first part of transitional feeding, the normal infant or young child gags or chokes mildly, with little distress or indication of alarm. A notable incidental videoradiographic observation in some neurologically impaired dysphagic children is that of regurgitation of pharyngeal content into the mouth by a simple constriction action of the pharynx; the content may then be expectorated or retained in the mouth until it is reswallowed. This pharyngo-oral regurgitation differs from choking or coughing in that it is not associated with expiration. It differs also from vomiting in that the esophagus is not emptied upward and the child's pharynx and mouth are not in a vomiting or retching position.

MATURE FEEDING IN CHILDHOOD

The graduations from transitional into fully mature feeding reflect the child's increasing autonomy and independent exploration of foods, leading to an omnivorous diet and independent use of feeding utensils. Drinking from a cup or glass is increasingly skilled. The actions of food prehension and biting and the various actions of the tongue, buccal wall, and mandibular muscles in chewing and bolus selection are stabilized and become more automatic. Maturation of the coordination of the facial muscles about the mouth is an important element of graduation into mature feeding. The buccinator muscle controls the expanding sulcus lateral to the molars. This function becomes more important as the infantile sucking pad and the panniculus in the cheek diminish, and with eruption of teeth and the change in form of the mandible, the mandible is increasingly separated from the maxilla. During chewing, the buccinator acts in a reciprocal manner with the transversely moving tongue to maneuver food on the molar table. The orbicularis oris and mimetic muscles are also changed in coordination pattern to achieve stable labial enclosure during intraoral food manipulation. This enclosure differs from that during suckle feeding, in which the lips are everted in pouting contour so that their inner aspect, adjacent to the pars villosa, approximates the nipple. During the suckle action, the lower lip, along with the tongue, mandible, and hyoid, is moved in relation to the nipple. During mature oral feeding in childhood, labial enclosure of oral content is in a vertical pattern. In the case of incisor malocclusion, overbite, or prognathism, the upper or lower incisors may be included in the labial seal. Failure to achieve this labial seal by any of its coordination mechanisms results in spill or drooling (Sochaniwskyj et al. 1986; Harris and Purdy 1987). The sensory resources of the oral area pertinent to chewing and biting are substantially increased by eruption of the teeth. During childhood, the mouth is enlarged and, more significantly, is changed in form by enlargement and eruption of the teeth and by changes in the dimensions and form of the mandible and midfacial skeleton (Bosma 1975, 1985) (Figure 6.9). The anatomically related structures of the tongue, hyoid, and larynx descend in relation to the facial skeleton and the cervical vertebrae. These changes in the facial and pharyngeal skeleton are related to changes in oral and pharyngeal feeding actions and also in the positional or postural

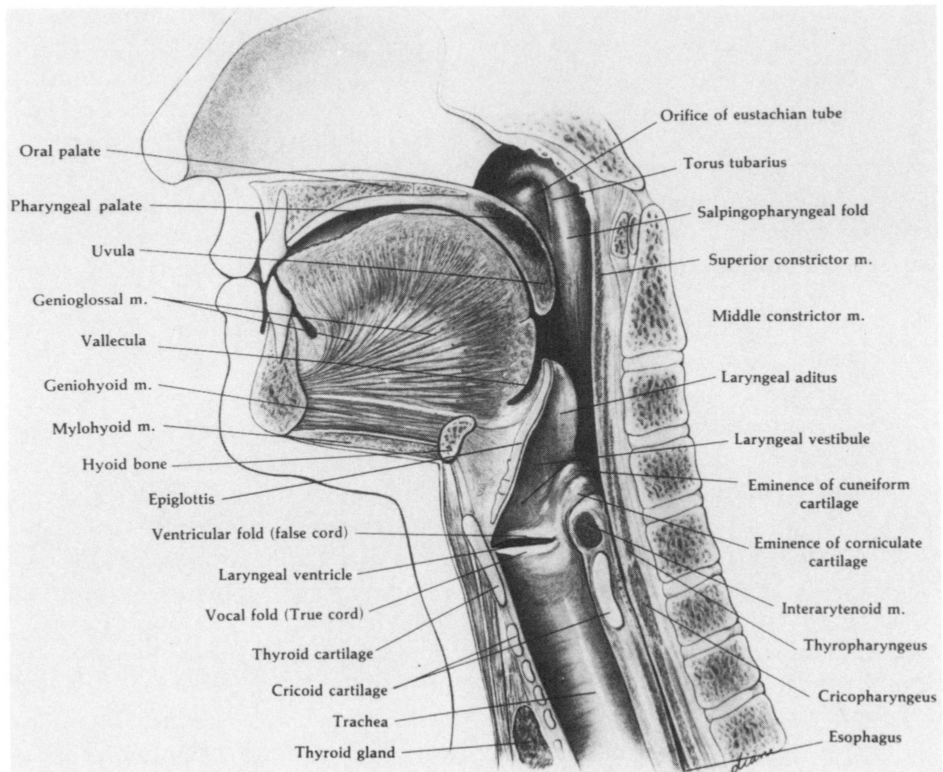

Figure 6.9 Midline section of the oral and pharyngeal area in an adult. This section, in comparison with that of Figure 5.7, demonstrates the result of postnatal growth of the oral and pharyngeal area. Note particularly the growth of the pharynx and larynx and the developmental descent of the larynx and adjacent pharynx in relation to the mandible and the cervical vertebrae.

actions of the head and neck and about the pharyngeal airway. These relations are reciprocal: the motor performances influence the form and position of the skeleton and related anatomy and the anatomic changes influence the displacements, but not the basic coordination pattern, of feeding and posture. The coordination pattern of pharyngeal swallow in the child who has achieved mature feeding is essentially similar to that in the adult, shown in Figure 6.10. The buccal space is enlarged by growth of the molars and their related alveolar structures and by diminution in the sucking pad and adjacent panniculus. Mastication and the lingual actions of selection and sizing of the bolus become more efficient. The entire suckle-feeding sequence is retained throughout life although, in normal individuals, its corollary reflexes of rooting and nipple latching are lost. Suckle feeding may continue to be a strategic mechanism of oral ingestion throughout life (Ramsey 1986).

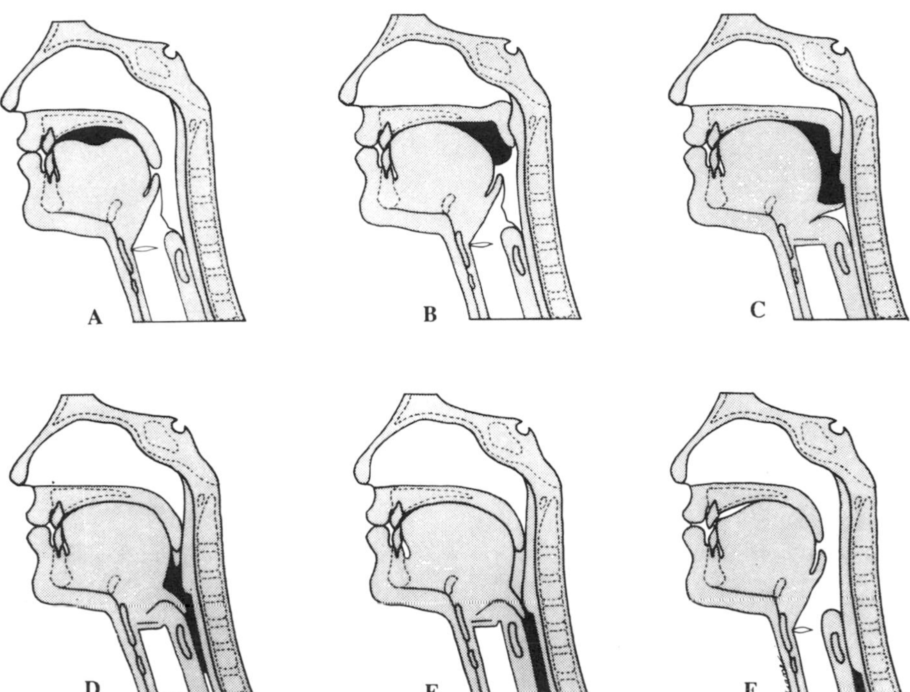

Figure 6.10 Summary schematic of the pharyngeal swallow of a large liquid bolus in an adult, as demonstrated by radiography in the lateral projection. A. The bolus is retained in the oral cavity by approximation of the velum with the tongue; nasal portal respiration can be continued. B. The bolus is conveyed through the faucial isthmus and into the oropharynx by the tongue. The velum is displaced upward and backward and is approximated by a protrusion on the posterior pharyngeal wall—the beginning of the pharyngeal peristaltic wave. C. The bolus extends into the laryngopharynx. The epiglottis is tilted downward, and the hyoid and larynx are fully displaced upward and forward. The peristaltic wave is descending in the constrictor wall. D. The bolus penetrates the opened pharyngoesophageal segment. The peristaltic wave has descended further. The upper portion of the palatopharyngeal isthmus has reopened. E. The bolus has nearly traversed the pharynx. The peristaltic wave has reached the hypopharynx. The oropharynx is beginning to reopen. F. The mouth, now empty, and the pharynx have returned to reference position. (From MW Donner, JF Bosma, D Robertson. Anatomy and physiology of the pharynx. Gastrointest Radiol 1985;10:196. Reprinted with permission from Springer-Verlag.)

FEEDING IMPAIRMENTS IN CHILDHOOD

The maturations of feeding actions and of the interaction of feeding and posture are of considerable significance in the feeding patterns and competencies of children whose feeding impairments originated in the fetus, the preterm infant, or the full-term infant. The impairments, which were manifested during transitional feeding, may simply be stabilized into lifetime patterns. This stabilization may occur at levels below the level of potential feeding competence.

Alternatively, the child who demonstrates oral or pharyngeal dysphagia during the time of transitional feeding is liable to different, possibly increasing, feeding problems at school age and puberty. These changes vary with the mechanisms of impairment. A malformation of the oral and pharyngeal area, of the medulla and pons, or adjacent cranial skeleton may result in increasing impairment. A pathologic process of the brain, musculature, or peripheral nerves may be progressive.

Increasing problems may result from social and environmental circumstances. Feeding efficiency may actually decline as the individual, along with his or her parents and caregivers, attempts to achieve the mature feeding patterns of the family or other associates by using feeding resources that are marginal or inadequate. The child and family may be unwilling to accept the available, and possibly more efficient, resources of suckle feeding or of pablum feeding by spoon or spout.

Embryopathy of the Oral and Pharyngeal Area

Most of the children who have embryopathy of the oral and pharyngeal area but have intact or adequate neurologic mechanisms for postural, respiratory, and feeding performances are expected to continue in the linked development of these performances and their effector anatomy.

In the child who has severe hypoplasia of the tongue, the physiologic compensations of the submental musculature, pharyngeal palate, and pharynx and the anatomic adaptations of the facial skeleton continue during childhood and pubertal growth in the facial and pharyngeal area. The repaired cleft palate functions well, preventing nasal regurgitation, until the time of spontaneous normal diminution of the adenoid mass, when nasal regurgitation may occur, along with hypernasality.

Embryopathy of the Medulla and Pons

The oral and pharyngeal feeding actions of the children who have embryopathy of the medulla and pons depend on possible further anatomic changes in the area of the malformation and on possible late changes in an Arnold-Chiari malformation (Caviness 1976; Warkany et al. 1981). The adaptations and compensations noted previously may be available for the irregularly disseminated muscle deficiencies and contractures that may be a part of nuclear hypoplasia.

Dyscoordination in the Oral and Pharyngeal Area

The dysphagia problems of the school-age child who has dyscoordination in the oral and pharyngeal area vary with the pattern of the disorder. The feeding problems and adaptations of those who have athetosis or choreoathetosis are similar to those of adults who have these disorders (see Chapters 3 and 9).

The dysphagia problems of school-age and pubertal children who have spastic disorder may increase. The hypertonus of the cervical extensors and the submental muscles and genioglossus, which become evident in some spastic quadriplegics in the time of transitional feeding, may be increasingly demonstrated in the child in the form of sustained hypertonus, with occasional surges during times of effort, as at meals. Increasing hypertonus, possibly associated with contracture of the craniocervical extensor and the mandible depressor muscles, may handicap oral and pharyngeal feeding actions by a secondary mechanism of malposition of oral and pharyngeal structures. Chew and bite may be absent or minimal. Tongue mashing may still sufficiently prepare soft and semiparticulate foods for the child's pharyngeal swallow; this adequacy may be inferred from the child's freedom from coughing and choking at mealtime, and, more significantly, by history, which indicates no chronic lower respiratory disorder or frank pneumonia. The competence of pharyngeal swallow, according to the criteria of its promptness of occurrence, the effectiveness of bolus transit, and the absence of penetration into the larynx or the palatopharyngeal isthmus, can be evaluated by videoradiography (Kramer 1989; Sivit 1990). These children's liability to laryngeal penetration and dispersion of food during swallow or regurgitation from the esophagus and stomach can be evaluated by scintigraphic tracing of radionuclide-labeled foods (Ham et al. 1985; Espinola 1986).

The children who have dyscoordination of the oral and pharyngeal stages of feeding may also have impaired control of respiration in general and of respiration adjacent to feeding. These abnormalities of respiration coincident with dysphagia have been physiologically described by Kenny et al. (1989a). Kenny and associates (1989b) also have developed a Multidisciplinary Feeding Profile that provides a description of the anatomy of the oral and pharyngeal area in bulbar dyskinetic children and the particulars of their feeding and respiratory performances. The Profile has been standardized (Judd et al. 1989) and can be used as a reference for describing these children.

The increasing nutritional needs of the child must be considered. We must keep in mind the need to frequently reassess feeding competence and routines. This reassessment must include estimation of nutritional state, at least by weight progression and thickness of skin folds in the areas least distorted by dyskinesia (Patrick and Gisel 1990). In dysphagic children who are liable to malnutrition, there is a constant possibility of supplementation of oral intake by intubation feeding, via a nasogastric or gastrostoma route, on a schedule that interferes minimally with the incentives, actions, and satisfactions of oral feeding. Clinicians who care for dysphagic infants and children are now well aware of the liability of intubation feeding to increase gastroesophageal reflux and esophageal and esophagopharyngeal regurgitation (Raventos et al. 1982; Mollitt et al. 1985).

Progressive Encephalopathy

Feeding competence may be impaired in progressive encephalopathy. The mechanisms, neurologic form, and patterns of progression are reviewed in pediatric neurology textbooks (Swaiman 1989; Menkes 1990; Brett 1991). The impairment may be a nonspecific diminution in appetite and other aspects of feeding incentive or a more specific impairment of the oral and pharyngeal feeding actions. The pattern and severity of feeding impairment reflects the involvement of the bulbar area in the pathologic process. In the simplest and most easily managed pattern, the encephalopathy spares the bulbar area, so that nutrition can be maintained by infant-patterned suckle feeding.

A special concern is that of interaction of feeding with seizures in those progressive encephalopathies that are epileptogenic. The pattern of these interactions varies. Children who have seizure-free intervals may be fed at those times; the success of feeding depends on the perceptions of the caregiver. Occasionally, partial seizures with preserved consciousness may be associated with feeding in transitional or mature pattern. If these partial seizures are manifested only in the limbs, it may be possible to continue feeding. If, however, partial seizures are evidenced in the bulbar innervation, as by nystagmus, by twitches of the facial muscles, or by apnea, then oral feeding should be interrupted. In occasional examples, partial seizures appear to be diminished during stable suckle feeding. If the child is pharyngeally dysphagic, pharyngeal content entering the larynx may elicit laryngospasm, possibly graduating into grand mal seizures. Conversely, persons liable to laryngospasm can sometimes sense an impending episode and can avoid the episode, and possible further seizure activity, by voluntary swallow. The subtlest correlation of feeding and seizure-like activity is that of syncope on swallowing, as reported in a 4-year-old child by Woody and Kiel (1986). Comparable episodes of syncope with bradycardia are described during esophageal swallow in adults (Levin and Posner 1972; Kalloor et al. 1977).

Static or Progressive Myopathy

The clinical pattern and sequence that result from progressive myopathy, such as that of nemaline or mitochondrial myopathy or muscular dystrophy (Swaiman 1989), is similar in many respects to that of the child with acute anterior poliomyelitis. In either circumstance, impaired feeding may be a sensitive indicator of bulbar impairment. Impairment of pharyngeal swallow may be life threatening. The progression of myopathic impairments may be irregular in the muscles of the face, mandible, or tongue or in the intrinsic and supporting muscles of the pharynx and larynx. Successive evaluations of feeding performance are essential. Optimally, these should include successive radiographic imaging at intervals determined by clinical changes in feeding competence or by calendar. On the basis of such evaluations, the clinician can modify the feeding routine, such as through exclusive use of suckle feeding by the use of a prosthesis to achieve a better match of the oral cavity to the atrophic or ptotic tongue, or by the use of intermittent sleep time or continual tube feeding.

Static or Progressive Peripheral Neuropathy

Familial dysautonomia (Riley 1974; Axelrod et al. 1974) is the type form of static or progressive peripheral neuropathy. It may be manifested by hypertonia and poor suckle in early infancy (Axelrod et al. 1987). Later in infancy and during transitional and mature feeding, feeding impairment results from deficiency of saliva and other secretions and from incoordination of pharyngeal and esophageal swallow (Silbiger et al. 1967). The syndrome is restricted to offspring of Eastern European Jewish ancestry and is identified by an absence of fungiform papillae on the tongue and by absence of local reaction to cutaneous injection of histamine. Other forms of congenital peripheral neuropathy (Axelrod and Pearson 1984) may be progressive and occasionally may be associated with self-mutilation of the lips, tongue, or hands and with increasing oral and pharyngeal feeding impairment.

Diminution in oral sensory input also may result from loss of teeth, chronic periodontal inflammation, or extensive orthodontic work. Another possible mechanism of diminution of oral mucosal sensibility is that of desiccation and chronic inflammation secondary to continuous, exclusive mouth breathing.

Acute Encephalopathy in Childhood

Acute encephalopathy with dysphagia may result from neurotrauma, tumor surgery, or encephalitis in a previously normal child. The circumstances and sequence of events in children are generally similar to those in adults. The acute occasion, in many instances, is associated with unconsciousness. If the initial impairment is severe or prolonged, the child may be fed by nasogastric intubation or gastrostoma and may be tracheotomized. Recovery of feeding and related oral and pharyngeal functions depends on the nature and severity of the lesion of the bulbar sensory and motor nuclei and of the bulbar and suprabulbar representations of oral and pharyngeal performances.

The feeding impairments that may occur as effects of acute encephalopathy in school-age or pubertal children differ from those of comparable central lesions in the fetus or young infant. The differences are both in the brain and the oral and pharyngeal area. The mature or nearly mature brain has less plasticity and therefore less potential for adaptation by surviving neural structures. The peripheral oral and pharyngeal structures presumably were formed by normal development until the time of the injury. A newly acquired impairment, as by poliomyelitis involving the muscles of the face, mandible, tongue, or pharynx, may actually produce a handicap because the oral and pharyngeal skeleton is anatomically normal. One must appreciate, however, that functional adaptation to the impairment of the skeleton and other structures may begin promptly after function is resumed. In this case of mismatch of performance with peripheral anatomy, use of an oral prosthesis may be helpful in regaining functional feeding. In experience with children recovering from acute bulbar poliomyelitic impairment of the mouth and pharynx (Bosma 1957a; Bosma

1957b; Bosma 1957c), we became aware of the varied succession of performance impairments and adaptive actions that reflect recovery of muscle strength, increase or release of muscle contracture, and increasing performance awareness and skill. In successive evaluations of children during recovery from feeding impairment due to acute suprabulbar central lesion, it is particularly important to evaluate infantile suckle and transitional puree feeding, since these early functions may be differentially retained and available.

COMMUNITY AND PUBLIC RESOURCES FOR THE FEEDING-IMPAIRED INFANT AND CHILD

The rapid evolution of the clinical area of infant and child feeding impairments reflects an increasing incidence of dysphagia in infants who have survived embryopathy, prematurity, or genetic or other pathologic mechanisms. But this evolution also reflects clinicians' increasing insight and effectiveness in evaluation and therapy of feeding impairments. These impairments are recognized as evidences of general disorder: the whole-child approach. The clinical history and general examination are concerned with neurologic and somatic development (Rogers and Campbell 1993; Rosenthal et al. 1995). As the evaluation converges on the feeding process, it may involve diverse specialties: developmental pediatrics, neurology, radiology, surgery, rehabilitation medicine, psychology, and occupational, speech and nutrition therapies.

In some centers, these specialties have matured into teams whose synthesized contributions are remarkably effective in evaluation and therapy of feeding impairments (Bryan and Pressman 1995). In most teams, the immediate effector persons are occupational and speech therapists.

The special measures required to ensure adequate hydration and nutrition of infants and children who have neurologic feeding impairments are now commonly available in the Western world. These measures range from physical modifications of food and adaptations of food delivery implements and feeding procedures to direct alimentation by nasogastric or gastrostoma tube. In some instances, nutrition by these special means is not adequate, so that the children demonstrate growth retardation and malnutrition (Gisel and Patrick 1988; Patrick and Gisel 1990). Nutritional failure demonstrated by successive observations of weight and skinfold thickness indicates a need for changes in feeding routine, supplemental feeding by intubation, or both.

The special feeding measures needed by these infants and children greatly increase the concerns and efforts of their parents or other caregivers. The home environment commonly requires adaptation of personnel and space and, in many instances, special facilities, such as those for food preparation and storage and for custom feeding equipment. Increasingly, these handicapped infants and children are placed in day care centers or special schools. Selection of the care center is greatly influenced by the child's feeding requirements. Those who have similar needs for feeding assistance, or for intubation, are commonly further grouped at mealtimes. Such community-based centers are usually created through the efforts of parents. These aggregations and related clinical and daily care are increased by federal and state sponsorship and arrangements under U.S. PL 99-457, An Act for Care for Handicapped Infants and Toddlers. We may anticipate that this further sponsorship and organization will result in more consistent reassessments and possible revisions and adaptations of feeding care, appropriate to changes in the child's feeding patterns and nutritional requirements. We reasonably anticipate that these aggregations of feeding-impaired infants and children, with an attendant increase in expertise in their evaluation and care, will result in greater efficiency and use of oral feeding. An essential element of these special schools and centers is successive evaluations of the competence of oral feeding, resulting in progressive changes in the choice of food texture, food delivery, or feeding mechanism in the center and in the home. Feeding competence can be sequentially evaluated by gross estimation of intake from notes of the caregiver at test feeding, and this information can be converted by a dietitian into an intake estimation. In problematic situations or for investigative purposes, a video-implemented, standardized, and quantified Gisel evaluation of feeding can be used (Gisel 1988a; Gisel 1991). Competence of current and recent intake can be inferred from the child's nutritional state and increments of weight plotted on a weight-for-age chart. This information can be the basis for making decisions about intubation (Gisel and Patrick 1988; Patrick and Gisel 1990), such as whether the intubation should be intermittent, as during night sleep, or continuous, and whether gastrostoma, with its attendant liabilities, is justified.

REFERENCES

Anderson GC, Marks EA, Wahlberg V. Kangaroo care for premature infants. Am J Nurs 1986;86:807.

Archambault M, Millen K, Gisel EG. Effect of bite size on eating development in normal children 6 months to 2 years of age. Phys Occup Ther Pediatr 1991;10:29.

Arvedson JC, Brodsky L. Pediatric Swallowing and Feeding: Assessment and Management. San Diego: Singular Publishing, 1993.

Ashmead DH, Reilly BM, Lipsitt LP. Neonates heart-rate, sucking rhythm, and sucking amplitude as a function of sweet taste. J Exp Child Psychol 1980;29:264.

Axelrod FB, Nachtigal R, Dancis NR. Familial dysautonomia: diagnosis, pathogenesis and management. Adv Pediatr 1974;21:75.

Axelrod FB, Pearson J. Congenital sensory neuropathies: diagnostic distinction from familial dysautonomia. Am J Dis Child 1984;138:947.

Axelrod FB, Porges RF, Sein ME. Neonatal recognition of familial dysautonomia. J Pediatr 1987;110:946.

Bamford O. Personal communication, 1991.

Barr RG, McMullan SJ, Spiess H, et al. Carrying as colic "therapy": a randomized controlled trial. Pediatrics 1991;87:623.

Benson JE, Lefton-Greif MA. Videofluoroscopy of Swallowing in Pediatric Patients: A Component of the Total Feeding Evaluation. In DN Tuchman, RS Walter (eds), Disorders of Feeding and Swallowing in Infants and Children: Pathophysiology, Diagnosis, and Treatment. San Diego: Singular Publishing, 1994.

Beraitis S, Kolb R, Sperling E, et al. Development of a child with long-lasting deprivation of oral feeding. Am Acad Child Psychiatry 1981;20:53.

Bernbaum JC, Peckham GJ, Pereira GR, et al. Nonnutritive sucking during gavage feeding enhances growth and maturation in premature infants. Pediatrics 1983;1:41.

Bernstein IL. Learned taste aversions in children receiving chemotherapy. Science 1978;200:1302.

Blackman L. Personal communication, 1991.

Blass EM, Teicher MH. Suckling. Science 1980;210:15.

Boix-Ochoa M, Canals J. Maturation of the lower esophagus. J Pediatr Surg 1976;11:749.

Bosma JF. Studies of the pharynx. I. Poliomyelitic disabilities of the upper pharynx. Pediatrics 1957a;19:881.

Bosma JF. Studies of the pharynx. II. Poliomyelitic disabilities of the lower pharynx. Pediatrics 1957b;19:1053.

Bosma JF. Residual disability of pharyngeal area resulting from poliomyelitis. JAMA 1957c;165:216.

Bosma JF. Anatomic and Physiologic Development of the Speech Apparatus. In DB Tower (ed), The Nervous System. Vol. 3. Human Communication and Its Disorders. New York: Raven, 1975.

Bosma JF. Sensorimotor examination of the mouth and pharynx. In Y Kawamura (ed), Frontiers of Oral Physiology. Vol 1. Basel: Karger, 1976;2:78.

Bosma JF. Postnatal ontogeny of performances of the pharynx, larynx and mouth. Am Rev Respir Dis 1985;131(suppl):S10.

Bosma JF. Anatomy of the Infant Head. Baltimore: Johns Hopkins University Press, 1986a.

Bosma JF. Development of feeding. J Clin Nutr 1986b;5:210.

Bosma JF, Hepburn LG, Josell SD, et al. Ultrasound demonstration of tongue motions during suckle feeding. Dev Med Child Neurol 1990;32:223.

Bosma JF, Truby HM, Lind J. Distortions of upper respiratory and swallow motions in infants having anomalies of the upper pharynx. Acta Paediatr Scand 1966;163 (suppl):111.

Boyle JT, Tuchman DN, Altschuler SM, et al. Mechanisms for the association of gastroesophageal reflux and bronchospasm. Am Rev Respir Dis 1985;131:S16.

Brett EM. Paediatric Neurology. Edinburgh: Churchill Livingstone, 1991.

Bruston WR. Mandibular Retrognathia. In RP Rickham, J Lister, IM Irvine (eds), Neonatal Surgery (2nd ed). London: Butterworth, 1978.

Bryan DW, Pressman H. Comprehensive team evaluation. In SR Rosenthal, JJ Sheppard, M Lotze (eds), Dysphagia and the Child with Developmental Disabilities: Medical, Clinical, and Family Interventions. San Diego: Singular Publishing, 1995.

Casaer P, Daniels H, Devileger H, et al. Feeding behaviour in preterm neonates. Early Human Dev 1982;7:331.

Catto-Smith AG, Machida H, Butzner JD, et al. The role of gastroesophageal reflux in pediatric dysphagia. J Pediatr Gastroenterol Nutr 1991;12:159.

Caviness VS Jr. The Chiari malformations of the posterior fossa and their relation to hydrocephalus. Dev Med Child Neurol 1976;18:103.

Cohen SR, Thompson JW. Variants of Mobius syndrome and central neurologic impairment. Lindeman procedure in children. Ann Otol Rhinol Laryngol 1987;96:93.

Colley JRT, Creamer B. Suckling and swallowing in infants. Br Med J 1958;12:422.

Cravioto J, Arrieta R. Stimulation and mental development of malnourished infants. Lancet 1979;2:899.

Daniels H, Casaer P, Devileger H, et al. Mechanisms of feeding efficiency in preterm infants. J Pediatr Gastroenterol Nutr 1986;5:593.

Daniels H, Devileger H, Minami T, et al. Infant feeding and cardiorespiratory maturation. Neuropediatrics 1990;21:9.

Davis CM. Results of the self-selection of diets by young children. Can Med Assoc J 1939;41:257.

Doty RW. Neural Organization of Deglutition. In CF Code (ed), Handbook of Physiology. Section 6: Alimentary Canal. Washington, DC: American Physiological Society, 1968;4:1861.

Dowling S. Seven infants with esophageal atresia: a developmental study. Psychoanal Study Child 1977;32:215.

Dubner R, Sessle BJ, Storey AT. The Neural Basis of Oral and Facial Function. New York: Plenum, 1978.

Erenberg A, Smith WL, Nowak AJ, et al. Evaluation of sucking in the breast-fed infant by ultrasonography [abstract]. Pediatr Res 1986;20:409a.

Espinola D. Radionuclide evaluation of pulmonary aspiration: four birds with one stone—esophageal transit, gastroesophageal reflux, gastric emptying, and bronchopulmonary aspiration. Dysphagia 1986;1:101.

Evans PR. Nuclear agenesis Mobius syndrome: the congenital facial diplegia syndrome. Am J Dis Child 1954;30:247.

Evans TJ, Davies DP. Failure to thrive at the breast: an old problem revisited. Arch Dis Child 1977;52:974.

Field T, Ignatoff E, Stringer S, et al. Nonnutritive sucking during tube feedings: effects on preterm neonates in an intensive care unit. Pediatrics 1982;70:381.

Geertsma MA, Hyams JS, Pelletier JM, et al. Feeding resistance after parenteral hyperalimentation. Am J Dis Child 1985;139:255.

Gisel EG. Chewing cycles in 2- to 8-year-old normal children: a developmental profile. Am J Occup Ther 1988a;42:40.

Gisel EG. Development of oral side preference during chewing and its relation to hand preference in normal 2- to 8-year-old children. Am J Occup Ther 1988b;42:378.

Gisel EG. Effect of food texture on development of chewing in children 6 months to 2 years of age. Dev Med Child Neurol 1991;33:69.

Gisel EG, Patrick J. Identification of children with cerebral palsy unable to maintain a normal nutritional state. Lancet 1988;1:283.

Gisel EG, Pollock NA. Eating skills: a review of current assessment practices. Occup Ther J Res 1988;8:38.

Goldblatt D, Williams D. I an sniling! Moebius' syndrome inside and out. J Child Neurol 1986;1:71.

Golubeva EL, Shuleikina KV, Vainstein II. The development of reflex and spontaneous activity of the human fetus during embryogenesis. Obstet Gynecol (USSR) 1959;3:59.

Grand RJ, Watkins JB, Torti FM. Development of the human gastrointestinal tract: a review. Gastroenterology 1976;70:790.

Gryboski JD, Thayer WT, Spiro HM. Esophageal motility in infants and children. Pediatrics 1963;31:382.

Gryboski JD. The swallowing mechanism of the neonate 1: esophageal and gastric motility. Pediatrics 1965;35:445.

Gryboski JD. Suck and swallow in the premature infant. Pediatrics 1969;43:96.

Gryboski JD. Gastrointestinal Problems in the Infant. Philadelphia: Saunders, 1975.

Guttman FM. On the incidence of hiatal hernia in infants. Pediatrics 1972;50:325.

Hack M, Horbar JD, Malloy MH, et al. Very low birth weight outcomes of the National Institute of Child Health and Human Development neonatal network. Pediatrics 1991;87:587.

Ham HR, Piepsz A, Georges B, et al. Evaluation of esophageal transit in children and in infants by means of krypton-81m. Pediatr Radiol 1985;15:161.

Harris SR, Purdy AH. Drooling and its management in cerebral palsy. Dev Med Child Neurol 1987;29:805.

Hays MR, Jordan RA, McLaughlin FJ, et al. Central ventilatory dysfunction in myelodysplasia: an independent determinant of survival. Dev Med Child Neurol 1989;31:366.

Heldt GP. Effect of gavage feeding on the mechanics of the lung, chest wall and diaphragm of preterm infants. Pediatr Res 1988;24:55.

Herbst JJ. Development of suck and swallow. In E Lebenthal (ed), Human Gastrointestinal Development. New York: Raven, 1989.

Holinger PC, Holinger LD, Reichert TV. Respiratory obstruction and apnea in infants with bilateral abductor vocal cord paralysis, myelomeningocoele, hydrocephalus and Arnold-Chiari malformation. J Pediatr 1978;92:368.

Humphrey T. Reflex Activity in the Oral and Facial Area of the Human Fetus. In JF Bosma (ed), Second Symposium on Oral Sensation and Perception. Springfield, IL: Thomas 1970;195.

Hyman SL, Porter CA, Page TJ, et al. Behavior management of feeding disturbances in urea cycle and organic acid disorders. J Pediatr 1987;111:558.

Illingsworth RS. Sucking and swallowing difficulties in infancy: diagnostic problem of dysphagia. Arch Dis Child 1969;44:655.

Illingsworth RS. Three months colic. Arch Dis Child 1954;29:165.

Illingsworth RS, Lister J. The critical or sensitive period, with special reference to certain feeding problems in infants and children. J Pediatr 1964;65:839.

Jelliffe D, Jelliffe E. Human Milk in the Modern World. New York: Oxford University Press, 1978.

Judd PL, Kenny DJ, Koheil R, et al. The multidisciplinary feeding profile: a statistically based protocol for assessment of dependent feeders. Dysphagia 1989;4:29.

Kalloor GJ, Singh SP, Collis JL. Cardiac arrhythmias on swallowing. Am Heart J 1977;93:235.

Kaslon K, Ruben RJ. Traumatically acquired conditioned dysphagia in children. Ann Otol Rhinol Laryngol 1978;87:509.

Kassen NY, Groen JJ, Fraenkel M. Spinal deformities and oesophageal hiatus hernia. Lancet 1965;1:887.

Kenny DJ, Casas MD, McPherson KA. Correlation of ultrasound imaging of oral swallow with ventilatory alterations in cerebral palsied and normal children. Dysphagia 1989a;4:112.

Kenny DJ, Koheil RM, Greenberg J, et al. Development of a multidisciplinary feeding profile for children who are dependent feeders. Dysphagia 1989b;4:16.

Klein PS. Nutritional Deprivation and Retardation of Cognitive Functions. In P Mittler (ed), Frontiers of Knowledge of Mental Retardation. Vol. 2. Biomedical Aspects. Baltimore: University Park Press, 1980.

Kramer SS. Radiologic examination of the swallowing impaired child. Dysphagia 1989;3:117.

Leeuw RD, Colin EM, Dunnebier EA, et al. Physiological effects of kangaroo care in very small preterm infants. Biol Neonate 1991;59:149.

Levin B, Posner JB. Swallow syncope. Neurology 1972;22:1086.

Logan WJ, Bosma JF. Oral and pharyngeal dysphagia in infants. Pediatr Clin North Am 1967;14:47.

Luschei ES, Goldberg LJ. Neural Mechanisms of Mandibular Control: Mastication and Voluntary Biting. In BV Brooks (ed), Handbook of Physiology. Vol. II. Washington, DC: American Physiological Society, 1981;1237.

Maller O, Turner RE. Taste in acceptance of sugars in human infants. J Comp Physiol 1973;84:496–501.

Marquis J, Pressman H. Radiologic Assessment of Pediatric Swallowing. In SR Rosenthal, JJ Sheppard, M Lotze (eds), Dysphagia and the Child with Developmental Disabilities: Medical, Clinical, and Family Interventions. San Diego: Singular Publishing, 1995;189.

McColley SA, Carroll JL. Pulmonary Complications of Impaired Swallowing. In DN Tuchman, RS Walter (eds), Disorders of Feeding and Swallowing in Infants and Children: Pathophysiology, Diagnosis, and Treatment. San Diego: Singular Publishing, 1994;209.

McCoy R, Kadowaki C, Wilks S, et al. Nursing management of breast feeding for preterm infants. Perinat Neonatal Nurs 1988;2:42.

Measel CP, Anderson GC. Non-nutritive sucking during tube feeding: effect on clinical course in premature infants. J Obstet Gynecol Neonatal 1979;8:265.

Meier P. A program to support breast-feeding in the special care nursery. Perinatology/Neonatology 1980;4:43.

Meier P, Anderson GC. Responses of small preterm infants to bottle and breast feeding. Am J Matern Child Nurs 1987;12:97.

Meier P, Pugh E. Breast feeding behavior in small preterm infants. MCN: Am J Matern Child Nurs 1985;10:396.

Menkes JH. Textbook of Child Neurology (4th ed). Philadelphia: Lea & Febiger, 1990.

Milla PJ. Feeding, Tasting and Sucking. In WA Walker, PR Duric, JR Hamilton, et al (eds), Pediatric Gastrointestinal Disease. Philadelphia: Decker, 1991.

Miller AJ. Deglutition. Physiol Rev 1982;63:129.

Mollitt DL, Golladay ES, Seibert JJ. Symptomatic gastroesophageal reflux following gastrostomy in neurologically impaired patients. Pediatrics 1985;75:1124.

Moroz SP, Beiko P. Relationship between lower esophageal sphincter pressure and serum gastric concentration in the newborn infant. J Pediatr 1981;99:725.

Morris SE. Development of oral-motor skills in the neurologically impaired child receiving non-oral feedings. Dysphagia 1989;3:135.

Morris SE. Pre-Speech Assessment Scale: a rating scale for the measurement of pre-speech behaviors from birth through two years. Clifton, NJ: JA Preston Corp, 1982.

Morris SE, Klein MD. Pre-Feeding Skills. A Comprehensive Resource for Feeding Development. Tucson, AZ: Communication Skill Builders, 1987.

Mueller HA. Facilitating Feeding and Pre-Speech. In PH Pearson, CE Williams (eds), Physical Therapy Services in the Developmental Disabilities. Springfield, IL: Thomas, 1972;283.

Newell SJ, Sarkar PK, Durbin GM, et al. Maturation of the lower oesophageal sphincter in the preterm baby. Gut 1988;29:167.

Pack AI. Acid: a nocturnal broncho-constrictor? Am Rev Respir Dis 1990;141:1391.

Packer RJ, Zimmerman RA, Bilanuik LT, et al. Magnetic resonance imaging of lesions of the posterior fossa and upper cervical cord in childhood. Pediatrics 1985;76:84.

Paludetto AR, Robertson SS, Martin RJ. Interaction between non-nutritive sucking and respiration in preterm infants. Biol Neonate 1986;49:198.

Patrick J, Gisel EG. Nutrition for the feeding-impaired child. J Neurol Rehab, 1990;4:115.

Peiper A. Cerebral Function in Infancy and Childhood. New York: Consultants Bureau, 1963.

Prensky AL. Malnutrition. In KJ Swaiman (ed), Pediatric Neurology: Principles and Practice. St. Louis: Mosby, 1989.

Ramsey WO. Suckle facilitation of feeding in selected adult dysphagic persons. Dysphagia 1986;1:7.

Raventos JM, Kralemann H, Gray DB. Mortality risks of mentally retarded and mentally ill patients after a feeding gastrostomy. Am J Ment Defic 1982;86:439.

Rickham PP, Ligter J, Irving IM. Neonatal Surgery (2nd ed). London: Butterworths, 1978.

Riley CM. Familial dysautonomia: clinical and pathophysiological aspects. Ann NY Acad Sci 1974;228:283.

Robin P. Glossoptosis due to atresia and hypotrophy of the mandible. Am J Dis Child 1931;48:541.

Rogers B, Campbell J. Pediatric and Neurodevelopmental Evaluation. In JC Arvedson, L Brodsky (eds), Pediatric Swallowing and Feeding: Assessment and Management. San Diego: Singular Publishing, 1993;53.

Rosenthal SR, Sheppard JJ, Lotze M. Dysphagia and the Child with Developmental Disabilities: Medical, Clinical, and Family Interventions. San Diego: Singular Publishing, 1995.

Rudolph CD. Feeding disorders in infants and children. J Pediatr 1994;125:S116.

Rybski DA, Almli RC, Gisel EG. Sucking behaviours of normal 3-day-old female neonates during a 24-hour period. Dev Psychobiol 1984;17:79.

Rybski DA, Gisel EG. Optimal and sub-optimal feeding behaviors of neonates. Phys Occup Ther Pediatr 1984;4:37.

Sarnat HB. Olfactory reflexes in the newborn infant. J Pediatr 1978;92:624.

Schaal B. Olfaction in infants and children in developmental and functional perspectives. Chem Senses 1988;13:145.

Selley WG, Ellis RE, Flack FC, et al. Coordination of sucking, swallowing and breathing in the newborn: its relationship to infant feeding and normal development. Br J Disord Commun 1990a;25:311.

Sessle BJ, Henry JL. Neural mechanisms of swallowing; neurophysiological and neurochemical studies on brain stem neurons in the solitary tract region. Dysphagia 1989;4:61.

Sieben R, Hamida MB, Shulman K. Multiple cranial nerve deficits associated with Arnold-Chiari malformation. Neurology 1971;21:673.

Silbiger ML, Pikielney R, Donner MW. Neuromuscular disorders affecting the pharynx (cineradiographic analysis). Invest Radiol 1967;2:442.

Sivit C. The role of the pediatric radiologist in the evaluation therapy of oral and pharyngeal dysphagia. J Neurol Rehab 1990;4:103.

Sochaniwskyj AE, Koheil RM, Bablich K, et al. Oral motor function, frequency of swallowing and drooling in normal children and in children with cerebral palsy. Arch Phys Med Rehabil 1986;67:866.

Sondheimer JM. Upper esophageal sphincter and pharyngeal motor function in infants with and without gastroesophageal reflux. Gastroenterology 1983;85:301.

Steiner JE. Facial Expressions of the Neonate Infant Indicating the Hedonics of Food-Related Stimuli. In JM Weiffenbach (ed), Taste and Development: The Genesis of Sweet Preference. Bethesda, MD: National Institutes of Health, 1977;173.

Stolovitz P, Gisel EG. Circumoral movements in response to three different food textures in children six months to two years of age. Dysphagia 1991;6:17.

Sullivan RM, Taborsky-Barba S, Mendoza R, et al. Olfactory classical conditioning in neonates. Pediatrics 1991;87:511.

Swaiman KF. Pediatric Neurology: Principles and Practice. St. Louis: Mosby, 1989.

Takagi Y, Irwin JV, Bosma JF. Prone feeding of infants with Pierre Robin syndrome. Cleft Palate J 1966;3:232.

Taubman B. Clinical trial of the treatment of colic by modification of parent-infant interaction. Pediatrics 1984;74:998.

Tuchman DN. Gastroesophageal Reflux. In DN Tuchman, RS Walter (eds), Disorders of Feeding and Swallowing in Infants and Children: Pathophysiology, Diagnosis, and Treatment. San Diego: Singular Publishing, 1994;231.

Tuchman DN, Walter RS. Disorders of feeding and swallowing in infants and children: pathophysiology, diagnosis, and treatment. San Diego: Singular Publishing, 1994.

Vane DW, Shiffler M, Grosfield JL. Reduced lower esophageal sphincter pressure after acute and chronic brain injury. J Pediatr Surg 1982;17:960.

Vice FL, Heinz JM, Giuriatti G, et al. Cervical auscultation of suckle feeding in newborn infants. Dev Med Child Neurol 1990;32:766.

Ward SLD, Nickerson BG, Vander Hal, et al. Absent hypoxic and hypercapneic arousal responses in children with myelomeningocele and apnea. Pediatrics 1986;78:44.

Warkany J, Lemire RJ, Cohen MM Jr. Mental retardation and congenital malformations of the central nervous system. Chicago: Year Book Medical, 1981.

Weinberg B, Christensen R, Logan W, et al. Severe hypoplasia of the tongue. J Speech Hear Dis 1969;34:157.

Wessel MA, Cobb JC, Jackson EB, et al. Paroxysmal fussing in infancy, sometimes called colic. Pediatrics 1954;14:421.

Widstrom AM, Marchini G, Matthiesen AS, et al. Non-nutritive sucking in tube fed preterm infants: effects on gastric motility and gastric contents of somatostatin. J Pediatr Gastroenterol Nutr 1988;8:517.

Wilkinson JD, Dudgeon DL, Sondheim JM. A comparison of medical and surgical treatment of gastroesophageal reflux in severely mentally retarded children. J Pediatr 1981;99:202.

Wilks S, Meier P. Helping mother express milk suitable for preterm and high-risk infant feeding. J Matern Child Nurs 1988;13:121.

Williams AJ, Williams MA, Walker CA, et al. The Robin anomalad (the Pierre Robin syndrome): a follow-up study. Arch Dis Child 1981;56:663.

Wilson JM. Oral-motor Function and Dysfunction in Children. Chapel Hill, NC: Division of Physical Therapy, 1977.

Wilson SL, Thach BT, Brouillette RT, et al. Coordination of breathing and swallowing. J Appl Physiol 1981;50:851.

Wolf L, Glass R. Feeding and Swallowing Disorders in Infancy. Tucson, AZ: Therapy Skill Builders, 1992;1.

Wolff PH. The serial organisation of sucking in the young infant. Pediatrics 1968;42:943.

Woody RC, Kiel EA. Swallowing syncope in a child. Pediatrics 1986;78:507.

7

Clinical Examination for Dysphagia

Robert M. Miller

A comprehensive evaluation of a patient known or suspected to have dysphagia involves a number of medical and allied medical disciplines. The evaluation is intended to assess factors that relate to swallowing function, not to diagnose the underlying disease, although it may either obviate or clarify the need for other studies. The word *dysphagia*, according to *Dorland's Illustrated Medical Dictionary,* is derived from the Greek *phagein*, meaning to eat. Conditions that could impair eating are numerous and diverse. Even considering the more limited definitions of dysphagia, such as "difficulty in swallowing," the complexity of comprehensively evaluating patients with such complaints can be appreciated.

A comprehensive evaluation for dysphagia should be considered a team evaluation, as no one discipline can assess in detail all phases of swallowing. Without attempting to enumerate all of the disciplines that might contribute to a comprehensive dysphagia evaluation (see Chapter 15), and recognizing that responsibilities and expertise vary from setting to setting, we present an outline of the relevant systems to be assessed and the methods available for evaluation in Table 7.1.

One component of a comprehensive dysphagia evaluation is the clinical examination for dysphagia (CED). The CED comprises a detailed description of the subjective complaint or problem, the acquisition of a relevant health history, pertinent clinical observations, and a focused physical examination. Although it is ideal to record all of these components in detail, circumstances may require clinicians to modify the examination to fit the situation and the needs of a given patient. At a minimum, the CED should allow the clinician to (1) screen for the presence or absence of a swallowing impairment, (2) contribute information regarding the possible etiology of the dysphagia relative to its anatomic and physiologic basis, (3) ascertain the relative aspiration risk for certain patients, (4) determine the need for an alternative means of nutritional management, and (5) recommend additional tests and procedures to diagnose and treat the dysphagia.

Disorders of swallowing may be found in diverse patient populations, e.g., among those who have had acute neurologic events and surgery of the head and neck. Dysphagia is also a manifestation of many subacute progressive neurologic diseases and may be an isolated symptom found in otherwise stable elderly patients. The CED needs to be modified and adapted to fit the clinical setting and patient population. The procedures for performing the CED outlined with-

Table 7.1 Comprehensive Evaluation for Dysphagia

Factors Influencing Swallowing	*Methods of Assessment*
Oral phase	
Mental status, judgment	Screen orientation, language, visual-motor perception, and memory
Muscles of facial expression	Examine for symmetry at rest and during movement
Muscles of mastication	Palpate and gently resist movement
Mucous membranes	Inspect
Dentition	Inspect
Lingual muscles	Inspect at rest and on protrusion; resist movement
Orofacial sensation	Subjective; identify stimulus qualities
Pharyngeal phase	
Palatopharyngeal closure	Observe at rest and during phonation; stimulate gag reflex
Pharyngeal contraction	Stimulate gag; motion radiography, electromyography
Extrinsic laryngeal muscles	Palpate larynx during swallow, auscultation
Intrinsic laryngeal muscles	Indirect laryngeal inspection or fiberoptic examination
Cricopharyngeus muscle	Motion radiography
Esophageal phase	
Morphology of the esophagus	Motion radiography and endoscopy
Esophageal motility	Manometry and motion radiography
Gastroesophageal sphincter function, hiatal hernia, and reflux	Manometry, motion radiography, gastroesophageal scintiscanning, acid perfusion, pH monitoring, endoscopy, and biopsy

in the chapter, therefore, should be viewed as general guidelines rather than a cookbook approach applied to every dysphagic patient.

WARNING SIGNS

Patients suspected of having swallowing dysfunction should undergo a CED as a minimum evaluation. Several warning signs should alert health professionals to the likelihood of dysphagia. The presence of a confused mental state or dysarthric speech in a patient with neurologic disease should be cause for special attention to the eating process. Since eating requires some degree of vigilance and planning, patients who exhibit poor judgment, perceptual impairments, or motor planning disorders following any form of brain damage are at risk for swallowing catastrophe. Similarly, dysarthric speech, characterized by slow, labored, or slurred articulation, nasal air emission, and hoarse or breathy voice, is a manifestation of the inherent weakness or incoordination of muscles common to both speaking and swallowing. An additional symptom suggestive of dysphagia is excessive drooling (sialorrhea), which is often due to motor or sensory impairments of the swallowing mechanism. Frequent episodes of coughing and choking on food and sputum should be considered a warning sign for dysphagia. Prolongation of meals, unexplained weight loss, effortful chewing, or difficulty in the oral preparation of a bolus may all signify swallowing difficulty.

A patient's complaint of pain or obstruction during swallowing should be taken seriously as a warning for dysphagia. A clinical finding on indirect laryngeal examination of the pooling sign, or accumulation of food debris in the valleculae or piriform sinuses, suggests that the swallowing mechanism has failed to completely clear the bolus from the pharynx into the esophagus. Excessive pooling and the potential for tracheal aspiration may be appreciated on radiographic studies of swallows.

EVALUATION

When beginning an examination for dysphagia, it is helpful to have a procedural outline or worksheet available (Table 7.2). This helps to ensure that important data are not overlooked during the assessment.

Subjective Complaints

The history begins with information regarding the present complaint. Frequently, the subjective description of the problem gives the examiner significant clues about its cause. In many instances, however, a history cannot be obtained from the patient because swallowing problems are frequently associated with altered mental states or severely impaired speech. In these instances, information may come from a professional observer, health care attendant, family member, or medical records. Specific questions would address such issues as the duration of the problem, the frequency of swallowing difficulty, intermittent versus constant presence, and factors and circumstances that exacerbate or alleviate the problem.

It is particularly important to determine the relative influence of solid, semisolid, and liquid foods on swallowing. In general, patients who suffer from neurologic conditions that weaken or result in dyscoordination of the swallowing mechanism complain that liquids are more likely to cause choking than solids or semisolids (Linden and Siebens 1983). Since fluids naturally spread as they move from the mouth through the pharynx into the esophagus, they require more precise channeling than solids, and therefore are more difficult for weak or uncoordinated motor mechanisms to control. Patients suffering from mechanical obstructive conditions such as strictures, tumors, or webs generally report no difficulty swallowing liquids. They are likely to complain about solid food sticking or lodging in the throat or esophagus. Patients with esophageal motility problems or primary neuromuscular abnormalities of the esophagus may report dysphagia

Table 7.2 Clinical Examination for Dysphagia

I. Subjective complaints
  A. Duration of the problem
  B. Frequency of swallowing difficulty
  C. Intermittent versus constant swallowing problem
  D. Factors exacerbating or relieving the problem
    1. Influence of solids, semisolids, and liquids
    2. Influence of hot and cold
  E. Associated symptoms
    1. Sensation of obstruction
    2. Mouth or throat pain
    3. Nasal regurgitation
    4. Mouth odor
    5. Choking or coughing while swallowing
    6. Pneumonia in the past
    7. Other respiratory symptoms (chronic cough, shortness of breath, asthmatic episodes)
    8. GE reflux (sensation of heartburn)
    9. Chest pain
  F. Ancillary symptoms
    1. Weight loss
    2. Eating habits
    3. Appetite changes/enjoyment
    4. Taste changes
    5. Dry mouth or saliva consistency changes
    6. Speech or voice changes
    7. Sleep disturbance
II. Medical history
  A. General health
  B. Family history
  C. Previous swallowing examinations
  D. Neurologic conditions
  E. Pulmonary disorders
  F. Surgeries
  G. Radiation
  H. Psychiatric/psychological history
  I. Current treatments
  J. Medications
    1. Current and past
    2. Prescriptive
    3. Over-the-counter
III. Clinical observations
  A. Feeding tube
  B. Tracheostomy (type of tube, cuff status)
  C. Nutrition/hydration status
  D. Drooling
  E. Mental status
    1. Attention

2. Orientation
3. Receptive/expressive language
4. Visual perceptual-motor function
5. Memory disturbance

IV. Clinical examination
  A. Speech function (voice, resonance, articulation)
  B. Weight
  C. Peripheral swallowing musculature and structures
    1. Muscles of facial expression
    2. Muscles of mastication
    3. Pathologic reflexes
    4. Oral mucosa
    5. Dentition
    6. Pharyngeal palatine musculature
    7. Tongue
    8. Sensation
    9. Intrinsic laryngeal musculature
    10. Extrinsic laryngeal musculature
  D. Test swallows

---

with both solids and liquids (Castell and Donner 1987). Although there is some correlation between the cause of the swallowing difficulty and the consistency of the bolus, caution is recommended to avoid being misled.

The differential effect of hot and cold food boluses may have diagnostic significance. For example, cold liquids are known to reduce primary esophageal peristalsis and produce distension of the distal esophagus. Esophageal spasms may be produced by ingestion of cold liquids (Jones and Donner 1989). For patients with myotonic dystrophy, swallowing cold liquids often elicits a myotonic contraction in the pharynx and interferes with subsequent swallows. For most other patients with neuromuscular oropharyngeal dysphagia, cold liquids are recommended to facilitate swallowing.

In detailing the history, specific questions should be asked that address symptoms frequently associated with dysphagia.

Obstruction

Although many clinicians associate subjective descriptions of obstruction with tumors, strictures, webs, and diverticula, obstruction is also a frequent complaint in patients with neurologic conditions that result in muscle weakness or incoordination and in those with esophageal motility disorders. The patient should be asked if food sticks and then directed to point to the level at which he or she senses the obstruction. Patients with cricopharyngeal dysfunction and those with a pharyngoesophageal (Zenker's) diverticulum usually describe the obstruction at the level of the thyroid cartilage (Jordan 1977). Those with pooling in the vallecula or piriform sinuses may also point to an area adjacent to the larynx as the site of obstruction. It should be noted, however, that the area in which the obstruction is sensed by the patient does not always correspond with the site of actual narrowing or blockage as demonstrated by radiography. Distal esophageal lesions, for example, may be referred to the lower neck (Edwards 1976).

The timing of an obstruction may be a more accurate indication of its level. When obstruction is felt within 1 or 2 seconds, it is most likely to be related to oropharyngeal dysfunction, whereas the sensation perceived after several seconds relates to an esophageal process.

A distinction should be made between the sensation of obstruction while swallowing and a "globus sensation" or the feeling of a foreign body. Patients with either complaint should be examined because there is a high incidence of abnormality in both groups. The globus sensation may be an early symptom of hypopharyngeal cancer or organic esophageal disease, such as hypertensive upper esophageal sphincter (Castell and Donner 1987) or reflux.

Complaints of intermittent obstruction should not be dismissed as psychological. Patients with organic lesions, such as those with Schatzki's ring, achalasia, and esophageal spasm, may report intermittent difficulties that are exacerbated during periods of stress (Pope 1989).

Mouth or Throat Pain

Odynophagia, or pain on swallowing, is rarely associated with dysphagia of central nervous system origin. Mouth or throat pain is more commonly related to infections (e.g., candidiasis, cytomegalovirus, or herpes), neoplasms, or mechanical obstructions in the oropharyngeal region.

Nasal Regurgitation

Patients should be asked about episodes of nasopharyngeal reflux—i.e., liquid or firm food moving up into the nasal cavity rather than down toward the esophagus. An occasional nasal penetration occurring in association with coughing is probably not significant. Frequent episodes of nasal regurgitation suggest some malfunction of the palatal and upper pharyngeal mechanism, or mechanical obstruction in the hypopharynx.

Mouth Odor

Foul mouth odors may be associated with a variety of conditions, including poor hygiene, oral retention of food, dental or periodontal disease, and oral-mucosal lesions that result in necrotic changes. An additional source for mouth odor is a Zenker's pharyngoesophageal diverticulum. In these cases, food trapped in the sac can putrefy and emit a foul odor. These patients may also describe episodes in which food returns to the mouth, sometimes hours after a meal.

Choking or Coughing

The patient with complaints regarding swallowing should be questioned about episodes of aspiration in which food or liquid tends to go into the windpipe. Coughing or choking frequently while eating is another manifestation of aspiration. Although sensations of aspiration can occur with a variety of conditions, it is probably most common in neuromuscular disorders of swallowing.

History of Pneumonia

Evidence of recurrent aspiration pneumonia may be associated with neuromuscular incoordination, weakness of the oropharyngeal swallowing mechanism, or esophageal dysfunction. It can result from a patient's inability to protect the airway due to selective muscle paralysis. Paralysis of the vocal folds is particularly significant. Recurrent pneumonia also can be found in patients who have mechanical obstructions of the deglutitory tract, severe gastroesophageal or pharyngeal-tracheal reflux, and achalasia. The occurrence of aspiration pneumonia is grossly related to the severity of dysphagia.

Other Respiratory Symptoms

Conditions related to either oropharyngeal or esophageal dysphagia can cause a number of respiratory symptoms. Chronic coughing may be a manifestation of a failed oropharyngeal swallowing mechanism, causing pooled secretions to intermittently spill into the airway. Cricopharyngeal dysfunction, either as an isolated impairment or when associated with esophageal reflux, may also contribute to chronic coughing. Nocturnal coughing is classically associated with achalasia (Castell and Donner 1987).

Clinicians are developing a keener appreciation of the relationship between the deglutitory mechanism and pulmonary functions. In patients with either mechanical obstruction or neuromuscular esophageal disorders, respiratory symptoms including episodic coughing, wheezing, sputum production, and dyspnea may be found. Reflux and lower esophageal sphincter (LES) dysfunction are known to be etiologic factors in chronic obstructive pulmonary disease. Evidence also suggests that cricopharyngeal dysfunction may either precede or be secondary to chronic obstructive pulmonary disease in some patients (Stein et al. 1990).

Gastroesophageal Reflux

Gastroesophageal (GE) reflux is usually identified by patients as a sensation of heartburn or acid regurgitation. Additionally, patients may complain of a globus sensation, hiccups, halitosis, a sour taste, dry throat, or pain in the throat or tongue.

GE reflux results from failure of the LES to prevent stomach contents from reentering the esophagus. Reflux is very common. The potential for symptomatic GE reflux is probably great in patients with a hiatal hernia, a condition that is present in about 67% of persons over 60 years of age (Straus 1979). It is also found in patients with peptic strictures, esophageal cancer, neuromuscular esophageal motor disorders, or loss of tone in the LES due to scleroderma (see Chapter 5).

Severe or persistent cases of GE reflux may lead to esophageal mucosal irritation, esophageal muscle and sphincter dysfunction, laryngeal mucosal ulceration or granulomata, aspiration of stomach contents (particularly during sleep), or some combination of these. Esophagitis, esophageal ulcer, and esophageal stricture are potential sequelae of reflux. Other less appreciated manifestations may be evident in the mouth and throat. Chronic pharyngitis, hoarseness, and loss of dental enamel may be evident. Among the pulmonary and cardiac symptoms related to reflux are exacerbation of asthma, chronic obstructive pulmonary disease, episodic apnea, bradycardia, and hypotension (Castell and Donner 1987).

Even when GE reflux cannot be appreciated on radiographic studies, the patient's report of symptoms associated with this condition should be taken seriously. When reflux is suspected, a trial of antireflux therapy can relieve pharyngeal symptoms of dysphagia (Jones et al. 1985).

Chest Pain

Chest pain may be a manifestation of an esophageal motor disorder. Pain that is not considered to be coronary in origin is one clue for diffuse esophageal spasm (Castell and Donner 1987). Intense esophageal pain is usually perceived substernally, with radiation into the back, jaw, neck, or down the left arm. It may be clinically indistinguishable from the pain of coronary artery disease (Pope 1977). Heartburn and a similar retrosternal burning perceived by patients with dilated esophagus due to achalasia are also important diagnostic clues.

Other Ancillary Symptoms

The previously mentioned symptoms are directly associated with an impairment at some level of deglutition, and the presence or absence of these symptoms offers diagnostic clues for the clinician. In addition to these major symptoms, questioning related to the following ancillary complaints allows one not only to discover additional diagnostic clues, but to assess how much the swallowing dysfunction has affected the patient in important ways. Although most of the major symptoms often can be related to a level of impairment along the deglutitory tract, a thorough evaluation demands exploration of complaints that the patient may not relate to the swallowing disorder, e.g., speech or voice changes.

Weight loss is one of the best barometers for assessing the effects of a swallowing impairment. It is usually related directly to impaired nutritional intake, although it may reflect the effects of an underlying disease process. Reported changes in weight become the clinician's yardstick for charting progressive dysphagia and assessing the effectiveness of a feeding management plan.

A change in eating habits may suggest to the clinician impairments that can be related to a specific stage of swallowing. For example, foods or food types may be avoided due to specific muscle weakness—e.g., lettuce is avoided with early pharyngeal weakness. Eating time may increase or the patient may eat smaller meals to compensate when swallowing initiation is delayed or there is deglutitory muscle fatigue. Enjoyment of meals is frequently affected as swallowing difficulty increases, and questions related to appetite and the pleasure derived from eating should be asked. When possible, it helps to receive a description of the patient's previous day's meals and an estimate of the amount of fluid intake per day.

Alterations of taste, mucosal dryness, and salivary consistency changes are known to affect appetite and may hinder the initiation of swallowing. Dysgeusia, the perversion of taste, and halitosis may be a consequence of poor oral hygiene and gingivitis. Thickening of secretions may reflect a patient's chronically dehydrated state due to impaired swallowing of liquids or be related to mouth breathing, salivary gland function, or medications. Debilitated patients with extreme oral and pharyngeal mucosal dryness may not be able to swallow on this basis alone. Certain syndromes associated with autoimmune disease, such as Sjögren's, have the affect of decreasing salivary output.

Since speech and swallowing depend on certain common neurologic, muscular, and anatomic factors, changes in speech or voice may parallel the development of swallowing difficulties. Patients should be asked if their speech has changed in any way—e.g., hoarseness or temporary loss of voice. A change in articulatory coordination or precision, interpreted by the patient as slurring or clumsy speech, usually reflects neurologic impairment. An isolated voice change may either be the consequence of neurologic, neoplastic, or inflammatory disorders or be related to GE reflux.

Dysphagia can cause sleep disturbance through a variety of mechanisms. Patients suffering from symptomatic GE reflux commonly suffer from sleep disturbance. In severe oropharyngeal dysphagia, patients may be unable to keep their airway clear of secretions while reclining or sleeping. Presumably, this is one of the factors, along with food regurgitation, that contributes to disruption of sleep in patients with a Zenker's diverticulum.

Medical History

Information relevant to a patient's swallowing and nutritional status can often be obtained from the general health history. Family history is important because a number of conditions have a known genetic basis; muscular dystrophy and Huntington's chorea, for example, have a hereditary predisposition. The results and findings from any previous swallowing examinations should be noted. Special attention should be paid to neurologic history; cerebrovascular accident, head trauma, central nervous system infection, demyelinating disease, and motor neuron disease are particularly pertinent to dysphagia. Since dysphagia has been implicated as a major factor contributing to the genesis and exacerbation of some pulmonary disorders, particularly chronic obstructive pulmonary disease, attention should be given to any pulmonary conditions (Stein et al. 1990). All prior surgery should be noted, particularly procedures involving the head and neck or gastrointestinal tract. When directed at the head and neck or mediastinum, radiation therapy can impair swallowing or exacerbate problems with deglutition.

Medications

Several medications influence swallowing. A list should be compiled of all medications currently prescribed and those taken regularly in the past. Sedative drugs or those that cause disorientation and confusion can significantly influence swallowing, particularly in brain-damaged patients. For example, slightly toxic doses of some anticonvulsants can add to the confusion of patients with brain trauma and cause decompensation of a previously marginal swallowing mechanism. Medications that potentially weaken muscles, such as some prescribed to reduce spasticity, may exacerbate existing swallowing problems. It is known that some moisture must be present in the mouth to elicit a swallow reflex, so medications with an action or side effect of diminishing secretions and thus drying the oral, nasal, and pharyngeal mucosae can adversely influence swallowing by delaying its initiation. Some medications, although they do not directly impair swallowing, may inhibit appetite or contribute to dehydration. Diuretics, often used to help control hypertension, can exacerbate problems of dehydration in the patient with dysphagia for liquids.

Many antipsychotic drugs can lead to extrapyramidal symptoms such as dystonia, motor restlessness, pseudoparkinsonism, and tardive dyskinesia. Persistent tardive dyskinesia may present as hyperkinesis of the face, jaw, tongue, and upper esophagus, each of which may interfere with the initiation and control of chewing and swallowing. In some cases, neuroleptic drugs cause dysphagia clinically indistinguishable from Parkinson's disease by blocking dopaminergic transmissions. For the psychiatric patient it may be difficult to determine the etiology for the swallowing impairment as it may be due to parkinsonism, tardive dyskinesia, anticholinergic drugs, or other preexisting neurologic conditions (Weiden and Harrigan 1986).

Certain over-the-counter medications and prescribed topical anesthetics used to relieve a sore throat or tickling cough have the potential to impair swallowing. Some denture powders also contain topical anesthetics that could disturb oral and pharyngeal sensation.

In general, drugs appear to have very little effect on the function of the esophagus and are not known to cause motor disorders of the esophagus (Christensen 1976). However, beta-adrenergic drugs, theophylline, alcohol, and tobacco have been reported to lower or overcome LES tone and promote reflux (Stein et al. 1990).

For debilitated patients and those with known dysphagia, pill-induced esophagitis is a concern. Common corrosive drugs like antibiotics, quinidine, iron, aspirin, and ibuprofen have the potential for causing caustic injury to the esophageal mucosa. This is of particular concern when taken in high concentrations, with little liquid, or in a supine position.

Clinical Observations

An experienced clinician will recognize innumerable clinical signs in the interview and examination process. Some of these observations clearly will be related to the deglutitory process and may influence performance on subsequent examination. The presence of a feeding tube, its site of insertion, and its size are significant. Attention should be given to any tracheostomy tube, its size, and the presence and status of a cuff. The patient's general nutritional state, whether appearing well nourished or cachectic with temporal wasting, should be noted. A clinical impression should be formed regarding the patient's relative hydration status. Clinical signs of chronic dehydration may include sunken eyeballs, dryness of mucosa, loss of skin turgor, hypotension, and elevated temperature. A thorough nutritional assessment, including laboratory measures, should be included in a comprehensive evaluation of the patient with dysphagia. Additional observations might include the presence of drooling or the presence of towels and tissues for the purpose of controlling secretions. The patient's general behavior and emotional state should be clinically judged and may be significant in the final diagnostic impression.

Mental Status

Specific attention should be given to assessing the patient's mental status and ability to cooperate. This is especially true when dealing with patients with known or suspected central nervous system lesions contributing to dysphagia. Larsen (1981) described the problems experienced by patients with left- or right-sided brain damage. With right-sided hemiplegia and aphasia, for example, patients may become overwhelmed or confused as they attempt to eat while engaging in conversation. Because of possible muscle spasticity in combination with the language disorder of aphasia, these patients are at risk for aspiration when trying to combine eating with speaking.

Conversely, Larsen describes right-sided brain-damaged patients as having problems with the praxis of eating—i.e., they are disturbed in organizing the motor sequence that would allow them to move food from plate to mouth. They are at risk of choking because of problems that relate to judgment, decisions about how much food to take in one bite and how much to chew. These problems are discussed in more detail in Chapter 9.

A screening psychometric-type test can be used to assess perceptual and language functions to anticipate the types of eating problems that could occur and apply the appropriate rehabilitation procedures. Such screening tests should include (1) questions regarding the patient's orientation; (2) a series of simple verbal and written commands to assess language comprehension; (3) a task that requires the patient to name common objects or geometric forms to assess simple expressive language; (4) a written task to evaluate the patient's ability to spell several common words or write a phrase from dictation; (5) a verbal problem-solving task requiring the patient to interpret the meaning of a sentence or proverb; and (6) a visual perceptual-motor task in which the patient reproduces forms, such as a square, triangle, and cross.

Physical Examination

In most cases, the description of the problem and background data dictates the appropriate course to follow in the physical examination. The detailed examination that follows may be used in whole or in part, as the case requires. Since dysphagia is almost never purely psychogenic, all patients with swallowing complaints should be examined thoroughly.

The purpose of this examination for the clinical assessment of swallowing is (1) to establish a possible cause of dysphagia; (2) to assess the patient's ability to protect the airway; (3) to determine the practicality of oral feeding or recommend alternative methods for nutritional management; (4) to determine the need for additional specific diagnostic tests, studies, or referrals; and (5) to establish baseline clinical data that can be used to chart changes in feeding function of patients with progressively deteriorating diseases (see Table 7.2).

Voice and Speech

The quality of a patient's speech should be assessed as a part of the swallowing evaluation. Speech is an extremely complex, overlearned behavior, and as such serves as a barometer from which the examiner can assess the status of the neuromuscular system that also serves swallowing. Patients should be asked to sustain a vowel, with the examiner noting duration, quality (hoarseness, breathiness, and harshness), pitch, and intensity. Articulation should be assessed for precision and speed. The use of oral diadochokinetic tasks (forced rapid alternating movements) using consonant-vowel combinations is recommended. Both hypernasal and hyponasal resonance qualities should be noted. Hypernasality suggests impaired palatopharyngeal function. Hyponasality implies filling of the nasopharynx or occlusion of nasal passages.

For patients with unimpaired voice and speech, the clinician may reasonably conclude that the swallowing problem either resides in the late pharyngeal stage (cricopharyngeal function) or is related to esophageal and LES function. One would expect the remaining physical examination to confirm the integrity of the peripheral sensory-motor swallowing mechanism. A final diagnosis in such cases would require additional radiographic swallowing studies.

Weight

Weighing the patient is vital when examination data are to be used for charting changes in progressive disease and when the clinician must assess the effectiveness of a nutritional management plan. These data also will be useful in developing an understanding of the severity of a swallowing problem.

Muscles of Facial Expression

Facial muscles should be inspected both at rest and during active movement, comparing movement of the two sides for symmetry. The patient should be asked to make grimacing and puckering movements. When possible, the muscles should be palpated for any weakness. The examiner should look particularly at the patient's ability to seal the lips, having the patient puff out the cheeks and hold the air while manual pressure is applied to the cheeks. Lip closure is important in preventing loss of food anteriorly during the oral phase of swallowing.

Muscles of Mastication

The masseter is the most powerful muscle of mastication. It originates at the zygomatic arch and inserts into the angle of the mandible. The temporalis, which adjusts the jaw up, forward, or back, originates at the squamous portion of the temporal bone and inserts at the anterior border of the ramus. These two muscles of mastication should be palpated as the patient bites and chews. Gentle resistance can be placed on the mandible to assess the strength of these muscles. Excessive resistance could result in dislocation of the temporomandibular joint. Clinicians recognize that it is almost impossible to swallow with the mouth open, so the ability to close the jaw is critical.

The grinding action that occurs in chewing is produced by two sets of muscles, the external and internal pterygoids. Their action can be appreciated by instructing the patient to move the mandible from side to side in a rotary action. Again, gentle resistance can be applied to assess the relative strength of these muscles.

Pathologic Reflexes

A number of brain stem–level primitive reflexes are associated with the chewing and swallowing mechanisms. Normally, these reflexes are inhibited in the adult by higher centers of the brain. Their presence in the adult patient suggests that these higher inhibitory centers are impaired. These pathologic reflexes are seen most commonly in patients with bilateral hemispheric or frontal lobe damage.

The suck reflex may be elicited either by tapping the upper lip with a reflex hammer or by stroking the vermillion border with a tongue blade. Movement of the lips in the direction of the stimulus is an abnormal response.

The bite reflex is often elicited in patients with severe neurologic lesions by touching the lips, teeth, or gums with a tongue blade and observing a strong closure of the jaw. This reflex can be particularly troublesome for the examiner, since it may prevent a good oral examination. Attempts to force a jaw open usually result in a stronger bite. The examiner should avoid strong resistance that could result in fracture or dislocation of the mandible. In some patients, spontaneous mouth opening will occur as a stimulus object, such as a spoon or food, is seen approaching the mouth. While the bite reflex can interfere with feeding management, this mouth-opening reflex can be used to aid in the feeding plan.

Oral Mucosa

The intraoral inspection should begin with an assessment of the mucosa. Dentures should be removed prior to this examination. Any pathologic lesions should be noted and proper diagnostic procedures followed to determine their nature. In many cases this procedure involves consultation with an oral surgeon or otolaryngologist for examination and biopsy.

Particular attention should be paid to the moisture present in the oral cavity. Extreme dryness of the oral and pharyngeal mucosa can virtually prevent voluntary and reflexive swallowing. Thick, tenacious mucus can inhibit swallowing. Any residual oral debris should be noted.

Dentition

The condition of natural teeth should be noted. Painful teeth can inhibit eating and lead to impaired nutritional states. It should be recognized that dental plates block sensory receptors in the palate and gums that contribute to the reflex stimulation of chewing. Dental consultation should be considered when dental or other oral disease or abnormality is suspected.

Pharyngeal Palate

The pharyngeal palatine musculature should be evaluated as a unit. In normal swallowing the palate should elevate and the pharynx constrict, allowing a properly masticated bolus to pass over the base of the tongue and enter the hypopharynx without regurgitation into the nasopharynx. Palatopharyngeal constriction should be assessed for symmetry during oral breathing, phonation, and tactual stimulation of the gag reflex. The gag reflex should be elicitable from either side, and the response should be compared on stimulation of each side. The gag is a highly variable reflex even among healthy persons. A diminished gag reflex is probably significant only when found in patients who have evidence of weakened or paralyzed pharyngeal palatine musculature, asymmetric gag reflexes, or other signs of cranial nerve dysfunction. Absence of a gag reflex does not automatically mean that the patient is unable to swallow or protect the airway (Linden and Siebens 1983).

Tongue

McConnel and associates (1988) compare the interaction of the tongue and pharyngeal muscles to that of a piston or plunger generating a propulsive bolus-driving force within a dynamic chamber. Lingual muscles should be examined for appearance and strength. In the edentulous or highly cooperative patient, palpation of the muscles can be revealing; atrophy, fasciculations, or abnormal movement should be noted. Recognizing that the tongue deviates toward the side of weakness, tongue strength can be grossly assessed by having the patient protrude the tongue. Tongue strength can also be evaluated by instructing the patient to push the tongue firmly against the inner cheek while the examiner resists the movement on each side.

Sensation

Chewing, salivary flow, and swallowing are all reflexes that depend in part on sensory stimulation. Sensations of hot, cold, pressure, and texture, carried by the trigeminal nerve, are known to stimulate chewing. Taste, which is carried by the facial and glossopharyngeal nerves, plays a role in stimulating salivary flow and, eventually, swallowing (see Chapter 2). If the gag reflex is absent, the patient drools, the mucosa is extremely dry, or food debris is retained in the mouth, some sensory loss involving oral structures may be suspected. Sensory loss alone is rarely the cause of dysphagia.

Many patients can detect and report sensory loss reliably, but in some instances clinicians may wish to test further. To evaluate functional swallowing, gross touch can be assessed on the face, lips, and buccal mucosa using a cotton

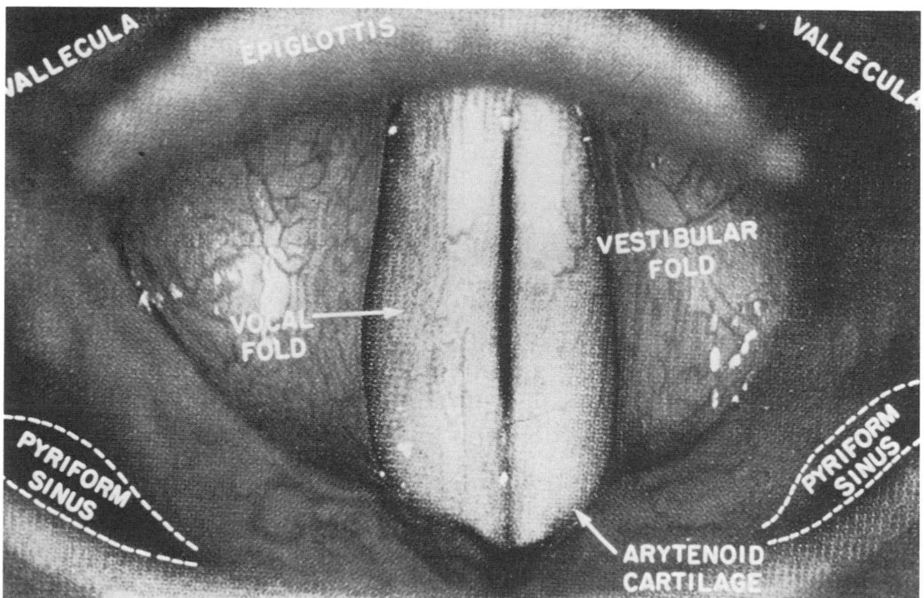

Figure 7.1 Structures visualized on mirror or fiberoptic examination of the larynx.

swab. Taste can be evaluated by having the patient identify a small sip of juice or the flavors of salt, sour, bitter, and sweet applied to various areas of the tongue with a moistened cotton swab.

Indirect Laryngoscopy

Indirect laryngoscopy should be performed whenever possible as part of the swallowing examination. A complete examination, as visualized in Figure 7.1, should include inspection of the base of the tongue, vallecula, epiglottis, piriform sinuses, vocal and vestibular folds, and infraglottic area. Otolaryngology consultation should be initiated if suspicious mucosal lesions are observed. The vocal cords should be evaluated for function, with observation of symmetry of movement during quiet breathing, forced inhalation, and phonation. Vocal cord function is essential in airway protection during the pharyngeal stage of swallowing and for coughing.

Presence of the pooling sign, detection of food debris or secretions in the vallecula or piriform sinuses, is an indication that the swallow reflex has been incomplete in clearing the bolus from the pharynx into the esophagus. When pooling is observed within the aditus of the larynx, the probability of tracheal aspiration is high.

Test Swallows

In normal swallowing, a bolus is worked into the oropharynx by muscles of the lips, tongue, and cheek. As the swallow reflex begins, the muscles sus-

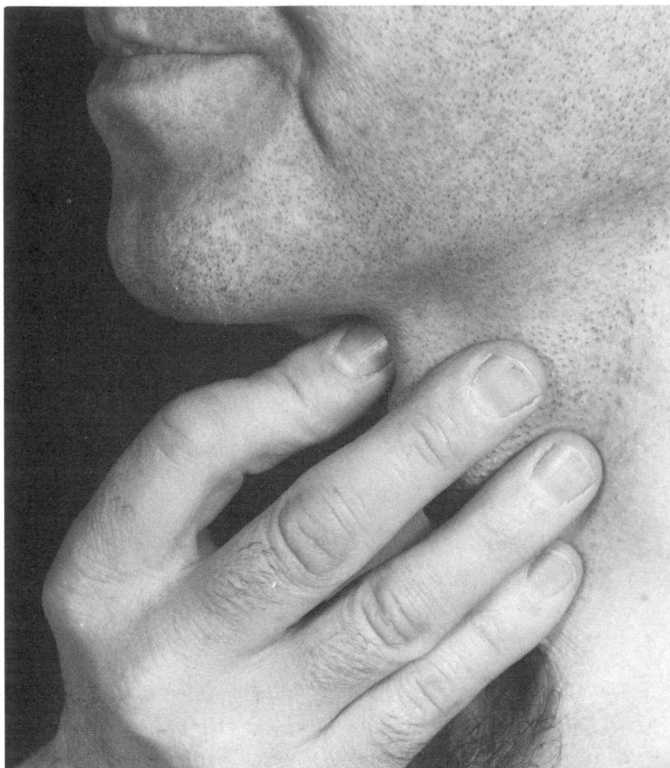

Figure 7.2 Manual stabilization technique of the larynx and hyoid bone.

pending the larynx contract and draw the larynx up to bury the epiglottis into the base of the tongue. The pharyngeal constrictors strip the bolus toward the cricopharyngeal sphincteric muscle, which opens ahead of the bolus and allows it to pass into the esophagus. An examiner can appreciate the moment of swallowing by placing a finger on the thyroid notch between the hyoid bone and the larynx and feeling the larynx move up and forward during the swallow (Figure 7.2). If the muscles are weak or the reflexes inadequate, the examiner's finger may fail to be deflected by elevation of the larynx. In this case, the cricopharyngeus may fail to open properly and the epiglottis will not be adequately inverted to occlude the airway, thus leaving the trachea unprotected.

On palpation of the laryngeal cartilages in some elderly patients, the larynx will be noted in an abnormally low position. This condition, laryngoptosis, may contribute to inadequate airway protection during swallowing.

Testing the adequacy of a swallow brings a certain degree of risk for aspiration. Coughing itself is not an indication that the patient is experiencing tracheal aspiration. In fact, the cough reflex is the final protective mechanism to prevent aspiration. The presence of an adequate cough reflex is necessary before an oral nutritional management program can be established. If the patient has lost or has an inadequate cough reflex, even test swallows with most foods and liquids are unsafe. Although a voluntary cough should be elicited and judged, the examiner should recognize that voluntary and reflexive coughs can be quite different in quality and effectiveness. Patients with cortical brain damage are frequently unable voluntarily to organize the motor behaviors necessary to produce a good cough, but their reflexive cough is intact. Conversely, in rare cases, patients can voluntarily cough, but because of an impaired sensorimotor complex, the reflexive cough is lost. Measurement of vital capacity is sometimes helpful in predicting the effectiveness of a cough reflex.

Initially, it is advisable to use a substance that is relatively safe if partially aspirated and to be absolutely certain that the patient is able to cough to protect the airway in case of aspiration. A spoonful of crushed ice is relatively safe and will provide a good medium for eliciting the chewing reflex because of its texture and cold stimulation to the receptors in the gums. The examiner should observe the chewing action and feel for laryngeal elevation to indicate that a swallow has occurred. Once it is determined that the patient adequately elevates the larynx and there is an adequate protective cough, the examination can proceed to using other substances with different textures and consistencies. During test swallows the examiner should take note of coughing, aspiration signs, or nasal regurgitation (see Chapter 9 for further discussion).

Some examiners attempt to demonstrate subtle weakness of the muscles and protective reflexes by testing swallowing under unfavorable circumstances. For example, it is known that the airway is more protected if a patient swallows with the head and neck flexed. Therefore, placing the patient in a posture with the neck extended and chin up may stress the swallowing musculature. Patients who can overcome this postural disadvantage are more likely to have an adequate swallow. Similarly, swallowing can be compromised by manually stabilizing the larynx and hyoid bone to bring out weakness of the muscles of laryngeal elevation (see Figure 7.2).

Swallowing reflexes are subject to fatigue and warm-up. Test swallows should be performed successively to evaluate for fatigability when the subjective complaint suggests this possibility. When the initial test swallow is judged to be inadequate due to coughing, additional tests may show improved function. This is particularly true when patients have pooled secretions in the valleculae and piriform sinuses. They may spill these secretions into the larynx when swallowing is stimulated initially but improve with subsequent swallowing efforts.

Aspiration is difficult to evaluate. If a patient is observed to experience some choking or respiratory distress that is not immediately relieved by coughing, it is probable that some aspiration has taken place. Some examiners listen with a stethoscope placed against the larynx during the swallow and have learned to perceive a characteristic sound of air mixing with liquids that suggests aspiration. Change in a patient's color, gurgling breath sounds, and extreme breathiness or loss of voice may indicate acute aspiration. Objectively, aspiration can be documented by radiographic studies. During test swallows the examiner should also note nasal regurgitation. This is more common when testing with liquids. Following each swallow, the oral cavity should be inspected for retention of food. Patients with damage to the parietal lobe of the brain and unilateral neglect commonly pocket food on the neglected side.

Test swallows for patients with tracheostoma tubes present distinctive problems. Tracheostoma tubes have a tendency to tether the larynx and trachea, resulting in inefficient laryngeal elevation and tilting (Bonanno 1971). Sasaki and associates (1977) pointed out that the laryngeal closure reflex is weakened and discoordinated when the upper airway is bypassed by tracheostomy. An airway diverted by tracheostomy does not retain its characteristic as a sealed, high-pressure cavity capable of inhibiting penetration by a foreign substance. The combination of the tethering effect, impaired protective laryngeal closure reflex, and the loss of a sealed high-pressure cavity leaves the larynx more susceptible to penetration, and the patient is less able to expel the material to prevent tracheal aspiration.

Patients who have cuffed tracheostoma tubes should be tested with the cuff deflated. The trachea above the cuff should be suctioned before the cuff is deflated. Before testing swallow, the tracheostoma tube should be plugged for several seconds to assess the patient's ability to breathe through the larynx as well as the voluntary laryngeal cough. As in other patients, laryngeal elevation should be felt during a swallow.

Ice chips provide an adequate stimulus to elicit the initial swallows. Aspiration should be checked by using a stimulus that is dyed with a contrast color that can be detected in the trachea. As the patient drinks approximately 10 ml of colored solution, the examiner observes for evidence of aspiration. In a patient with inadequate swallowing and an unprotected airway, the solution may show up immediately in the trachea. The trachea should be suctioned and the contents examined for evidence of the colored solution. Color contrast solutions such as methylene blue tend to coat the entire oropharyngeal mucosa, and it is not unusual to find a very small amount of blue-tinged secretion in the tracheostoma several minutes after a test swallow. This is a very common finding and usually is not associated with inadequate swallowing (Cameron et al. 1973).

Greenbaum (1976) suggested a protocol for the decannulation of the patient who has a cuffed tracheostoma tube. The patient is required to drink 4 oz of methylene blue–dyed water at intervals of 15 minutes for an hour. The trachea is then thoroughly suctioned, and secretions are inspected for evidence of blue coloration. If this test result is negative, the cuff is deflated for meals and at other times, with close supervision for 24 hours. Greenbaum added that even though a positive test result suggests aspiration, it is not automatically a contraindication to decannulation if the patient demonstrates adequate swallowing during meals with the cuff deflated. Conversely, it has been illustrated that failure to detect dyed material in the tracheostoma does not completely rule out aspiration (Thompson-Henry and Braddock 1995).

Just as tracheostoma tubes can interfere with the swallow reflex and the protective reflexes in the larynx, nasogastric feeding tubes have the potential to interfere with normal swallowing by altering sensations in the pharynx and deflecting the bolus. A tube passing transnasally may force the patient to breathe from the mouth, thus drying mucosa and additionally impairing normal reflexes. Some patients may be further decompensated by even a mild degree of dehydration. The examiner must be cognizant of all mechanical and metabolic factors that impede swallowing and the protective reflexes. In some cases, before final decisions can be made to proceed with oral feeding plans, the patient's swallowing should be assessed with tracheostoma and nasogastric tubes removed, the mucosa moist, and the patient adequately nourished and hydrated.

Repeat Indirect Laryngoscopy

After testing a patient's swallow reflex, a repeat indirect examination of the larynx should be performed. Here again, evidence of excessive pooling of debris in the vallecula or piriform sinuses suggests that swallowing has not completely cleared the bolus from the hypopharynx. Tracheal aspiration also might be appreciated by this repeat examination when the debris is visualized within the aditus of the larynx or subglottally. Langmore and associates (1988) have described a protocol for the fiberoptic endoscopic examination of swallowing safety that can be used to assess patients with oropharyngeal-stage dysphagia. Their procedure allows for laryngeal inspection before, during, and immediately following swallows of liquid and pureed food boluses.

ADDITIONAL STUDIES

The CED is not intended to be a definitive diagnostic evaluation for dysphagia; rather, as we stated at the outset, it is one component of a comprehensive dysphagia evaluation. However, in some cases the findings of the CED will be consistent with a previously diagnosed condition, and this examination will be sufficient to establish an effective management and treatment plan. The CED should allow the clinician to determine the need for additional studies and specify those that are required to diagnose specific impairments of swallowing and related functions.

To make a proper judgment regarding the need for other studies of swallowing, clinicians must have considerable experience in conducting and interpreting a CED and in providing management for patients with dysphagia. A working knowledge of studies that may be appropriate for the evaluation of swallowing and related functions is essential. Dynamic radiographic swallows, ultrasound, manometry, manofluorography, electromyography, endoscopy, a variety of reflux tests, and nutritional assessment all have a place in the comprehensive evaluation of dysphagia.

Dynamic radiographic studies of swallowing, either cineradiography or videotaped modifications of barium swallows, are the best procedures available for visualizing the deglutitory muscles during function. Dynamic radiography is required for all cases of dysphagia in which the CED suggests that the problem is directly related to, or complicated by, a cricopharyngeal, esophageal, LES, or gastric impairment. Radiographic studies are necessary when the CED fails to determine the cause of dysphagia, the findings are not consistent with a previously diagnosed condition, and the examination suggests multiple factors are contributing to the dysphagia. Radiography should be used in cases of unexplained aspiration pneumonia, and it may be useful to help determine the effectiveness of compensations in preventing aspiration.

Before automatically proceeding to radiography after the CED, one can reasonably ask whether the results are likely to alter the diagnosis or management in a given case. For patients with dysphagia caused by a well-documented etiologic event—e.g., stroke—or when the symptoms and findings are consistent with a previously diagnosed disease, radiography may not be indicated unless the result is to be used as the determining factor in deciding on methods for nutritional management. For acute conditions necessitating intensive care unit observation, spinal cord injury cases, and many patients with limited mobility or limited access to appropriate radiographic equipment, the CED may be the only method available to assess swallowing, and the patient's management is determined on the basis of this protocol alone.

REFERENCES

Bonanno PC. Swallowing dysfunction after tracheostomy. Ann Surg 1971;174:29.

Cameron JL, Reynolds J, Zuidema GD. Aspiration in patients with tracheostomies. Surg Gynecol Obstet 1973;136:68.

Castell DO, Donner MD. Evaluation of dysphagia: a careful history is crucial. Dysphagia 1987;2:65.

Christensen J. Effects of drugs on esophageal motility. Arch Intern Med 1976;136:532.

Edwards DA. Discriminatory value of symptoms in the differential diagnosis of dysphagia. Clin Gastroenterol 1976;5:49.

Greenbaum DM. Decannulation of the tracheostomized patient. Heart Lung 1976;5:119.

Jones B, Donner MW. How I do it: examination of the patient with dysphagia. Dysphagia 1989;4:162.

Jones B, Ravich WJ, Donner MW, et al. Pharyngoesophageal interrelationships: observations and working concepts. Gastrointest Radiol 1985;10:225.

Jordan PH. Dysphagia and esophageal diverticula. Postgrad Med 1977;61:155.

Langmore SE, Schatz K, Olsen N. Fiberoptic endoscopic examination of swallowing safety: a new procedure. Dysphagia 1988;2:216.

Larsen GL. Chewing and Swallowing. In N Martin, N Holt, DJ Hicks (eds), Comprehensive Rehabilitation Nursing. New York: McGraw-Hill, 1981;174.

Linden P, Siebens AA. Dysphagia: predicting laryngeal penetration. Arch Phys Med Rehabil 1983;64:281.

McConnel FMS, Cerenko D, Hersh T, et al. Evaluation of pharyngeal dysphagia with manofluorography. Dysphagia 1988;2:187.

Pope CE. Motor disorders of the esophagus. Postgrad Med 1977;61:118.

Pope CE. Heartburn, Dysphagia, and Other Esophageal Symptoms. In MH Sleisenger, JS Gordtran (eds), Gastrointestinal Disease (4th ed). Philadelphia: Saunders 1989;200.

Sasaki CT, Suzuki M, Horiuchi M, et al. The effect of tracheostomy on the laryngeal closure reflex. Laryngoscope 1977;87:1428.

Stein M, Williams AJ, Grossman F, et al. Cricopharyngeal dysfunction in chronic obstructive pulmonary disease. Chest 1990;97:347.

Straus B. Disorders of the Digestive System. In I Rossman (ed), Clinical Geriatrics (2nd ed). Philadelphia: Lippincott 1979;266.

Thompson-Henry S, Braddock B. The modified Evan's blue dye procedure fails to detect aspiration in the tracheostomized patient: five case reports. Dysphagia 1995;10:172.

Weiden P, Harrigan M. A clinical guide for diagnosing and managing patients with drug-induced dysphagia. Hosp Community Psych 1986;37:396.

8

Radiologic Evaluation of Swallowing

Olle Ekberg

To evaluate swallowing, radiology is crucial. It allows evaluation of both the function and the structure of the organs involved. During swallowing of a radiopaque bolus (such as barium), movements of anatomic structures as well as bolus transportation can be studied in detail. On the dysphagia team, the radiologist should act as a consultant to the other team members, selecting from different imaging modalities—videofluorography, cineradiography, computed tomography, magnetic resonance imaging, ultrasound, and nuclear medicine—according to specific patient needs or disease entity. Choice of the correct imaging technique depends on the answers needed to clinical questions. Therefore, the radiologist's responsibility goes beyond performing and interpreting the barium swallow. The radiologist should contribute knowledge from other fields of radiology, such as neuroradiology, tying together information from different studies in addition to performing dynamic or static barium swallows. The radiologist also is responsible for technical aspects such as exposure technique and the identification and reduction of image artifacts. Even when a modified barium swallow is directed by a speech-language pathologist, it is important that a radiologist be responsible for the quality of the imaging procedure. As a swallow-team member, the radiologist must also be aware of the limits of radiology for assessing the course and treatment of function and structure. In the interest of the individual patient, it is important that both the radiologist and the speech-language pathologist be knowledgeable about the performance and interpretation of this "interdisciplinary" barium study.

Swallowing can be divided into four stages: oral, pharyngeal, pharyngoesophageal segment (PES), and esophageal. This subdivision is based primarily on anatomic considerations. However, there is overlapping function. The oral stage participates in ingestion as well as some events in the pharynx and in the voluntary initiation of pharyngeal swallow. The PES stage basically pertains to the inferior pharynx and the upper cervical esophagus. However, it should be understood that although physiologic dysfunction is the most frequent abnormality in the neurologically impaired patient, the coincidental presence of a morphologic abnormality is common (Goldstein and Zornoza 1978; Thompson et al. 1978). Therefore, a meticulous search for structural abnormalities is important strategically, as these abnormalities may add to swallowing problems.

Radiologically, swallowing can be described in terms of (1) displacement of a defined anatomic structure and (2) bolus movement. Moreover, there is a close relationship among the oral, pharyngeal, and PES components of swallow. The relation between these three components and the esophagus is less obvious (Ekberg and Lindgren 1986). Therefore, all patients with dysphagic symptoms referred from the mouth, neck, or chest should undergo a complete radiologic evaluation (Halpert et al. 1985; Jones et al. 1985; Jones and Donner 1988; Levine and Rubesin 1990). However, swallowing dysfunction may be asymptomatic, especially in demented or mentally impaired individuals. The observation by a caregiver that a patient has difficulty swallowing also should lead to a radiologic investigation. Other important indications for radiologic studies of swallowing are recurrent pneumonia, cough that may be due to chronic aspiration, and unintentional weight loss.

Radiologic evaluation is an extension of the physical examination and should be included as part of the sensory-motor examination of the oral cavity, pharynx, PES, and esophagus. The pharynx can be examined only partly during conventional neurologic evaluation (radiologic evaluation is required to document its entire dimension). Most neurologically impaired patients with swallowing dysfunction do not undergo a radiologic swallowing study, even though there may be a reason to suspect dysphagia, such as voluntary restriction of diet choices, prolonged meal times, and postprandial heartburn. One of the explanations for this discrepancy is that swallowing dysfunction is frequently not discovered at bedside evaluation (Linden and Siebens 1983; Splaingard et al. 1988). Further, some patients do not cough while aspirating and therefore are unlikely to be referred for a swallowing study. Another category of indication for radiologic swallowing studies is treatment planning. Even if there is a transition between diagnostic studies and treatment planning, these two studies have different focuses. All diagnostic procedures should be performed by the radiologist. In subsequent studies, the interaction with a speech-language pathologist is crucial in planning treatment. Therefore, swallowing studies fall into either of two categories: (1) diagnostic examination or (2) therapeutic examination.

Patients referred for diagnostic evaluation of swallowing fall into either of two subcategories: (1) mild or moderate dysphagia or (2) severe dysphagia.

Mild or Moderate Dysphagia

Patients in this category usually have dysphagia of unknown etiology when referred for the radiologic study. They present with a feeling of "something getting stuck" while swallowing, or they cough during or after swallowing. Patients in this category have no feeding problem and are not losing weight. Patients may complain of having to cut food finely, of avoiding certain difficult-to-particulate foods, or of having to eat slowly. The majority of these patients do not have a neurologic diagnosis when referred for the radiologic evaluation of deglutition. However, the majority do have swallowing dysfunction secondary to neurologic disease.

Severe Dysphagia

Patients with severe dysphagia have a severe feeding problem, and the presence of swallowing dysfunction is easily recognized. The purpose of the radiologic study is to assess the type and degree of feeding impairment, including airway protection and concomitant morphologic abnormalities. Treatment evaluation is usually needed. The videoradiographic study is inherently concerned with therapy, particularly if the study includes trials of adapted physical character of bolus, changes in posture as compensations for deficits, or both.

RADIOLOGIC EXAMINATION TECHNIQUE

The radiologic examination takes advantage of the interaction between imaging radiation and materia. However, this interaction also has a potential harmful effect and may cause damage. Therefore, it is important to always perform the examination in a way that keeps radiation to a minimum. Even more important is to avoid an unnecessary examination. However, if the indication for the radiologic examination is correct, the advantages of the study always exceed the risk to the patient.

Feeding can be evaluated radiographically in most patients. Only patients who cannot be immobilized during deglutition need to be excluded. The effectiveness and contribution of the radiologic study with a patient who is resistant or has severe impairment depend on the patience and skill of the radiologist. The study may determine whether the patient will be orally fed and, eventually, whether the patient goes home or to a long-term care facility. In patients who are difficult to examine, such as those with psychoses or mental retardation, sedation before the study is contraindicated as the results will be invalid.

The examination of the mild-to-moderate and the severely dysphagic patient focuses on two different goals. In patients with mild or moderate dysphagia, one should look for the "worst swallow" (focusing on techniques to decompensate oral and pharyngeal deglutition). In patients with severe dysfunction, the primary concern is with treatment, focusing on techniques to elicit the "best swallow" as a method of compensation.

Cineradiography is optimal for monitoring minor dysfunction by reason of its excellent image delineation. For other patients, especially those who have severe impairment, videoradiography is preferable. Video allows a longer observation time because of lower radiation doses, is readily available, and is less expensive.

The examination should start with the patient in an upright position, either standing or sitting on the elevated foot plate of the x-ray stand (Figure 8.1). Patients who cannot be seated without support may be seated in a specially designed chair that fits on the footplate, or be seated in a wheelchair. Chairs may need to be narrow (17–19 inches) to fit between the table top and the fluoroscopy unit. An erect position is ideal, but if the patient is unable to cooperate, any recumbent position can be used. However, such positioning makes assessment of function difficult because of the unfamiliar, oblique projection of the foodway.

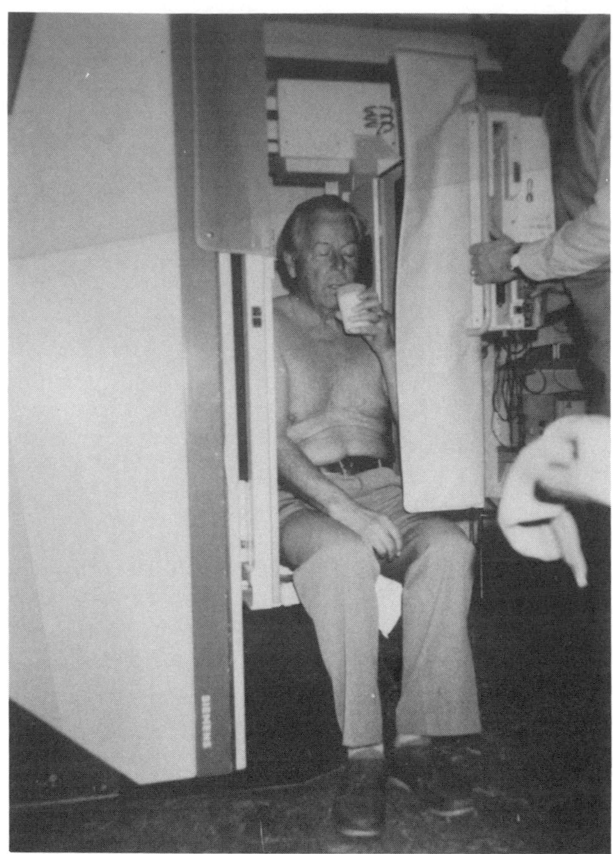

Figure 8.1 For radiologic evaluation of oral and pharyngeal swallow, the patient can be seated on the footplate of the x-ray stand.

Examinations of the Oral Cavity, Pharynx, and Pharyngoesophageal Segment

The examination begins in the lateral projection with a brief assessment of the velopharynx during phonation. The patient is instructed to say "candy" and "eeee." Evaluation of vocal cord mobility during phonation and breathing can be made after repositioning the patient to the frontal projection. Both observations are done without barium. Ideally, the swallowing study should start with boluses of high-density barium (250% weight to volume). It is important that the entire examination be videorecorded and audiorecorded. Use of an audio track increases the information substantially. Ingestion should be from a cup, spoon, straw, or, when applicable, any feeding device to which the patient is accustomed. In a patient with severe oral impairment, the pharyngeal phase may be elicited by injecting a small barium bolus (1–3 ml) directly into the pharynx through a soft tube. This may be placed into the pharynx via either the mouth or a nostril. Such techniques, however, are used only for examination and not for feeding. The patient should be allowed to self-feed or be gently assisted as necessary. The patient should keep the ingested barium in the mouth until instructed to swallow. This interval should be 10–15 seconds and is intended to reveal failure of containment of the bolus. Three ingestions and swallows are observed. The patient is instructed to take a mouthful of barium. For the diagnostic examination, the size should be a normal bite size or slightly larger. The patient should be able to swallow it during one swallow attempt. It should be noted if the bolus swallowed is smaller than the volume ingested; in such cases, considerable residue may be left in the mouth after swallow (Ekberg et al. 1988).

Severely impaired patients may reach the fluoroscopy suite without proper physical evaluation or medical histories. In a setting with a patient who is unable to self-feed and follow instructions, it is advisable for the radiologist to observe the patient swallowing water before positioning the patient on the x-ray table. Water is often accepted by the patient. Forced feeding should be avoided. If the patient or examiner is unable to get the water into the mouth, it is unnecessary to place the patient on the x-ray table. This water swallow test will serve as a screening device, saving much time and effort (Feinberg 1990). However, some patients may claim they are unable to swallow water, but can ingest barium for evaluation of function and structure. These patients may be found among those with a history of acute dysphagia and a suspicion of foreign bodies (Ekberg 1983a).

The first three bolus ingestions can be used to assess the oral stage and part of the pharyngeal stage. The field of view should include the lips, the laryngeal vestibule (to detect penetration of barium), and the pharynx. An additional three swallows should be observed, centering the field over the pharynx and the PES. It is important to have the patient lower and move the shoulders posteriorly because they may obscure the PES. The patient is then moved into the frontal position, and two swallows including the oral cavity and two swallows including the pharyngoesophageal (PE) segment are observed. The previously mentioned schedule is a minimum of projections. If additional information is needed, more swallows should be recorded. After these swallows there usually is good coating of the mucosa of the oral cavity and pharynx, and double-contrast views should be obtained with the patient phonating ("eeee"), or during slow expiration through almost closed lips, or during modified Valsalva. These double-contrast radiograms should allow detection of mucosal abnormalities as well as mass lesions (Ekberg and Nylander 1985; Rubesin et al. 1987; Rubesin and Glick 1988). Films in lateral, frontal, and both oblique positions should be obtained (Figure 8.2).

Most patients tend to swallow with the head bent forward because it helps close the laryngeal vestibule (allowing for airway protection). However, patients with poor tongue control often extend the neck to propel the bolus posteriorly into the pharynx. Some dysphagic patients who do not have airway penetration with the head in the neutral position may penetrate when the head is extended. Few patients show the reverse phenomenon of being able to compensate for poor laryngeal closure when swallowing with the head extended (Ekberg 1986b; Jones and Donner 1988).

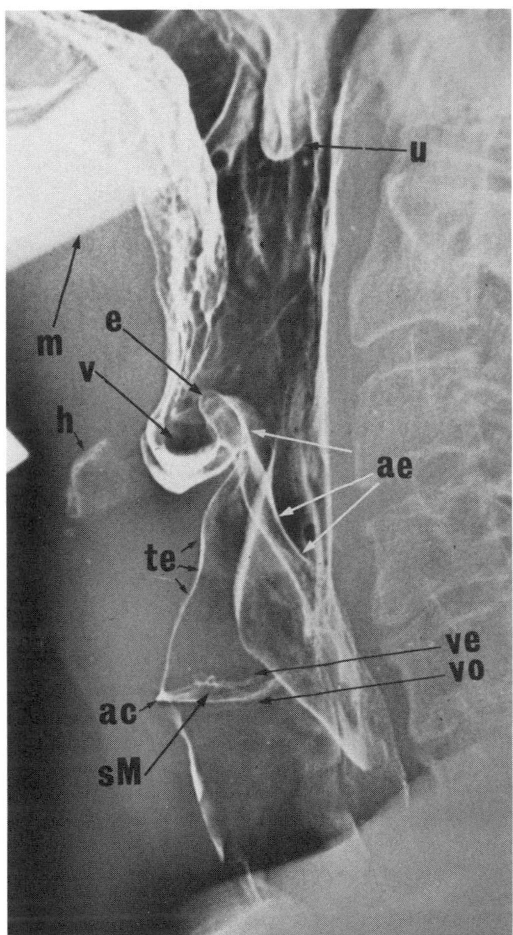

Figure 8.2 Lateral radiogram of the neck after barium swallow with coating of the mucosa. Contrast medium has reached the laryngeal vestibule and the proximal trachea. Anatomic landmarks are well visualized. (ac = anterior commisure; ae = aryepiglottic fold; e = epiglottis; h = hyoid bone; m = mandible; sM = sinus Morgagni; te = tubercle of the epiglottis; u = uvula; v = vallecula; ve = ventricular fold; vo = true vocal fold. (Reprinted with permission from O Ekberg. Closure of the laryngeal vestibule during deglutition. Acta Otolaryngol 1982;93:123.)

Therefore, the head should be in the neutral position. The easiest way to decompensate pharyngeal swallow is to tilt the head backward. Another method is to increase the bolus size. In some circumstances the unfamiliarity of the radiography room may create enough stress to exacerbate pharyngeal dysfunction. This is best appreciated during the first swallow in the lateral projection for visualization of the laryngeal vestibule. Attempts to decompensate the swallow are not part of the normal routine, but may be made with patients who complain of swallowing in these positions or those who are symptomatic with studies in the neutral position.

Patients evaluated for severe dysfunction often have concomitant impairment such as hemiparesis and cognitive impairment that may interfere with positioning or cooperation. It is important to note that observations of anatomic details and structural displacement are the most crucial in mild or moderately severe dysphagia, while attention to bolus transport is the focus of attention in patients with severe dysphagia. Therefore, any projection for the severely compromised patient is often sufficient to obtain the needed information. A radiologic examination should determine whether severely dysphagic patients can achieve pharyngeal swallow competence by any adaptation of food or feeding. For treatment planning, the patient first should be examined in the position in which feeding occurs, followed by suggested changes in position, bolus size, or amount. Evaluation of pharyngeal function as well as closure of the laryngeal vestibule is difficult if the examination is performed in the oblique projection or in other nonstandard routines. Alteration in swallow during compensatory maneuvers by the patient or those suggested by the therapist is notoriously difficult to evaluate. This is often due to low barium content of the bolus and obliteration of views. Therefore, it is important to standardize the examination as much as possible to validate observations of changes in function between studies on different occasions. Successive examinations should preferably be made by the same radiologist employing familiar routines. The radiologist who completes the study is the one who should provide the written report. Consultations on radiographic studies obtained by other radiologists and from other hospitals may be meaningless if not accompanied by thorough details about technique.

Some examinations may start with a consistency of barium known to be more efficiently and safely swallowed. Usually in severe pharyngeal dysfunction this is barium of high density, with subsequent graduations of thick to thin fluid.

For evaluation of treatment strategies, the radiologist is assisted by the speech-language pathologist. The speech-language pathologist should be familiar with the patient's feeding problem and have performed a clinical evaluation. Both should be trained to implement a feeding care plan based on the diagnostic and treatment components of the examination. The precise description of the appropriate textures to be used is discussed in the chapters on physical evaluation and treatment.

Esophagus

The examination should start with the patient in a standing position with double-contrast technique (Ott 1988; Levine and Rubesin 1990). The patient should swallow an effervescent agent, followed by 20 ml of water. The patient is instructed not to burp or belch and is then positioned in a left posterior oblique position and asked to gulp rapidly a cup (120 ml) of barium (250% weight to volume). This will open the lower esophageal sphincter, allowing the carbon dioxide to rise and distend the esophagus (Figure 8.3). At least four spot films, covering the length of the esophagus, should be rapidly exposed. Because peristalsis causes the esophagus to collapse immediately after passage of the barium, timing of the exposure during the relatively brief period of distention is important. To fully document abnormalities, additional swallows may be necessary.

For functional evaluation of the esophagus the patient is then placed in a recumbent position, usually prone (Figure 8.4). The patient drinks from a cup

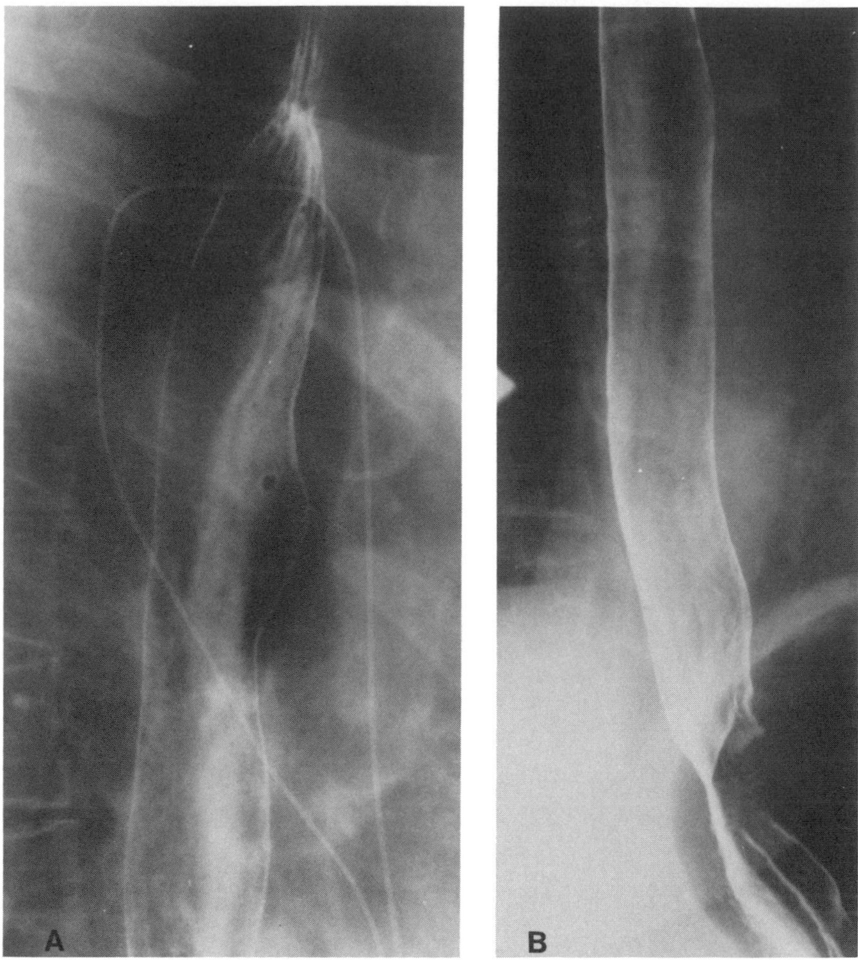

Figure 8.3 Double-contrast examination of a normal esophagus. A. Proximal part. B. Distal part.

through a straw. The patient is instructed to make one swallow at a time, as the examiner follows the tail of this bolus into the stomach. As new swallows abolish ongoing esophageal peristalsis, it is important to instruct the patient to swallow just once. If necessary, the patient should be instructed to open the mouth immediately after the first swallow because this makes an additional swallow difficult. Three to five single-bolus swallows are observed. Following these swallows, the patient is instructed to gulp the remainder of the barium. This distends the esophagus, and films should be obtained of the lower esophagus and gastroesophageal region. With air and barium in the stomach, the fundus and body of the stomach are screened to reveal structural lesions. Lesions in the gastric

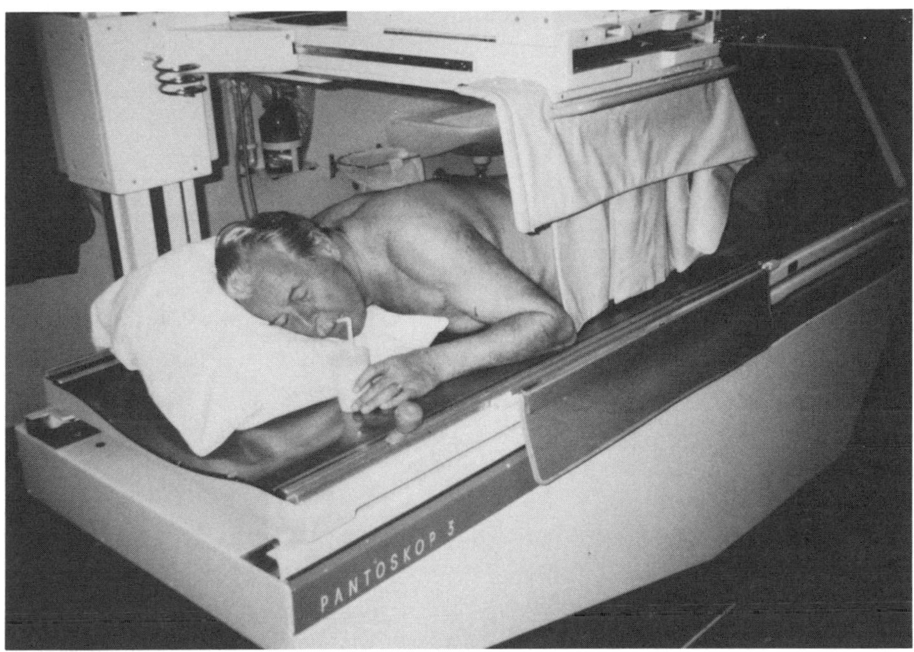

Figure 8.4 For functional evaluation of the esophagus the patient has to be placed in a recumbent position, usually prone.

fundus may produce symptoms of obstruction (Jones and Donner 1988; Levine and Rubesin 1990). In one study, dysphagia was the predominant presenting symptom in five patients with carcinoma of the stomach (Halpert et al. 1985). Because patients are not fasting for this study, detailed evaluation of the stomach is not possible. The examination ends by testing for gastroesophageal reflux. This is done with the patient positioned first on the left side and then on the back so that barium pools in the gastric fundus.

The gastroesophageal junction is then monitored as the patient turns to the right, coughs, and performs a straight-leg-raising or Valsalva maneuver to increase the intra-abdominal pressure and elicit reflux. In patients with gross aspiration, the esophageal component of the evaluation is limited. All diagnostic examinations also must include the esophagus, preferably at the same time as the oral and pharyngeal study. It is not enough to briefly observe the bolus dropping down into the stomach after the pharyngeal swallow. The esophagus must be examined carefully in every patient to detect the cause of dysphagia. In patients with pharyngeal abnormalities it is important to rule out accompanying lesions in the esophagus, which may add to, or be the source of, pharyngeal dysfunction. Patients with pharyngeal carcinoma have a significantly increased risk of coincident esophageal carcinoma (Goldstein and Zornoza 1978; Thompson et al. 1978). Boluses of varied texture and viscosity might be added to the study, but have limited value in the diagnostic evaluation of the esophagus.

Additional Techniques

In several circumstances the previously mentioned routine is changed. The most common change is to manipulate the bolus consistency. This may be done for the diagnostic portion of the examination and is always done during the therapeutic part. As a test for how thin liquids are managed in the oral cavity and pharynx, a barium suspension of 140% weight to volume is used.

Paste has an extremely high viscosity and is used to study pharyngeal and esophageal function. Paste is seldom seen to penetrate the laryngeal vestibule. In patients with poor primary peristalsis during liquid swallow, the extremely cohesive bolus of paste is regularly transported uninterrupted. Crackers soaked in high-density barium can be used to test oral function to assess mastication and bolus formation.

Barium tablets that are 13 mm in diameter plus water or 140% weight-to-volume barium can be used to assess strictures. It is not necessary to use barium tablets if a stricture of less than 13 mm has been revealed with liquid barium. For the same purpose, a bagel bread sphere with a diameter of 10 mm can be used together with 5 ml of low-density barium (Curtis et al. 1987). If barium tablets are unavailable for assessment, half of a standard marshmallow can be used (Kelly 1961; Somers et al. 1986). An acid barium suspension with a pH of 1.7 has been advocated as a screening test for acid-induced esophageal pain (Jones and Donner 1988). The acid barium also can induce abnormal peristalsis. It is prepared by mixing 100 ml of barium suspension and 0.5 ml of concentrated hydrochloric acid (37%). The patient is studied first with a standard barium suspension in the prone position and then with the acid barium. A positive acid barium test result is present when normal peristalsis is replaced by segmental nonperistaltic contractions. After this test, 15 ml of antacid is given to neutralize remnants of acid barium left in the esophagus. The result is negative when esophageal function is unaffected.

When barium sulfate penetrates the lower airways, it is readily expectorated within a few days and produces few pulmonary complications. When massive, aspiration of barium may be fatal (Gray et al. 1989). Nonambulatory patients and those with known pulmonary disease can benefit from chest physical therapy to promote pulmonary drainage (Gray et al. 1989). If barium is retained in the lungs, it causes a benign short-term foreign body reaction within hours. Eventually, minimal fibrosis may follow after days or months (McAlister and Askin 1983; Ginai et al. 1984). Another variation in technique might include the use of water-soluble contrast medium such as meglumine diatrizoate (Gastrografin). Iodinated aqueous contrast media, however, produce a more intense acute inflammatory reaction with edema. Therefore, their use is contraindicated in patients with massive aspiration due to the risk for pulmonary edema if the contrast medium reaches the alveola. Barium sulfate, therefore, is the contrast medium of choice for the gastrointestinal tract, including the oral cavity, pharynx, and esophagus, except for patients with a known or suspected perforation. The latter are often patients with postsurgical resections with a suspected anastomotic leak. Iodinated contrast media have low radiodensity, do not coat the mucosa, and give suboptimal visualization of pathology. The only reason not to use barium to visualize a fistula is that barium trapped internally would cause difficulties in subsequent radiologic studies. With adequate technique, however, including spot films before injection of new barium during the repeat study, these difficulties can be overcome.

SWALLOW INTERPRETATION

The oral, pharyngeal, PES, and esophageal stages of swallowing are precisely scheduled and symmetric and are readily appreciated radiographically (Ekberg and Nylander 1982; Curtis et al. 1985). Interpretation is in slow motion by swallowing stage, following a precise scheme of sequenced observations.

Oral Stage

A normal person can follow the instruction to drink from a cup and to take a bolus of appropriate size in a coordinated way. Liquid barium is not masticated or blended in the oral cavity. The bolus should be well contained in the oral cavity (Ekberg and Hillarp 1986; Hamlet et al. 1988). On instruction to swallow, the bolus should immediately be brought onto the posterior tongue. In the anteroposterior view the tongue dorsum is grooved to cradle the bolus in the swallow-preparatory position (Hamlet et al. 1988). Delay in transfer and jerky tongue or jaw movements are abnormal.

Pharyngeal Stage

Pharyngeal swallow is then initiated. During eventual oral processing of the bolus, there is superior, inferior, and some anteroposterior movement of the hyoid bone. At the voluntary initiation of pharyngeal swallow, however, the hyoid bone moves distinctly superiorly and anteriorly. There is also a distinct apposition of the thyroid cartilage and the hyoid bone. The larynx and pharynx with the PES moves superiorly (Palmer et al. 1988). Peristaltic pharyngeal swallow is probably cued by bolus passage through the faucial isthmus between the tongue and the palate. Radiologically, it is convenient to use the beginning of the anterior hyoid movement as the starting point of pharyngeal swallow.

The tongue thrust propels the bolus posteriorly into the pharynx and farther down into the PES and cervical esophagus, assuming the pharyngeal constrictor wall has normal compliance. The palatopharyngeal isthmus is closed by elevation of the muscular palate and constrictor convergence, which is mostly medialward of the lateral walls. No regurgitation of barium into the nasopharynx occurs in the normal patient (Figure 8.5).

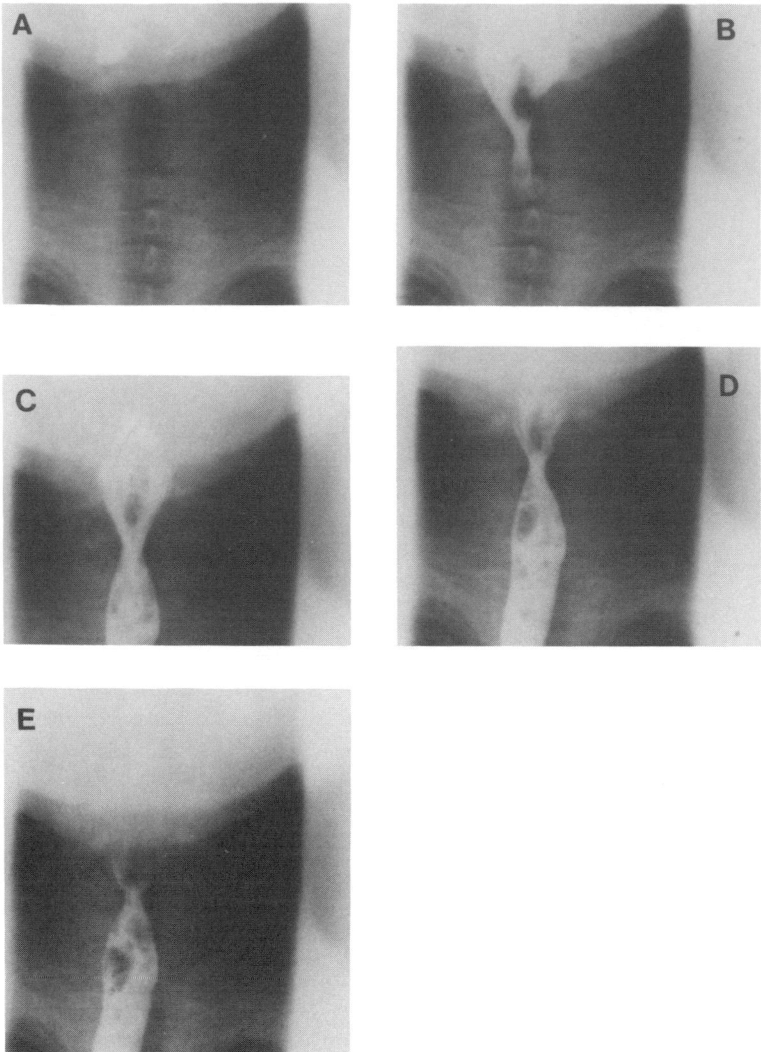

Figure 8.5 Cine sequence in (A–E) anterior and (F–J) lateral projections. The barium bolus is transported from the oral cavity into the cervical esophagus in a symmetric and synchronous way. The epiglottis is tilted down and the laryngeal vestibule is closed. The pharyngeal constrictor wave clears the pharynx of barium.

Closure of the Airways

Closure of the airways occurs at four anatomically distinct and functionally separate levels: (1) the epiglottis, (2) the subepiglottic portion of the laryngeal vestibule, (3) the supraglottic portion of the laryngeal vestibule, and (4) the vocal folds (Ardran and Kemp 1952; Ardran and Kemp 1956a). The airways also are pro-

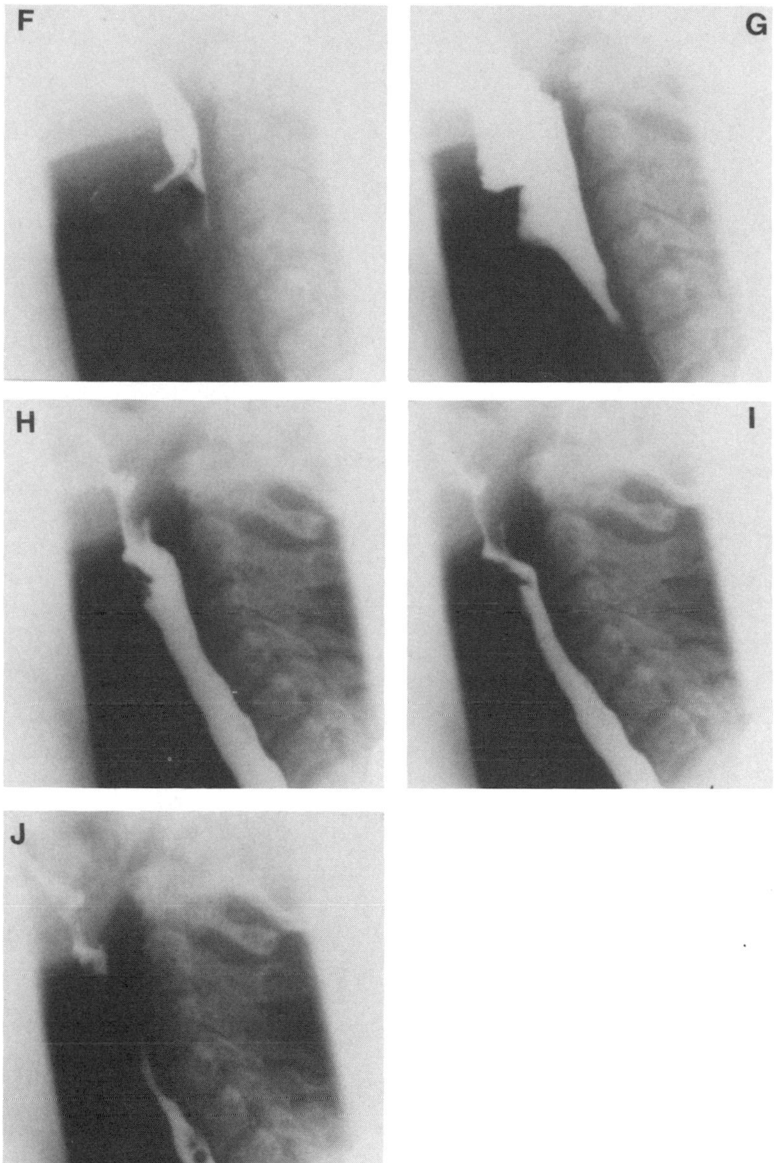

tected by an apposition of the thyroid cartilage toward the hyoid bone, leading to closure of the laryngeal vestibule. The vocal folds normally close before initiation of pharyngeal swallow and simultaneous with elevation of the larynx. The closure is best assessed in the anteroposterior view. Closure of the airways starts at the vocal folds and progresses in superior direction in a manner resembling peristalsis (Figure 8.6).

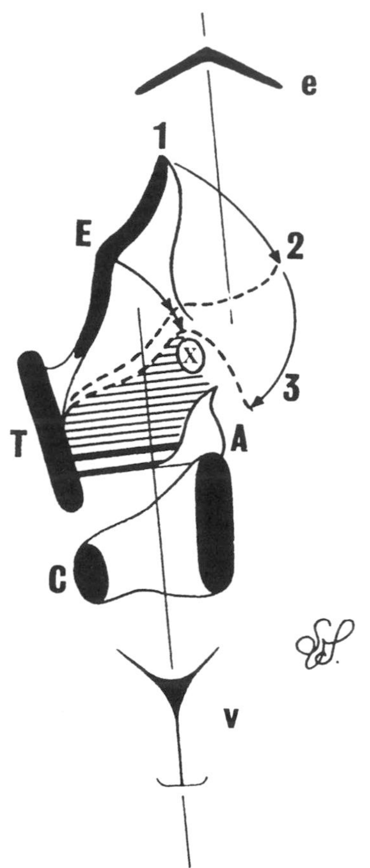

Figure 8.6 Schematic drawing of epiglottis and adjacent structures, seen from the left. The epiglottis is reproduced in its three different positions: 1 = resting upright position; 2 = transverse position; 3 = final down-tilted and inverted position. Hatched area represents closed supraglottic portion of the laryngeal vestibule. (A = arytenoid cartilage; C = cricoid cartilage; E = epiglottis; T = thyroid cartilage; e = horizontal position, free lip of epiglottis seen in coronal plane; v = closed vestibule seen in coronal plane; x = corniculate cartilage. (Reprinted with permission from O Ekberg. Epiglottic dysfunction during deglutition in patients with dysphagia. Arch Otolaryngol 1983;109:376.)

Epiglottis

During resting conditions between swallows, the epiglottis is kept in an upright position (Ardran and Kemp 1967; Ekberg and Sigurjònsson 1982). During swallowing, the epiglottis first attains a horizontal position and then an inverted position (see Figure 8.6). The first movement of the epiglottis (from an upright resting to a horizontal position) is passive and occurs synchronously with the elevation of the larynx. This movement is due to the anterior movement of the hyoid bone and the approximation of the thyroid cartilage to the hyoid bone. The epiglottis is bilaterally fixed by the pharyngoepiglottic plicae and during laryngeal elevation and thyrohyoid approximation tilts to the transverse position, with these plicae as turning points (or fulcrum). During this movement the epiglottis maintains its hollow form, with its concavity in the cranial direction. The second movement of the epiglottis is from the transverse plane to the position where it is flipped into the esophageal inlet. During the latter movement, the epiglottis changes its shape to an inverted caudal, concave form. The inferior surface of the epiglottis is then pressed over the arytenoids. According to Fink and colleagues (1979), this movement can be explained by either compression from side to side or by contraction of the thyroepiglottic muscles. The latter theory is compatible with the synchronous downward tilt of the epiglottis and compression of the subepiglottic portion of the laryngeal vestibule. The final contraction of the aryepiglottic musculature closes the superior laryngeal inlet more effectively, acting like the string in a tobacco pouch. The downward tilting of the epiglottis occurs inconsistently in relation to peristalsis in the pharyngeal constrictors and in relation to the bolus location. It is also obvious that the epiglottis may or may not tilt down, regardless of bolus size. However, during dry swallows, the epiglottis usually tilts down only to the horizontal position.

Laryngeal Vestibule

The vestibule can be described as a bent tube, with an angle of about 45 degrees. This angulation divides the vestibule anatomically into a cranial (subepiglottic) and a caudal (supraglottic) segment. This subdivision also is valid from a functional point of view (see Figure 8.6). Just before initiation of pharyngeal swallow (seen as the beginning of an anterior movement of the hyoid bone), the pharynx and larynx elevate and the thyroid cartilage comes into apposition to the hyoid bone by contraction of the thyrohyoid muscles. This apposition, together with contraction of the thyroarytenoid muscles (pars ventricularis), closes the supraglottic segment of the vestibule. At this time the arytenoids also are apposed by contraction of the interarytenoid muscles. Somewhat later and simultaneous with the final descent of the epiglottis, the subepiglottic segment of the vestibule closes. This is affected by an apposition between the fixed portion of the epiglottis and the arytenoids and is due to contraction of the thyroepiglottic muscles and to further elevation of the larynx. The two segments of the vestibule are thereby closed in two separate and distinct anatomic planes, which form a right angle to each other. The supraglottic segment closes in a sagittal and vertical plane, while the subepiglottic segment closes in a sagittal and horizontal plane.

Pharyngeal Constrictors

In the normal individual, the tongue sweep, including the posterior bulging of the tongue base, is followed by forward bulging of the posterior pharyngeal wall in a wavelike manner, starting superiorly and traversing inferiorly. The forward bulging wave normally is faint or absent in the superior constrictor area. A more conspicuous bulge, however, is regularly seen in the middle and inferior constrictors. This wave is much easier to observe in the frontal projection when the lateral pharyngeal walls are seen to oppose and form a wedge-crescent shape, with an acute angle superiorly. In the lateral projection the displacement of the anterior pharyngeal wall is more pronounced than the displacement of the posterior wall. The anterior wall displacement has three components. The most superior third is caused by the posterior bulge of the back of the tongue and is effected by the following muscles: constrictor superior, hyoglossus, styloglossus, and glossopalatinous. The middle third corresponds to the hypothyroid segment, including the inverted epiglottis and arytenoids brought posteriorly by the stylohyoid muscle and the middle pharyngeal constrictor. This posterior displacement occurs somewhat earlier than the activity in the constrictors posteriorly and laterally. The inferior component is at the level of the cricoid lamina. The posterior bulge of the cricoid is effected by the following muscles: the inferior constrictor, the stylopharyngeus, and the pharyngopalatinus. Abnormal pharyngeal clearance may be due to weakness in any of the previously described six components, three of which are anterior and three of which are posterior and lateral.

Normal pharyngeal constrictor activity is reflected in several ways during swallowing. Normal tone keeps the pharynx as a relatively straight tube without flaccidity and outpouchings. This allows the tongue to create sufficient force on the bolus, propelling it down into the esophagus. Contraction of the constrictors is then seen as a peristaltic wave, stripping the barium from the pharynx and leaving only a thin coating on the mucosa. This peristaltic wave is always conspicuous in the frontal view and is regularly seen in the lateral view as a few-millimeter-deep, smooth indentation traversing inferiorly.

Monitoring the pressure gradients generated from the oral cavity, pharynx, and PES has revealed the importance of the tongue thrust and the compliance of the pharyngeal constrictors (McConnell et al. 1988a; Dodds 1989; Richter and Castell 1989). Moreover, the simultaneous recording of pressure and structural movement as well as bolus position again emphasizes the importance of laryngeal and pharyngeal elevation during swallowing.

Pharyngoesophageal Segment

The PES is composed of the most inferior portion of the inferior constrictor, the cricopharyngeus, and the most superior portion of the cervical esophagus. Between swallows, the PES provides a barrier to air reaching the esophagus during inspiration and keeps refluxed or regurgitated material from the stomach and esophagus from entering the pharynx. During swallow the PES opens by a combined effect of cessation of muscle tone, elevation by the anterior movement of the hyoid bone and larynx, and the intraluminal pressure of the bolus (Kahrilas et al. 1988; McConnell et al. 1988a; McConnell et al. 1988b). During normal conditions there should be no indentation of the cricopharyngeal muscle posteriorly into the barium column when the PES is well distended. Some impingement may normally be seen early during the transport of the bolus through the PES. The PES also takes part in a peristalsis-like contraction with the constrictor muscles. The contracting wave continues uninterrupted from the oropharynx through the cricopharyngeus. In most persons there is a slight delay before the peristaltic contraction continues into the cervical esophagus.

Esophagus

Normal esophageal function is seen as a peristaltic wave, elicited by pharyngeal peristalsis, traversing from the cervical esophagus. During liquid barium swallows, normally only a thin coat of barium covers the mucosa. However, loss of peristaltic activity at the level of the aortic arch, where the transition between striated and smooth muscle occurs, is regularly seen and should not be considered abnormal.

Influence of Bolus Type and Head Positioning

Compared with a low-density barium bolus, the high-density barium preparations have a slightly slower oral and pharyngeal bolus transit time not recognizable during fluoroscopy (Dantas et al. 1989). However, the effect on upper esophageal sphincter function is significant. The sphincter opening and closing is later. The duration of sphincter opening is longer, the flow rate is lower, and the maximal anterior hyoid movement is greater. The sagittal sphincter diameter is also greater (Dantas et al. 1989).

Solids (tablets) and semisolids (marshmallows) are supposed to reveal strictures in the esophagus. The bolus is halted above and then helps to distend the narrow segment. Especially with the tablet, the exact size of the narrowing can be assessed.

Evaluation of chewable food like crackers is difficult because such foods require processing, chewing, and containment. With this stimulus, only a gross assessment of oral cavity and pharyngeal clearance, penetration, and aspiration can be made.

ABNORMAL SWALLOW

In terms of what abnormalities can be expected on the four different anatomic levels, a rule of thumb is that dysfunction is by far the principal abnormality in the oral cavity and pharynx. In those with motility dysfunction of the PES, structural abnormalities may coexist. In the esophagus, structural abnormalities predominate (Ekberg and Wahlgren 1985a; Ekberg and Wahlgren 1985b).

Oral Stage

In patients with neurologic disease, oral dysfunction regularly predominates over pharyngeal dysfunction (Ardran and Kemp 1956b; Ardran et al. 1957; Murray 1962; Donner and Siegel 1965; Donner and Silbiger 1966; Silbiger et al. 1967; Bosma and Brodie 1969a; Bosma and Brodie 1969b; Calne et al. 1970; Ekberg and Wahlgren 1985a; Ekberg and Wahlgren 1985b; Veis and Logemann 1985; Robbins et al. 1986; Ekberg et al. 1986a; Ekberg et al. 1986b; Kim et al. 1987; McConnell et al. 1988a; McConnell et al. 1988b; Horner et al. 1988; Robbins and Levine 1988; Dantas et al. 1989). Rapid ingestion or the inability to

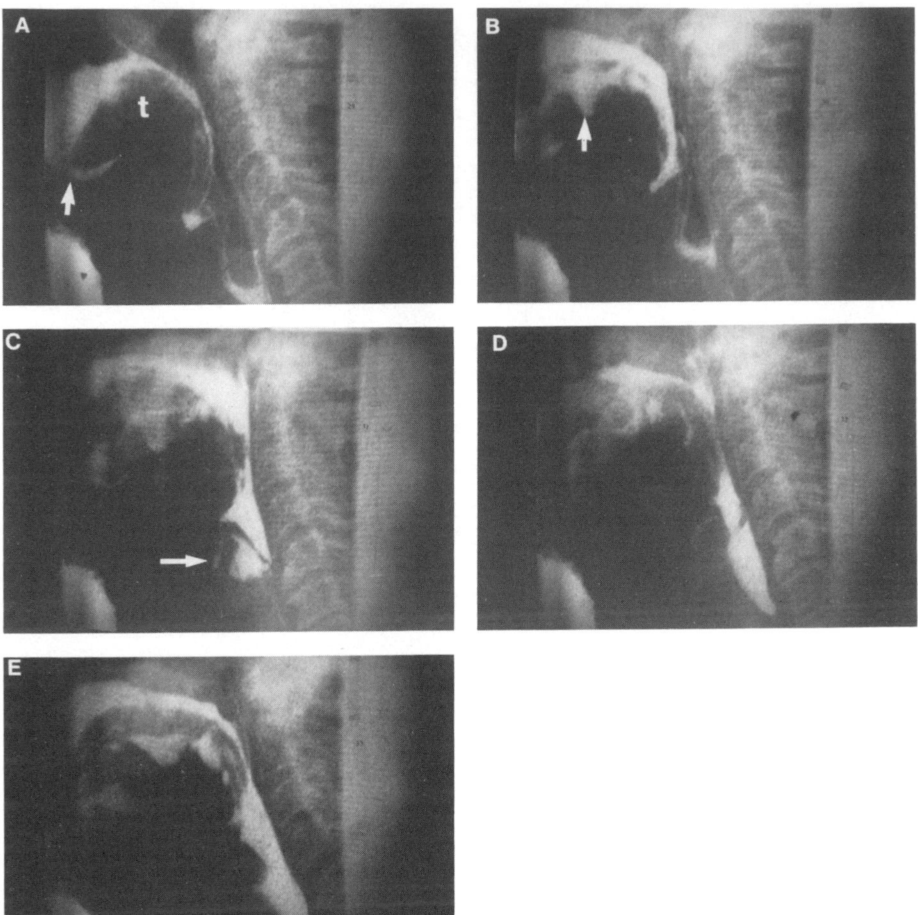

Figure 8.7 Oral dysfunction. A 73-year-old man who had undergone resection of a part of the tongue and the floor of the mouth due to carcinoma. A, B. After having ingested the barium, part of the liquid bolus flows anteriorly and laterally over the tongue (t). C. The barium flows posteriorly into the pharynx without being gathered as a bolus. A large amount of barium reaches into the pharynx without any initiation of pharyngeal swallow. Barium also reaches into the open laryngeal vestibule (arrow). The epiglottis, however, is partly inverted. D. Due to the defective elevation of the PES, it does not open and barium is trapped in the pharynx. E. When the patient elevates the mandible with his hand, the PES opens and there is elicitation of pharyngeal swallow.

restrict size of oral content may produce severe abnormalities. In the same way, defective containment characterized by leakage of barium is abnormal. This may occur either anteriorly through the lips, laterally into the buccal pouches, or posteriorly into the pharynx, where it potentially may reach the airways if the laryngeal vestibule is not closed (Figure 8.7). Uncoordinated, jerky movements of the tongue and jaw or chewing gestures are abnormal when a liquid bolus is held in the oral cavity. Delayed transfer of the bolus within the oral cavity into a ready-to-swallow preparatory position is abnormal. An abnormal tongue thrust can be difficult to appreciate and is characterized by slow and weak posterior movement of the posterior tongue. Usually there is lack of effacement of the valleculae as well as retention in this region. Abnormalities in the oral phase of swallowing, including impaired lingual movement or soft tissue defects, generally lead to delayed oral transit and clearance of the oral bolus with retention of barium. Premature spill of barium into the pharynx may be accompanied by failed initiation of swallow, aspiration, or both. The pharyngeal phase may be delayed but, once initiated, is normal.

Patients with uncoordinated, weak, or jerky tongue movements commonly cannot correctly position the bolus on the tongue. Accordingly, the tongue cannot displace the bolus posteriorly. There is a strong correlation between an abnormal anterior movement of the hyoid bone and overall abnormal oral and pharyngeal functions as well as defective opening of the PE segment (Dodds 1989). Abnormal initiation of the pharyngeal stage of swallow is easily appreciated when the bolus is conveyed into the pharynx without the pharynx being elevated and without occurrence of constrictor activity. Lack of anterior displacement of the hyoid bone is a conspicuous indicator of a serious abnormality. Demonstration of dissociation between the oral and pharyngeal stages depends on observation of structural displacement. Except for this failure of voluntary elicitation of pharyngeal swallow, the oral as well as the pharyngeal stages of swallow basically appear radiologically normal.

The wide range of normalcy can be observed during chewing and swallowing of a mixture of solid and liquid, especially while talking, when the barium or solid is brought into the pharynx while chewing and without tongue propulsion. In this circumstance, what happens to the bolus is more important than observing pharyngeal wall displacement. It is commonly difficult to distinguish a leak (whether due to defective sensory input or weak musculature) from compensatory delivery of the bolus into the pharynx.

Barium reaching superiorly into the nasopharynx is consistent with defective closure of the velopharynx secondary to either soft palate dysfunction or defective function of the superior pharyngeal constrictor. Medialward movement of the lateral pharyngeal walls is more pronounced and easy to appreciate than is anterior movement of the posterior constrictor wall. Compensation may be in the form of a Passavant's ridge, a protrusion similar to that seen as a compensatory maneuver in speech or in patients with cleft palate.

Pharyngeal Stage

Abnormal hyoid movement is seen either as lack of anterior displacement or as total absence of movement. The latter is rare. Motion also may be delayed in relation to bolus positioning—i.e., the bolus is in the pharynx before (>1 second) hyoid elevation. This is an indicator of dissociation between the

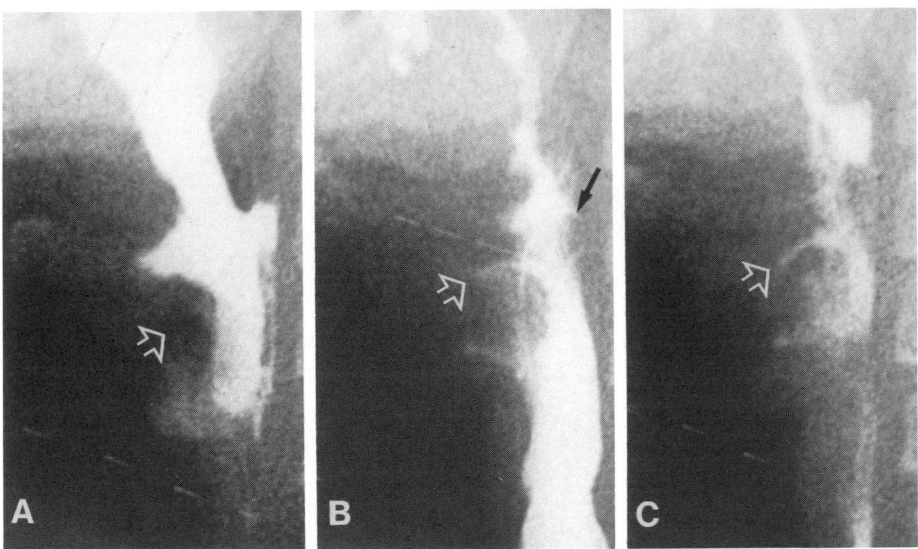

Figure 8.8 A–C. Sequence from a cineradiographic examination in lateral projection during barium swallow. Defective tilting down of the epiglottis that is halted in a horizontal position (i.e., the second stage of tilting down is missing). (Arrow = tip of the epiglottis). There is delayed closure of the laryngeal vestibule and barium contrast medium reaches into the subepiglottic portion (open arrow). (Reprinted with permission from O Ekberg, G Nylander. Cineradiography of the pharyngeal stage of deglutition in 150 individuals without dysphagia. Br J Radiol 1982;55:253.)

oral and pharyngeal stages and is a frequent cause of misdirected bolus. Absence of thyrohyoid apposition is always abnormal and is often coincident with airway penetration.

Defective elevation of the larynx and pharynx is usually due to abnormal hyoid bone elevation, abnormal thyrohyoid apposition, defective contraction of palatopharyngeal muscles, or any combination of these factors.

Abnormal vocal fold apposition is seen in patients with involvement of the recurrent laryngeal nerve.

Epiglottis

Abnormal movement of the epiglottis is common and always indicates pharyngeal dysfunction.

Defective secondary movement of the epiglottis from a horizontal to an inverted position is common (Figure 8.8). This is seen as the epiglottis remaining in the horizontal position (Curtis and Sepulveda 1983; Ekberg 1983b). However, in a variety of abnormalities the epiglottis tilts down incompletely. This might indicate a variable degree of incoordination of muscle function or a varying degree of paresis. Immobility of the epiglottis is seen as absence of the first movement. However, there is movement that is regularly transmitted from the back of the tongue. Therefore the epiglottis is never completely immobile.

Laryngeal Vestibule

Defective closure of the supraglottic portion of the laryngeal vestibule causes the bolus to reach the airways (see Figure 8.8). In the majority of patients with abnormal closure of the supraglottic portion of the laryngeal vestibule, closure is accomplished too late. The barium reaches into the lumen of the vestibule and is expelled either superiorly into the pharynx or inferiorly into the trachea beyond the vocal folds (Ekberg 1982; Curtis and Sepulveda 1983) (Figure 8.9). Complete absence of closure of the supraglottic vestibule is rare and is seen only in patients with a defective thyrohyoid apposition. The closure of the supraglottic portion of the laryngeal vestibule is crucial to protection of the airways. When the bolus extends beyond this point, it is a matter of chance whether it is expelled or reaches the trachea (Ekberg and Hilderfors 1985). Defective closure of the subepiglottic portion of the laryngeal vestibule is usually interpreted as delayed closure. A majority of these patients propel the bolus into the pharynx beyond the superior inlet of the laryngeal vestibule too early in relation to its closure. In these patients, it is more appropriate to identify the abnormality as an oral propulsion disorder instead of a laryngeal closure deficiency. Closure of the subepiglottic portion often is normal, but delayed. However, in half of the patients in whom contrast medium reaches into the subepiglottic portion, closure is never complete (Curtis et al. 1984). With nonclosure of the subepiglottic space, it is obvious that patients who inspire after swallowing may aspirate the retained contrast medium.

Pharyngeal Constrictors

Pharyngeal constrictors play a crucial role in swallowing (Ardran et al. 1957; Ekberg and Nylander 1981). If constrictor muscles are paretic, the pharyngeal chamber undergoes an abnormal expansion during the compression phase of swallow. This lack of compliance may result in impaired transit of bolus from the oral cavity into the esophagus, even if the tongue acts normally (Figure 8.10). Defective action of the pharyngeal constrictors leads to retention of barium in the pharynx. This constrictor activity is best evaluated in the frontal projection. As the middle pharyngeal constrictor is the most commonly involved, retention characteristically occurs at the level of the superior laryngeal inlet and may lead to aspiration after swallowing. Unilateral constrictor paresis is rare (Donner and Siegel 1965). Since the barium is asymmetrically transported (in the anteroposterior view), it may mimic a pharyngeal tumor on the normal side (Thulin and Welin 1954).

Discovery of misdirection of the barium into the larynx, trachea, or both should not lead to interruption of the study. However, some patients have mas-

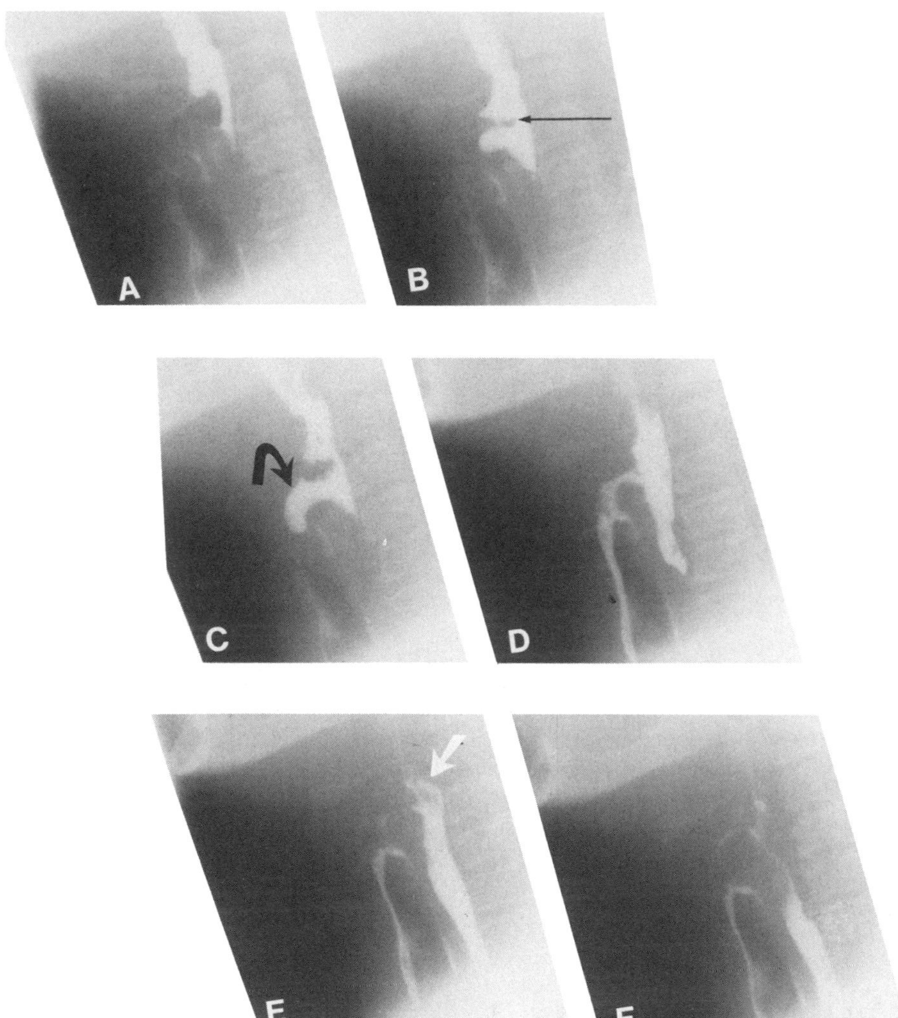

Figure 8.9 A–F. Sequence from a cineradiographic examination in lateral projection during barium swallow. Late closure of the laryngeal vestibule. The liquid barium reaches into the pharynx while the vestibule is still open. Part of the barium bolus reaches into the vestibule (C, bent arrow), the epiglottis is halted in a horizontal position (B, thin arrow). E. Late during swallowing, the laryngeal vestibule is closed. F. Pharyngeal constrictor activity clears the barium from the pharynx. (Reprinted with permission from O Ekberg, L Wahlgren. Pharyngeal dysfunctions and their interrelationship in patients with dysphagia. Acta Radiol Diagn 1985;26:659.)

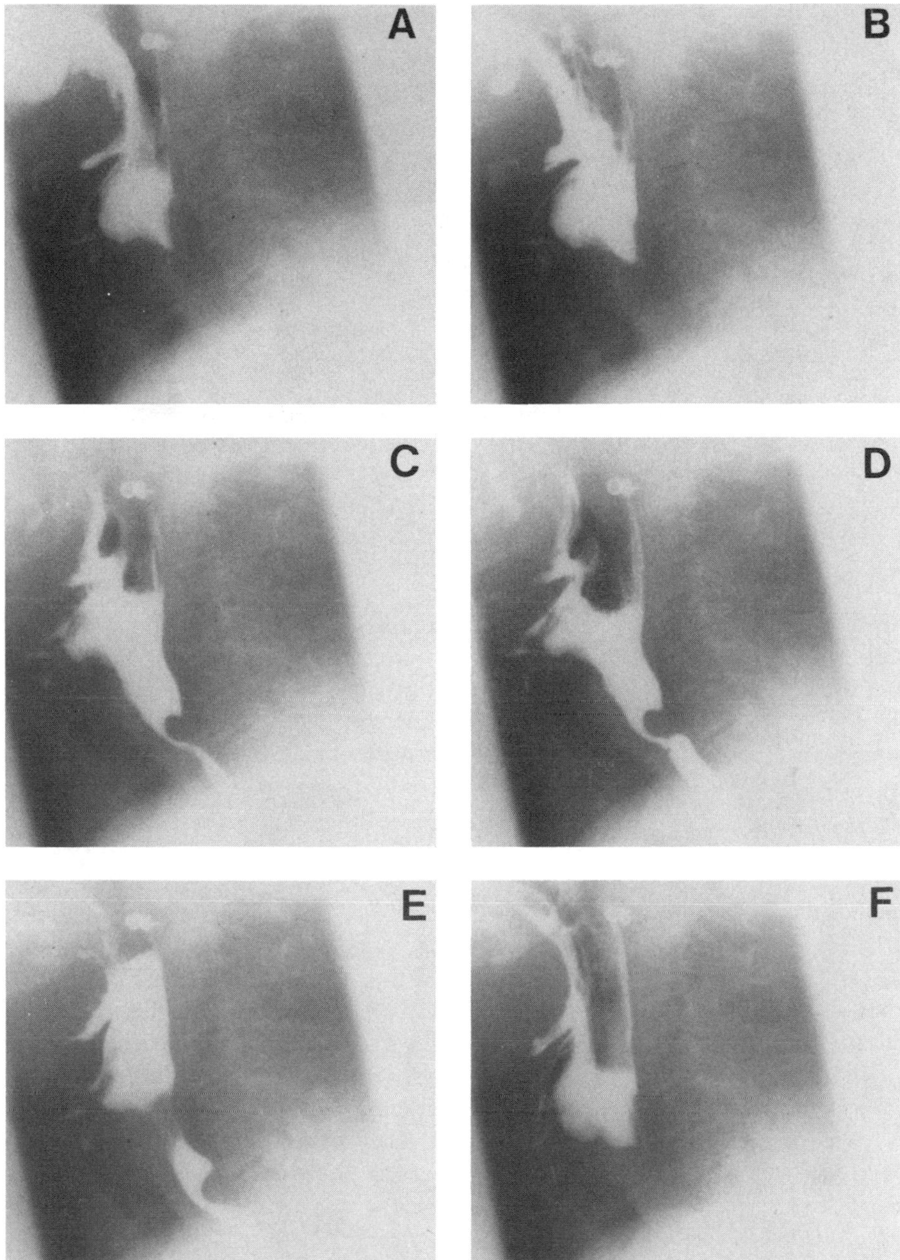

Figure 8.10 Cineradiographic examination in lateral projection during barium swallow. Multiple pharyngeal dysfunction. There is paresis of the middle and inferior pharyngeal constrictors. The epiglottis is not tilting down, allowing the contrast medium to reach the laryngeal vestibule and trachea. There is defective opening of the cricopharyngeal muscle.

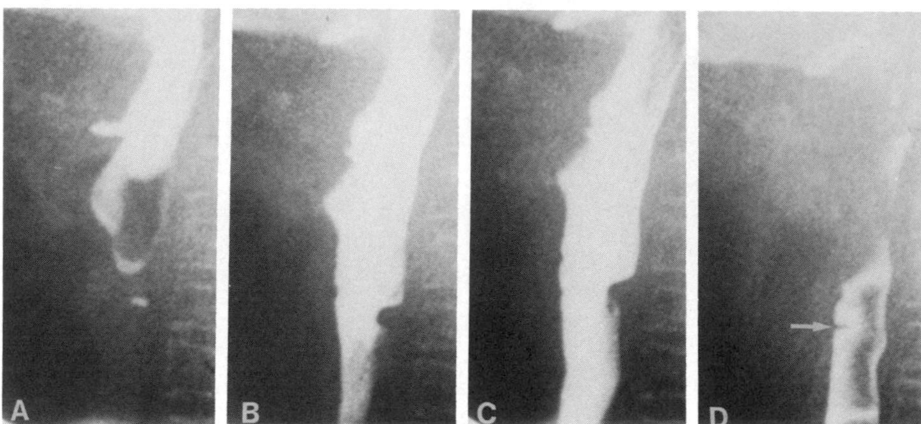

Figure 8.11 Delayed opening of the PES. The cricopharyngeal muscle is seen as a posterior inbulging. There is also a small cervical esophageal web (D, white arrow).

sive penetration into the trachea, and in these patients a very limited study is sufficient to answer the clinician's immediate question regarding possible oral feeding. It is important to elucidate the underlying pathophysiology in these patients. Therefore, a few swallows should be obtained in the lateral projection, even if the first swallow was aspirated. The hazard of acquiring bronchopneumonia secondary to a misdirected barium bolus produces little morbidity.

Pharyngoesophageal Segment

Failure of the PE segment to open may be seen in neurologic disease, but it is generally not accompanied by abnormal pharyngeal bolus transport (Curtis et al. 1984; Ekberg et al. 1986a). Failure of the cricopharyngeal muscle to open or elongate may be due to (1) defective relaxation, (2) defective distensibility, (3) hypertrophy or hyperplasia, or (4) fibrosis. The posterior bar intruding into the barium that is created by contraction of the cricopharyngeus muscle is seldom an isolated dysfunction. It commonly is associated with abnormal motor function in the segment above (i.e., the inferior pharyngeal constrictor), in the segment below (i.e., the cervical esophageal region), or in both (Figure 8.11). Therefore, even though the cricopharyngeal indentation is the most conspicuous, it may be only one aspect of severe motor dysfunction in the adjacent PE segment (Ekberg 1986a).

In dysphagic patients, cervical esophageal webs are relatively common (Clements et al. 1974; Ekberg et al. 1986b) and often are present together with cricopharyngeal indentation (Ekberg and Wahlgren 1985b). However, webs may be the only abnormality (Figure 8.12). The web is easy to dilate during endoscopy.

Less common are diverticula in the PES. A Zenker's diverticulum is located in the posterior midline, superior to the cricopharyngeus muscle (Figure 8.13).

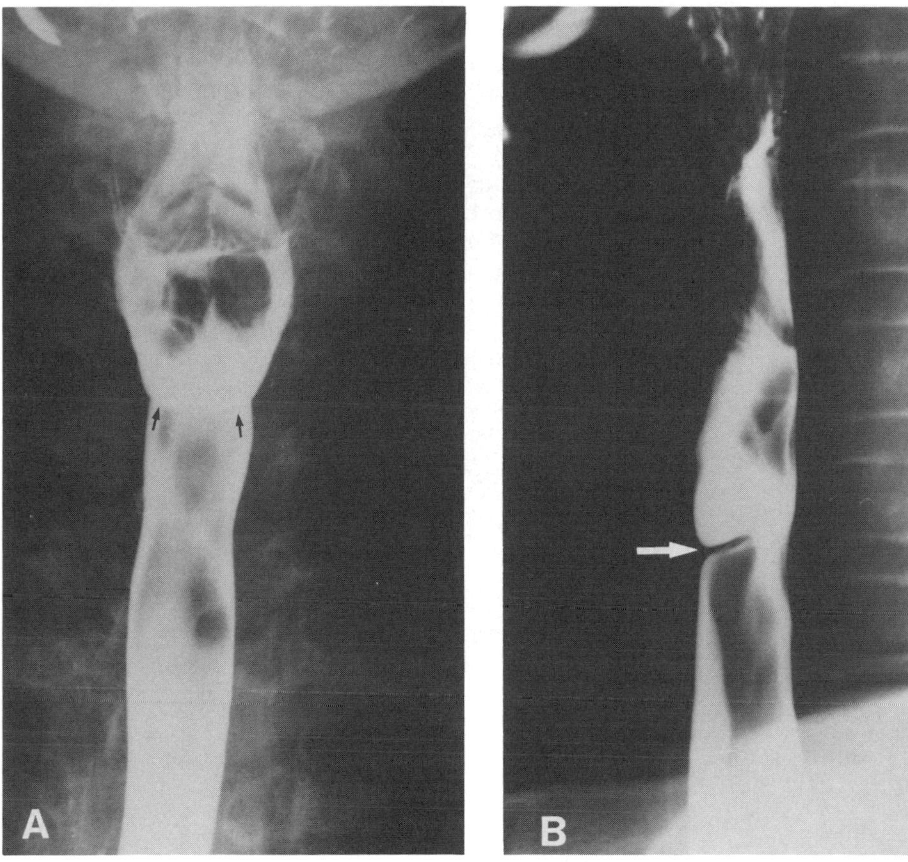

Figure 8.12 A. Anteroposterior view. B. Lateral view of the pharynx during barium swallow. There is a deep web in the anterior wall (white arrow).

When large, they regularly protrude to the left of midline. A Killian-Jamieson type diverticulum is located laterally and inferior to the insertion of the cricopharyngeus muscle on the cricoid cartilage (Ekberg and Nylander 1983) (Figure 8.14).

Structural abnormalities in the pharynx and PES are common. When suspected following radiography, endoscopy should be done. The importance of double-contrast technique in this circumstance is emphasized because superficial lesions are likely to be obscured without it. Benign tumors in the pharynx include cysts in the vallecula, which usually are asymptomatic unless large or infected. Carcinoma of the epiglottis and piriform sinus may be of considerable size before producing symptoms. Laryngeal carcinoma often spreads beyond the larynx into the pharynx. The carcinoma is likely to have produced hoarseness well before dysphagia.

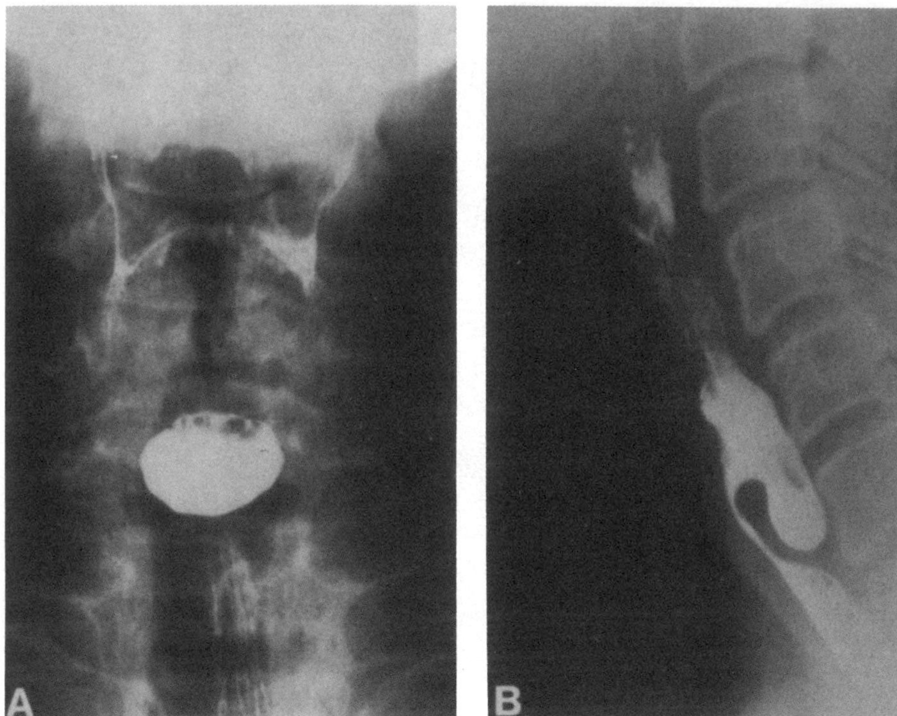

Figure 8.13 A. Anteroposterior projection. B. Lateral projection. Zenker's diverticulum.

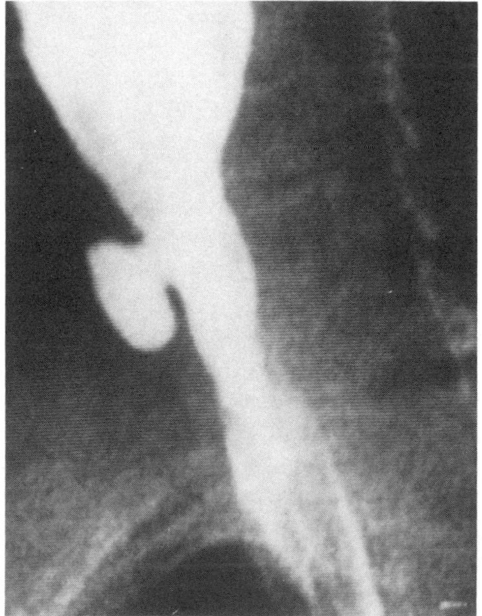

Figure 8.14 Cine frame from an examination during a barium swallow in the oblique projection. There is a 2-cm diverticulum of the Killian-Jamieson type that protrudes obliquely and anteriorly to the right.

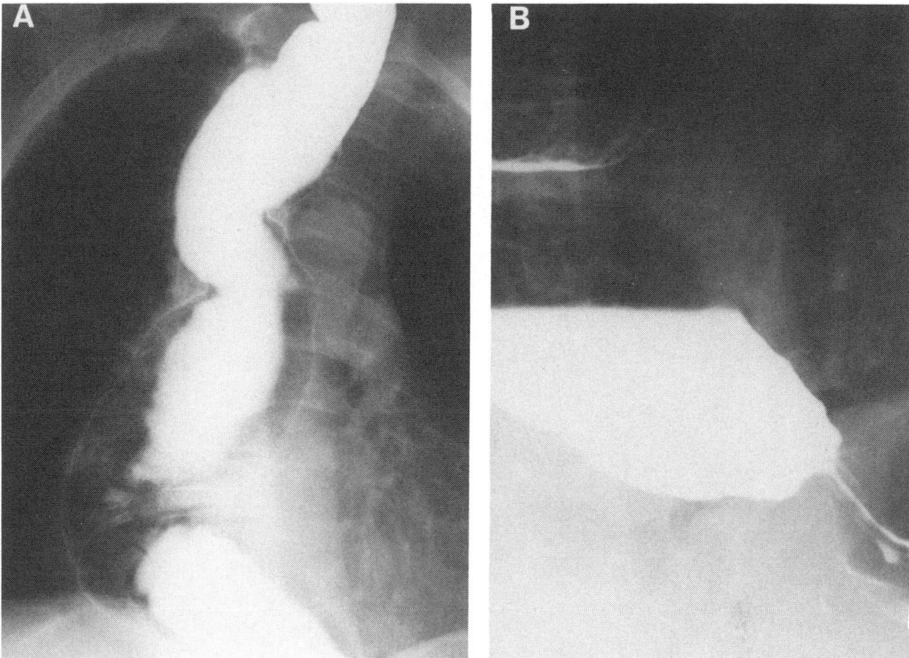

Figure 8.15 A. Thoracic esophagus. B. Lower esophageal sphincter segment. In a patient with achalasia the esophagus can be dilated and tortuous. During swallowing, the barium accumulates in the distal esophagus above the lower esophageal sphincter.

Adapted and compensated swallow may have the same radiologic appearance, but in the majority of patients is difficult to demonstrate. Therefore, a normal radiologic study may not rule out pharyngeal dysfunction (Buchholz et al. 1985).

Esophagus

Abnormal motor function of the esophagus is radiologically demonstrated as absent or defective primary peristalsis or as increased or vigorous contractions (see Chapter 5). The opening of the lower esophageal sphincter may be abnormal either in closing or opening. Therefore, radiographic dysfunction falls into one of five major categories. Achalasia is seen as absence of peristalsis with defective opening of the lower esophageal segment. The latter is seen as a "bird beak" narrowing (Figure 8.15). The esophagus is often dilated and sometimes tortuous. The etiology is unknown but seems to imply defective innervation of the esophageal musculature.

In scleroderma, a disease of smooth muscle, primary peristalsis is absent; however, the lower esophageal segment is open and gastroesophageal reflux may be severe.

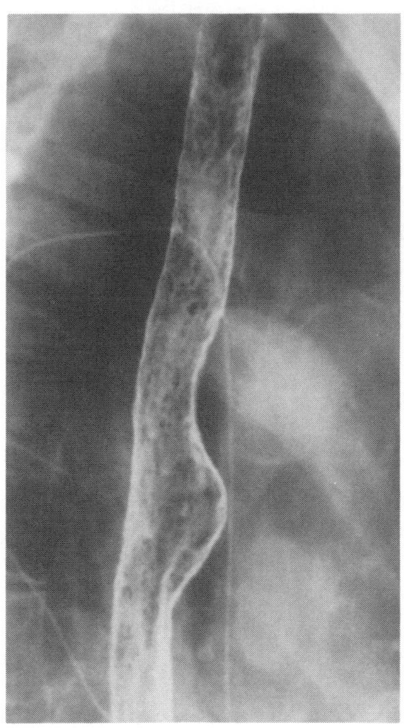

Figure 8.16 *Candida* esophagitis. There are multiple-millimeter protrusions from the esophageal mucosa. These protrusions are arranged in rows. The distension of the esophagus is limited.

Diffuse esophageal spasm is seen as nonpropulsive vigorous contractions as well as weak or absent primary peristalsis. "Nutcracker" esophagus is one variety of diffuse esophageal spasm and has a pathognomonic manometric appearance with very high pressures. However, the radiologic appearance may be that of normal bolus transit.

Gastroesophageal reflux may commonly cause cervical dysphagia (Jones et al. 1985). Ekberg and Lindgren (1986a) found that 12% of patients without gastroesophageal reflux and 40% of patients with reflux had cricopharyngeal indentation. Other pharyngeal dysfunctions were not common among patients with gastroesophageal reflux. This finding supports the assumption of a possible relationship between gastroesophageal reflux and cricopharyngeal function. The pathogenesis of this relationship, however, is unclear. Peptic strictures are common and may be severe. Peristalsis is weak or absent in the distal esophagus, and this causes prolonged contact between the acid and the mucosa.

Morphologic abnormalities of the esophagus include inflammatory lesions that may be caused by infections such as *Candida* (Figure 8.16) or by chemicals such as acid reflux. It has been suggested that dysphagia should be produced during gastroesophageal reflux only if the pH is below four and in the presence of esophagitis (Triadafilopoulos 1989). Benign (leiomyoma) and malignant tumors (squamous cell carcinoma) (Figure 8.17) also must be considered.

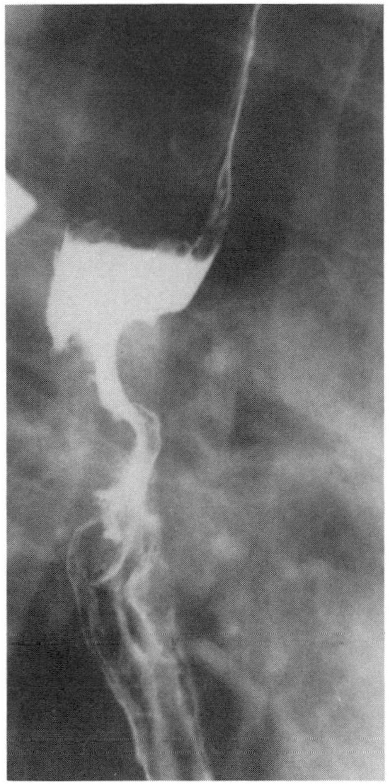

Figure 8.17 Carcinoma of the esophagus. In the midesophagus there is a short irregular stricture with overhanging edges. During endoscopy adenocarcinoma was revealed.

The immunocompromised patient with oral and pharyngeal candidiasis is seen with increasing frequency. During double-contrast examination, *Candida* appear as a surface that is mottled, nodular, or both.

It is important to detect structural abnormalities in the esophagus in these patients. Infectious esophagitis secondary to *Candida* or herpes may be the cause of dysphagia. However, they may occur in patients with other functional abnormalities of the swallowing apparatus and therefore be overlooked if the potential of the radiologic study is not fully used.

A distal esophageal ring (Schatzki's type) is another cause of intermittent dysphagia, particularly during solid bolus swallow. A ring with a diameter of more than 20 mm is rarely symptomatic. A diameter less than 13 mm nearly always causes dysphagia. Radiologic demonstration of this mucosal ring requires distention of the esophagogastric region above or beyond the caliber of the ring.

Course of Swallowing Disorders

The course of dysfunctions and their consequences in terms of dysphagic symptoms often do not correlate. Deterioration or progression of dysphagia is, as a rule, well compensated. Only by attempting to decompensate swallow can one reveal the progression, as when the radiologist intentionally elicits decompensation by extension of the neck or by giving a large bolus at a faster rate (Buchholz et al. 1985).

It is important to remember that repeat studies of pharyngeal function in patients suspected of progressive disease can be very important. Disability might go undetected if a repeat study is not considered.

REFERENCES

Ardran GM, Kemp FH. The protection of the laryngeal airway during swallowing. Br J Radiol 1952;23:406.

Ardran GM, Kemp FH. Closure and opening of the larynx during swallowing. Br J Radiol 1956a;29:205.

Ardran GM, Kemp FH. Radiologic investigation of pharyngeal and laryngeal palsy. Acta Radiol Diagn 1956b;46:446.

Ardran GM, Kemp FH. The mechanism of the larynx II: the epiglottis and closure of the larynx. Br J Radiol 1967;40:372.

Ardran GM, Kemp FH, Wegelius C. Swallowing defects after poliomyelitis. Br J Radiol 1957;30:169.

Bosma JF, Brodie DR. Disabilities of the pharynx in amyotrophic lateral sclerosis as demonstrated by cineradiography. Radiology 1969a;92:97.

Bosma JF, Brodie DR. Cineradiographic demonstration of pharyngeal area myotonia in myotonic dystrophy patients. Radiology 1969b;92:104.

Buchholz DW, Bosma JF, Donner MW. Adaption, compensation and decompensation of the pharyngeal swallow. Gastrointest Radiol 1985;10:235.

Calne DB, Shaw DG, Spiers AS, et al. Swallowing in parkinsonism. Br J Radiol 1970;43:456.

Clements JL, Cox GW, Torres WE, et al. Cervical esophageal webs—a roentgen-anatomic correlation. Am J Roentgenol 1974;121:221.

Curtis DJ, Cruess DF, Berg T. The cricopharyngeal muscle: a video-recording. Am J Roentgenol 1984;146:497.

Curtis DJ, Cruess DF, Dachman AH. Normal erect swallowing: normal function and incidence of variations. Invest Radiol 1985;20:717.

Curtis DJ, Cruess DF, Willgress ER. Abnormal solid bolus swallowing in the erect position. Dysphagia 1987;2:46.

Curtis DJ, Sepulveda GV. Epiglottic motion: video recording of muscular dysfunction. Radiology 1983;148:473.

Dantas RO, Dodds WJ, Massey BT, et al. The effect of high- vs. low-density barium preparations in the quantitative features of swallowing. Am J Roentgenol 1989;153:1191.

Dodds WJ. The physiology of swallowing. Dysphagia 1989;3:171.

Donner MW, Siegel L. The evaluation of pharyngeal neuromuscular disorders by cinefluorography. Am J Roentgenol 1965;94:299.

Donner MW, Silbiger ML. Cineradiofluorographic analysis of pharyngeal swallowing in neuromuscular disorders. Am J Med Sci 1966;251:600.

Ekberg O. Defective closure of the laryngeal vestibule during deglutition. Acta Otolaryngol 1982;93:309.

Ekberg O. Cineradiography in 45 patients with acute dysphagia. Gastrointest Radiol 1983a;8:295.

Ekberg O. Epiglottic dysfunction during deglutition in patients with dysphagia. Arch Otolaryngol Head Neck Surg 1983b;109:376.

Ekberg O. The cricopharyngeus revisited. Br J Radiol 1986a;59:875.
Ekberg O. Posture of the head and pharyngeal swallow. Acta Radiol Diagn 1986b;27:691.
Ekberg O, Hilderfors H. Defective closure of the laryngeal vestibule: frequency of pulmonary complications. Am J Roentgenol 1985;145:1159.
Ekberg O, Hillarp B. Radiologic evaluation of the oral stage of swallow. Acta Radiol Diagn 1986;27:533.
Ekberg O, Lindgren S. Gastroesophageal reflux and pharyngeal function. Acta Radiol Diagn 1986;27:421.
Ekberg O, Lindgren S, Schultz T. Pharyngeal swallowing in patients with paresis of the recurrent nerve. Acta Radiol Diagn 1986a;27:697.
Ekberg O, Malmquist J, Lindgren S. Pharyngeal webs in dysphageal patients. Fortschr Rontgenstr 1986b;146:75.
Ekberg O, Nylander G. Pharyngeal constrictor paresis in patients with dysphagia: a cineradiographic study. Clin Radiol 1981;33:253.
Ekberg O, Nylander G. Cineradiography of the pharyngeal stage of deglutition in 150 individuals without dysphagia. Br J Radiol 1982;55:253.
Ekberg O, Nylander G. Lateral diverticula from the pharyngoesophageal junction area. Radiology 1983;146:117.
Ekberg O, Nylander G. Double contrast examination of the pharynx. Gastrointest Radiol 1985;10:263.
Ekberg O, Olsson R, Sundgren-Borgstrom P. Relation between bolus-size and pharyngeal swallow. Dysphagia 1988;3:69.
Ekberg O, Sigurjonsson SV. Movement of the epiglottis during deglutition: a cineradiographic study. Gastrointest Radiol 1982;7:101.
Ekberg O, Wahlgren L. Dysfunction of pharyngeal swallowing: a cineradiographic investigation in 854 dysphagic patients. Acta Radiol Diagn 1985a;26:389.
Ekberg O, Wahlgren L. Pharyngeal dysfunctions and their interrelationship in patients with dysphagia. Acta Radiol Diagn 1985b;26:659.
Feinberg M. Aspiration and the elderly. Dysphagia 1990;5:61.
Fink BR, Martin RW, Rohrman CA. Biomechanism of the human epiglottis. Acta Otolaryngol 1979;87:554.
Ginai AZ, Lenkate FJW, ten Berg RGM, et al. Experimental evaluation of various available contrast agents for use in the upper gastrointestinal tract in case of superficial leakage effects on lung. Br J Radiol 1984;57:895.
Goldstein HM, Zornoza J. Association of squamous cell carcinoma of the head and neck with cancer of the esophagus. Am J Roentgenol 1978;9:791.
Gray C, Sivaloganathan S, Simpkins KC. Aspiration of high-density barium causing pulmonary inflammation: report of two fatal cases in elderly women with disordered swallowing. Clin Radiol 1989;40:397.
Halpert RD, Spickler E, Feczko PJ. Dysphagia in patients with gastric cancer and a normal esophagram. Radiology 1985;154:589.
Hamlet SL, Stone M, Shawker TH. Posterior tongue grooving in deglutition and speech: preliminary observations. Dysphagia 1988;3:65.
Horner J, Massey EW, Riski JE, et al. Aspiration following stroke: clinical correlates and outcome. Neurology 1988;38:1359.
Jones B, Donner MW. Examination of the patient with dysphagia. Radiology 1988;167:319.
Jones B, Ravich WJ, Donner MW, et al. Pharyngoesophageal interrelationships: observations and working concepts. Gastrointest Radiol 1985;10:225.
Kahrilas PJ, Dodds WJ, Dent J, et al. Upper esophageal sphincter function during deglutition. Gastroenterology 1988;95:52.
Kelly JE Jr. The marshmallow as an aid to radiologic examination of the esophagus. N Engl J Med 1961;265:1306.

Kim WS, Buchholz D, Kumar AJ, et al. Magnetic resonance imaging for evaluating neurogenic dysphagia. Dysphagia 1987;2:40.
Levine MS, Rubesin SE. Radiologic investigation of dysphagia. Am J Roentgenol 1990;154:1157.
Linden P, Siebens AA. Dysphagia: predicting laryngeal penetration. Arch Phys Med Rehabil 1983;64:281.
McAlister WM, Askin FB. The effects of some contrast agents in the lung: an experimental study in the rat and dog. Am J Roentgenol 1983;14:245.
McConnell FMS, Cerenko D, Jackson RT, et al. Clinical application of the manofluorogram. Laryngoscope 1988b;98:705.
McConnell FMS, Cerenko D, Mendelsohn MS. Manofluorographic analysis of swallowing. Otolaryngol Clin North Am 1988a;21:625.
Murray JF. Deglutition in myasthenia gravis. Br J Radiol 1962;35:43.
Ott DG. Radiologic evaluation of esophageal dysphagia. Curr Problem Diagn Radiol 1988;17:1.
Palmer JB, Tanaka E, Siebens AA. Motions of the posterior pharyngeal wall in swallowing. Laryngoscope 1988;98:414.
Richter JE, Castell JA. Esophageal Manometry. In: Gelfand DW, Richter JE, eds. Dysphagia: diagnosis and treatment. New York: Igaku-Shoin 1989;83.
Robbins J, Levine RL. Swallowing after unilateral stroke of the cerebral cortex: preliminary experience. Dysphagia 1988;3:11.
Robbins JA, Logemann JA, Kirschner HS. Swallowing and speech production in Parkinson's disease. Ann Neurol 1986;19:283.
Rubesin SE, Glick SN. The tailored double-contrast pharyngogram. CRC Critical Rev Diagn Radiol 1988;28:132.
Rubesin SE, Jessurun J, Robertson D, et al. Lines of the pharynx. Radiographics 1987;7:217.
Silbiger M, Pikielney R, Donner MW. Neuromuscular disorders affecting the pharynx. Invest Radiol 1967;2:442.
Somers S, Stevenson GW, Thompson G. Comparison of endoscopy and barium swallow with marshmallow in dysphagia. J Can Assoc Radiol 1986;37:72.
Splaingard ML, Hutchins B, Sutton LD, et al. Aspiration in rehabilitation patients: videofluoroscopy vs. bedside clinical assessment. Arch Phys Med Rehabil 1988;69:637.
Thompson WM, Oddson TA, Kelvin F, et al. Synchronous and metachronous squamous cell carcinoma of the head, neck, and esophagus. Gastrointest Radiol 1978;3:123.
Thulin A, Welin S. Radiographic findings in unilateral hypopharyngeal paralysis. Acta Otolaryngol 1954;116(suppl):288.
Triadafilopoulos G. Nonobstructive dysphagia in reflux esophagitis. Am J Gastroenterol 1989;84:614.
Veis SL, Logeman JA. Swallowing disorders in persons with cerebrovascular accident. Arch Phys Med Rehabil 1985;66:272.

9

General Treatment of Neurologic Swallowing Disorders

Robert M. Miller and Michael E. Groher

An early and accurate diagnosis and evaluation of patients suspected of having dysphagia secondary to neurologic disease are essential for the design of safe and effective treatment. The neurogenic causes of dysphagia are numerous (see Chapter 3), and it is important that the dysphagia specialist become familiar with the clinical pathologic mechanisms of certain disease processes. This should include a thorough understanding of effects on the neuromuscular system, clinical course and expected prognosis, changes that medical or surgical intervention might bring, and potential effects on the patient's learning skills. The interaction of these factors should determine the proper approach to management.

The most challenging aspect of neurologically based swallowing disorders is that patients with similar pathologic processes develop swallowing disorders that differ in severity and in schedule. For instance, all patients with amyotrophic lateral sclerosis (ALS) do not develop similar patterns of dysphagia and therefore do not require identical therapy. In some ALS patients, dysphagia is a significant problem at first diagnosis. In others it is not evident until the later stages of the disease, and even then, its clinical manifestations may differ among individuals. Even though dysphagia with significant aspiration may be part of a well-known set of clinical signs for a particular neurologic disease, it may not manifest itself in an identical manner and may be demonstrated at unpredictable times. And when dysphagia becomes apparent, patients with identical causative conditions require different treatment approaches due to disease severity; previous medical history; willingness to cooperate, learn, or both; and present state of health. Successful management depends on an awareness of such disparities.

These introductory comments alert the reader to the fact that the treatment concepts presented in this chapter should not be generalized. The approaches described are to be used only as guidelines for treatment. Overgeneralization may result in inflexibility in dealing with patients who require a great deal of adaptation of treatment. Unfortunately, every patient will not benefit from our suggestions, but with continued investigation and the application of individualized clinical problem solving, those with neurogenic dysphagia can be managed effectively. Specific neurofacilitative approaches to deglutition management that often are used as precursors to oral intake are covered in detail in Chapter 10.

TREATMENT OF DYSPHAGIA PARALYTICA

Diseases that affect the lower motoneurons of the brain stem or their peripheral connections to the swallowing muscles may render the musculature needed for swallow either weak or paretic. There may be several disorders of cranial innervation so that the ability to swallow is incapacitated. The facial nerve, hypoglossal nerve, or both may be involved. The cough reflex, which is mediated by the ninth and tenth cranial nerves, may be so impaired that the patient cannot expel accumulated secretions or a bolus that has penetrated the larynx. Cineradiography may demonstrate failure of the cricopharyngeus muscle to relax, thus incapacitating pharyngeal swallow. The principal causes of dysphagia secondary to lower motoneuron involvement are discussed in Chapter 3.

Because the respiratory centers are located in the brain stem, and because of patients' failure to adequately control their own secretions, those with dysphagia paralytica may require a tracheostoma. Increased respiratory rates (>30) also may interfere with the time requirement for airway closure during swallow. The critical medical condition in the acute stages often requires intravenous and subsequent nasogastric or bypass feeding to support life.

Although one of the goals of a swallowing management program is to avoid the prolonged use of nasogastric tube feedings, these are particularly important in the initial stages of medical management because they supply the nutrients that may eventually give the patient the strength to begin receiving nutrition orally. As metabolic balance is achieved, critical protective reflexes may return and a swallowing treatment plan can be implemented.

Such a feeding program should not begin until the physician feels the patient's acute medical status warrants it. The swallowing evaluation must demonstrate that the patient has an adequate protective and productive cough reflex and can elevate the larynx during a swallow (see Chapter 7). Ideally, the cannula will be removed, as the tracheostoma tube may interfere with normal laryngeal elevation and cricopharyngeal relaxation (Bonanno 1971). The presence of the tube also may alter the pressure gradient needed in a normally closed system to move a bolus rapidly from the mouth to the esophagus.

Swallowing management and treatment of patients with dysphagia paralytica are based on five major concepts: (1) establish an effective means of communication, (2) use a safe and stimulating diet in an effort to trigger a weak reflex, (3) capitalize on intact voluntary cortical drive to facilitate swallowing, (4) strengthen weakened oral and pharyngeal musculature, and (5) attempt surgical intervention.

Communication

Before diet and muscle-strengthening exercises can be considered, it greatly facilitates the clinician's work if a viable communication system is established between patient and staff. Due to the weakened articulatory muscles, patients with dysphagia paralytica often cannot produce intelligible speech even though

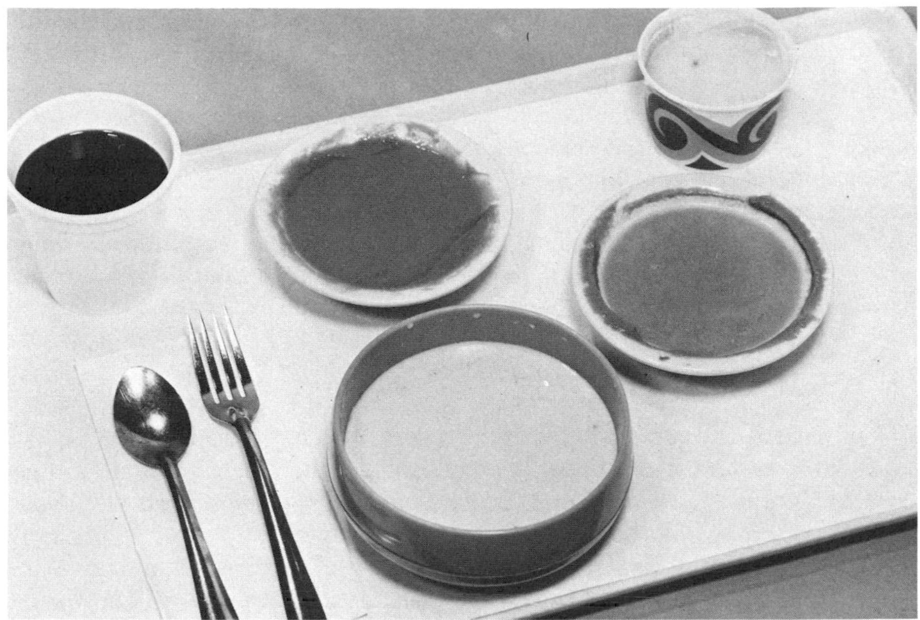

Figure 9.1 Typical puréed food consisting of strained vegetables, thinned applesauce, soup, and coffee. All items are liquid and appear unappetizing in addition to their bland flavoring.

their mental abilities with respect to language remain intact. Electronic communication aids, "silent spokesman" boards, and yes-no question strategies are all commonly employed modes of communication that aid in the patient's treatment. More elaborate computer interface systems can be used if recovery is prolonged. It is very beneficial to the clinician if the patient can express difficulties and successes that occur during swallowing remediation.

Diet

If the swallow reflex is absent or very weak, patients with brain stem pathology need maximal dietary stimulus to give the reflex the best chance to respond. A diet that enhances the sensations of taste, temperature, texture, and pressure is recommended rather than the traditional puréed foods (Curran and Groher 1990). Unless special care is taken in the preparation of puréed foods to amplify the sensations that stimulate chewing and swallowing, they may prove to be more difficult to swallow because they lack these qualities (Figure 9.1). Purées are difficult to control in the oral cavity when the musculature is weakened, and the patient with lower motoneuron weakness finds it difficult to form the bolus necessary to trigger a swallow. For the same reason, fluids often are harder to control than semisolids. Some patients with dysphagia paralytica who also have accompanying cricopharyngeal dysfunction may find that if the reflex is elicited, softer foods and liquids pass into the esophagus more easily, while solids are obstructed at this level due to failure of the sphincter to relax or because of premature sphincter closure. In selected cases, larger boluses may improve the function of this sphincter.

In general, patients with lower motoneuron dysphagia should avoid foods such as applesauce, which falls apart as it passes through the pharynx, fresh white bread or bananas that are sticky and tend to hang up, and chocolate or ice cream that increases heavy mucus retention, which can in itself become an interference.

Muscle Strengthening

If patients demonstrate that they are unable to take liquids safely, and solids fail to reach the esophagus, they perhaps can be taught to swallow a gastric feeding tube orally (Campbell-Taylor et al. 1988) (Figure 9.2). We prefer a red rubber urinary catheter because of its ease of insertion and tolerance in the oropharynx. It is not long enough to penetrate the lower esophageal sphincter, which minimizes reflux, but it should only be used for patients with known competent distal esophageal function. Because the gag reflex already is diminished or absent, the patient may find oral insertion of the feeding tube easy to do. Stimulation of the tongue and pharyngeal muscle bundles by the tube during oral passage may activate contraction of weakened muscles. By reciprocal action, enhancement of contraction of the inferior constrictor allows the cricopharyngeus to relax. The patient can not only self-administer nutrition, but he or she strengthens the muscles needed for swallowing with an easily retrievable bolus. Intermittent passage of the tube allows the patient to receive nutrition, water, and medication and avoids the constant irritation of a nasogastric tube. With recovery, sensation and active reflexes in the pharynx may return. If the patient reports nausea during orogastric tube passage or while the tube is in place, the procedure should be discontinued until the cause is determined. Emesis must be avoided because of the potential for aspiration of stomach contents.

Passage of an oral tube can be used as an exercise for swallowing in which the patient uses the tongue and facial muscles to move the tube back and attempts to elevate the larynx. In patients with paralysis of swallowing due to progressive degenerative neurologic diseases such as ALS or exacerbation of myasthenia gravis, exercises for strengthening are contraindicated. For them, the feeding tube can be passively inserted and used as a tool for nutritional management.

For those with swallowing reflex delay, thermal stimulation may enhance the swallowing reflex. In 25 patients with pharyngeal swallow reflex delay, thermal stimulation at that anterior faucial arch before swallow improved total transit time in 82% while ingesting liquid and in 100% while ingesting a paste consistency (Lazzara et al. 1986). Rosenbek et al. (1991) studied the long-term consequences of thermal application on the reduction of oropharyngeal dysphagic symptoms in seven neurologically impaired subjects using a single-subject

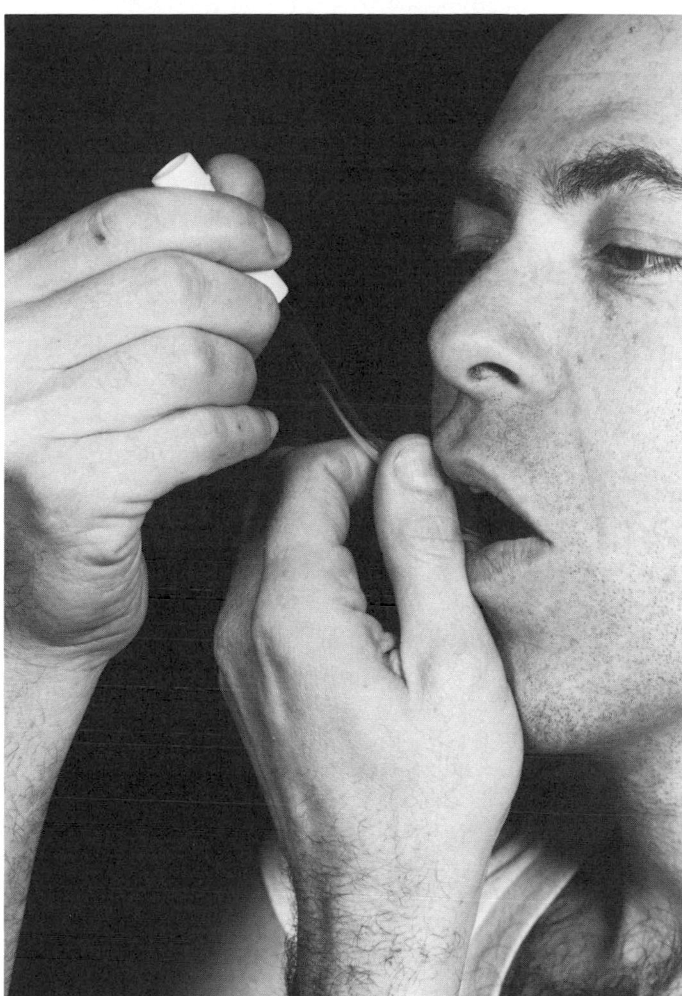

Figure 9.2 Patient passing a feeding tube through his mouth. This serves as a convenient way to take nutrition and helps to exercise weakened oral and pharyngeal musculature.

withdrawal (ABAB) paradigm. Measures of improvement were taken from descriptions of videoradiographs and actual timed sequences. They concluded that the efficacy of thermal stimulation with this design could not be denied or supported but could positively change some aspects of swallow performance.

Intellectual Controls

Most of the patients with dysphagia paralytica retain intellectual functions and some voluntary (upper motoneuron) control of the swallowing musculature, which can be used to advantage during feeding. Once the treatment plan has advanced to the point of using food and liquid to stimulate swallowing, the patient's attention can be focused on fully appreciating the taste, feel, and temperature of the bolus. Once the bolus has moved posteriorly in the oral cavity, the patient should concentrate on swallowing. This often triggers a reflex when the bolus alone fails to activate the weakened muscles (Larsen 1976). Some patients can be taught to hold a full breath consciously during each swallow and produce a gentle voluntary cough on completion of the swallow. This procedure may help protect the airway.

Surgical Alternatives

At times it is appropriate to consider surgical intervention either to improve the chances of the patient swallowing and protecting the airway or to provide an alternative route by which the patient can receive food and water. If radiography demonstrates that the cricopharyngeus has failed to relax, the patient may be a candidate for a myotomy of this sphincter. If the problem is unilateral vocal fold paralysis and associated ineffectiveness of cough and inability to seal the airway, injection of the paralyzed fold with an absorbable gelatin or a vocal fold medialization procedure can be considered (Crary and Golasky 1996; Kraus et al. 1996; Isshiki 1990).

It is important to remember that many patients with brain stem pathology, such as those with end-stage demyelinating diseases, will not improve or show increased strength in the swallowing musculature. As a consequence, they will not take food orally and a surgical alternative must be considered. In most cases we favor the feeding esophagostomy (English et al. 1970) over the gastrostomy because the patient can sit upright while eating, which aids in proper digestion; the tube can be removed between feedings, which is to the patient's psychological advantage; skin care is minimal; and the procedure is easily reversible should the patient's neurologic status improve. Percutaneous endoscopic placement also should be considered, although patients with bulbar pathology may be at respiratory risk when the esophagoscope is in place.

If a patient is incapable of protecting the airway from aspiration and recurrent aspiration pneumonia is a problem, considerations for surgery might include laryngeal closure (Montgomery 1975), tracheoesophageal anastomosis (Lindeman 1975), or even laryngectomy (Smith et al. 1965). Each of these procedures sacrifices voice but eliminates aspiration. Alternative forms of communication then become a primary consideration. (See Chapter 14 for a full discussion of surgical issues and procedures.)

TREATMENT OF PSEUDOBULBAR DYSPHAGIA

Of the patients with neurologic disease whom we have examined for dysphagia, the majority have pseudobulbar dysphagia. Typically, this is the result of bilateral upper motoneuron involvement. The patient frequently has had bilateral capsular infarctions, the first of which may cause transitory dysphagia, and successive infarcts cause further dysphagia. This does not seem unusual when

Table 9.1 Differences Between Pseudobulbar Dysphagia and Paralytic Dysphagia

Factor	*Paralytic Dysphagia*	*Pseudobulbar Dysphagia*
Pathology	Lower motoneuron	Upper motoneuron
Swallow reflex	Absent or very weak	Present, slow, or uncoordinated
Intellect	Intact	May be impaired
Oral strength	Poor	May be normal or uncoordinated
Affect	May be labile	Lability is common
Speech	Flaccid dysarthria	Spastic, hypokinetic, or hyperkinetic dysarthria

we remember the distinctive bilateral representation of swallow coordination. In the acute stages of single hemispheric stroke, dysphagia also may be present, and its effects are hemisphere-specific (Robbins and Levine 1988). Following the acute phase, most patients can expect improvement (Barer 1989). Pseudobulbar dysphagia also can be an effect of diffuse cerebrocortical disease. Older patients may have no other demonstrable neurologic deficits, but there is usually a pattern of "soft signs" of central nervous system disintegration together with decompensation in meeting daily needs. Cineradiologic swallows in such patients may be similar to those in patients who have specific demonstrable neurologic deficits. The overall pattern shows occasional penetration of swallowed material into the pharyngolaryngeal spaces with varying degrees of aspiration and reflex delay.

In pseudobulbar dysphagia, the musculature for swallowing may be somewhat weak and uncoordinated. This condition is distinguished from dysphagia secondary to involvement of the lower motoneurons in that patients retain a swallowing reflex even though it may be difficult to stimulate or initiate voluntarily (Table 9.1). On physical examination, signs such as positive bilateral extensor movements of the great toe (Babinski's sign) are found and are consistent with involvement of the upper motoneurons. Disinhibition of oral reflexes is considerable, as evidenced by active rooting, sucking, and biting reflexes that frequently interfere with feeding. Palatal and gag reflexes may be present and may be hyperactive. Speech may be harsh and unintelligible, and language expression and comprehension may be impaired. Because pseudobulbar dysphagia frequently results from bilateral damage to upper motoneurons, patients may lose the cortical controls of swallowing. Loss of learning potential and a reduced ability to make sound judgments may also be found in clinical testing. Disorientation and perceptual deficits may be present as well. Part of therapeutic management is directed toward compensating for these deficits (Miller and Groher 1982).

The loss of intellectual control over swallowing may be superimposed on uncoordinated performance. Because of the wide variance in the contribution of each of these factors, the clinician must be able to use different combinations of treatment strategies. The challenge is to employ the proper combination of intellectual controls in an effort to give the swallow reflex a maximal chance of triggering.

Loss of these intellectual controls translates behaviorally into (1) forgetting to chew and swallow, usually secondary to reduced environmental awareness or distractibility; (2) poor judgment characterized by excessive bite sizes or a rapid eating rate, making it most difficult to swallow an overly large bolus; (3) failure to adequately clear the oral cavity before the next bite (the phenomenon of squirreling or pouching of food contents may be related to sensory loss); (4) failure to understand feeding directions secondary to aphasia; (5) different degrees of parietal and frontal lobe pathology that interfere with the patient's perception of the food tray or result in inability to sequence the motor acts for feeding; (6) an attempt to eat and talk simultaneously, risking aspiration; (7) generalized failure to appreciate the importance of eating, which is often interpreted as lack of motivation, depression, or failure to cooperate; and (8) inability to organize and initiate a volitional swallow (Miller and Groher 1982).

Patients with pseudobulbar dysphagia frequently have a nasogastric tube already in place when a feeding plan is initiated. As stressed earlier, before beginning the program, it is desirable to have the patient in an optimal state of nutrition and hydration. The decompensating effects of nutritional deficiency and dehydration on bilaterally brain-damaged patients can be marked. Some become so decompensated that once they are fed by nasogastric or intravenous routes their ability to swallow improves dramatically. A team should include a physician and dietitian to monitor progress to give the patient the best chance to succeed when oral feeding trials begin.

First Feeding Trial

As soon as the patient is medically stable, appropriately alert, and cooperative, the first trial feeding can begin. Ideally, this is attempted with the nasogastric tube out, although there is no evidence that patients are not decompensated by small-bore nasoenteric feeding tubes. The trial should not be attempted immediately after a nasogastric feeding, which eliminates the hunger drive as an important motivator. The presence of a large (>14 French) tube during oral feeding has four negative effects: (1) it is a mechanical interference in a neurologically impaired system; (2) it partially blocks normal nasal air flow, which makes it more difficult to swallow; (3) its presence in the nasal cavity often forces the patient to mouth-breathe, which dries the oral mucosa and interferes with swallowing; and (4) it can cause food to adhere to it and fall off at an unexpected time and perhaps be aspirated.

Some patients with pseudobulbar dysfunction swallow well enough to protect the airway but fail to maintain an adequate nutritional state. Fatigue, distractions, and dietary factors may contribute to inadequate intake. Intermittent use of the nasogastric tube in the evening can supplement intake. Clinicians should watch for evidence of irritation of the nasal mucosa that can occur with frequent passage of a feeding tube.

Selection of Foods

As with dysphagia paralytica, the principle of maximal stimulation to trigger the reflex should be applied to patients with pseudobulbar dysphagia. "Easy to chew does not mean easy to swallow" (Larsen 1976). We recommend using foods that maximally stimulate sensory receptors and are of such consistency that they can be swallowed as a single bolus.

Patients with pseudobulbar dysphagia typically report that liquids are more difficult to swallow than solids. Complaints of problems controlling liquids are most believable for patients whose swallowing mechanisms lack the proper timing and reflex elicitation due to neurologic impairment. Slow, spastic muscles are particularly susceptible to having liquids unpredictably spill into the pharynx. Fruit juices are somewhat better because they are flavorful. We have had greater success with liquids when they are first frozen into slush form. The slush consistency provides temperature and texture and helps to form a more predictable and therefore more manageable bolus. Another medium for facilitating intake of liquids is gelatin desserts, particularly when they are prepared with less water than usual (finger gelatin) or blenderized to the consistency of whipped cream. Food in these forms does not melt rapidly and is moderately manageable in the mouth and pharynx. Additionally, commercially prepared thickeners that can be added to any fluid may be used to control fluids. Some alter fluid texture significantly and may be rejected by the patient. None have been tested for tolerance by the lungs following aspiration.

Most of these patients do best with solid foods of soft consistency. If possible, it helps to select foods in this category that the patient enjoys. If this information is unavailable from the patient, a family member or friend usually can provide it. Foods that the patient enjoys serve as motivators and are easier to swallow because of their appeal. The clinician always should try to make the first few bites significant, and using the patient's favorite foods can help. Selecting the proper semisolid and thickening fluids for those with pseudobulbar dysphagia significantly reduced the occurrence of aspiration pneumonia in patients with known histories of this complication (Groher 1987).

Food items that have proved to be effective in eliciting swallowing are medium-soft boiled eggs, cottage cheese, and sliced canned peaches (Larsen 1976). Bergman (1982) listed foods that are tolerated best in the early stages of treatment: mildly sweet and salty foods; gelatin; poached, boiled, or scrambled eggs; clear soups; broccoli, beets, carrots, peas, and beans; egg and tuna salad; and gravy. She goes on to list foods that are difficult to eat, including such items as hamburger patties, plums, prunes, mashed potatoes, cola-flavored carbonated beverages, all crackers except biscuits, and onions. We recommend that medications be given in custard, jelly, or blenderized flavored gelatin rather than in an applesauce mixture because of the latter's tendency to fall apart during swallowing. Sticky foods, dry substances, mucus producers, and boluses that fall apart should be avoided.

The patient may tend to use poor judgment by attempting to wash down a solid bolus with liquids. This can lead to aspiration if the bolus has either been inadequately masticated or has become lodged in the valleculae. Even mixing liquids with solids in a single bite can confuse the sensory receptors of brain-damaged patients and result in a choking episode.

Intellectual Controls

Selecting the correct diet must be combined with providing the intellectual controls the patient may lack. Therefore, all beginning feedings require direct assistance aimed at providing the necessary cortical inputs to get a patient swallowing safely.

The first step in providing these controls is to reduce the number of environmental distractions that tend to draw the patient's attention from eating. The first set of distractions is patient-generated. For instance, discomfort due to an improperly positioned arm can focus attention away from eating. If the patient is in pain, prescribed analgesics should be taken well before the meal so that the patient feels their comforting effect by mealtime. All prosthetic aids should be working and fitting properly or they are a constant source of distraction. Patients with heavy mucus secretions should have thorough suctioning before meals. Papain, found in most meat tenderizers or in tablet form at health food stores, can be used on a swab to thin thickened secretions. The oral cavity may need to be cleaned with a fresh swab or toothbrush to stimulate saliva flow and provide needed moisture. In short, the patient should be as comfortable as possible before eating.

The second set of distractions comes from outside sources such as other patients, staff, televisions, and radios. Turning off the television and radio, pulling curtains, and closing doors or facing the patient toward the wall all help the dysphagic individual concentrate on swallowing. The importance of minimizing these distractions in preparation for swallowing should not be overlooked. We have seen patients who complain at initial feedings about discomfort from leg braces, hand splints, condom catheters, or intravenous apparatus, making it impossible to focus their attention on feeding. Clinicians who have made the effort to rehabilitate patients with bilateral brain pathology can attest to the importance of reducing distractions as a prerequisite to learning.

Feeding Process

After the patient has been properly settled in an upright position, head slightly forward with neck flexed, the feeding process can be initiated (Figure 9.3). (See Chapter 10 for additional detail.) The clinician should avoid long explanations of what is to be expected and accomplished; these explanations often confuse brain-damaged patients, particularly those with language deficits. For the same reason, the clinician should avoid excessive verbal and gestural cuing during feeding. In most cases, the patient knows the person is there to assist with feeding, and that is sufficient.

The feeding process begins with the patient or feeder loading the utensil with a medium-sized bite (about 15 cc). Bites smaller than this may not create

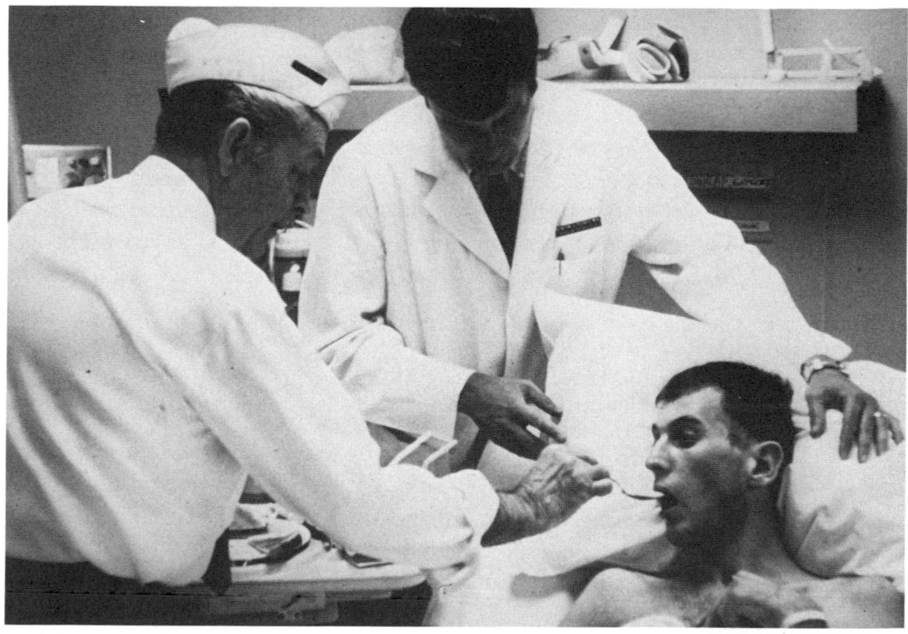

Figure 9.3 Bedridden patient is positioned properly for oral intake with the assistance of a trained volunteer.

enough pressure to trigger the reflex easily. It often helps to let the patient see and smell the bolus before placing it midway into the oral cavity. This helps to prepare the mechanism for swallowing and is not unlike what happens with normal eating. What the patient does with the bolus should be immediately assessed, including elicitation of a swallow reflex (by palpation or auscultation), postswallow residuals and phonatory integrity, and attention to change in the respiratory baseline. The proper bolus size and amount can be determined with dynamic radiography that samples the effect of these variables on the pharyngeal swallow. No evidence suggests, however, that successful ingestion of one bolus size predicts effective swallow of larger or smaller boluses.

Cognitive cues must be provided as necessary. Some patients need verbal or gestural cuing to chew; some need to be told when to swallow; others need to be reminded that food has remained in their mouth and that it must be swallowed before another bite is taken. At this point, it is important to let the patient know when the desired sequence of motor behaviors has been performed (Hargrove 1980). Constant reinforcement of correct behaviors helps the patient retain what has been learned.

The clinician should carefully observe each swallow, paying particular attention to the moment of laryngeal elevation. If the patient prematurely tires or loses interest, no attempt should be made to force feed, because this will only frustrate both clinician and patient (Hargrove 1980). If the patient progresses satisfactorily, the clinician should begin to eliminate specific cues and observe for evidence of compensations in behavior and improved judgment while eating. Some patients will not make these generalizations, and family members or other attendants must be trained to provide the proper input at each meal.

Patients who demonstrate active biting and rooting reflexes that can interfere with placement of utensils often do well if they are allowed to feed themselves. If motor control does not allow this, we recommend a trial with finger foods in measured bites that can be placed in the mouth without utensils or reflex inhibition techniques as described in Chapter 10.

Many patients need an excessive amount of time to complete a meal. Because of the time factor, foods tend to become cold and unappetizing and therefore less stimulating. Patients in this stage of swallowing management benefit from receiving smaller portions more frequently or from early tray scheduling.

MYASTHENIA GRAVIS

Because myasthenia gravis involves the striated musculature, it may compromise swallowing. Commonly, it shows a predilection for the bulbar nuclei, with accompanying dysphagia.

An estimated 33% of patients with myasthenia have significant deglutitory disorders due to fatigue following mastication (Murray 1962; Silbiger et al. 1967).

Because of this tendency for the musculature to fatigue easily after repeated exercise, patients typically do well at the beginning of a meal but tire at the end (Merritt 1967). Mastication and swallowing may be normal and then deteriorate to the point at which there is total loss of the ability to chew and swallow. Continued attempts at feeding past this point can lead to significant aspiration.

Murray (1962) demonstrated by cinefluoroscopy that tongue movements were slow and weak and continued to weaken with additional attempts at swallowing. Holding the bolus on the tongue was particularly troublesome. He studied 23 patients with disease ranging from mild to severe. Most had barium residual in the oropharynx and valleculae because the tongue failed to arch backward and down into the pharynx. Patients with moderate to severe disease could not clear the valleculae on repeated attempts. There was no evidence of myasthenia affecting the cricopharyngeal sphincter, a finding that Silbiger and colleagues (1967) and Donner and Siegel (1965) supported. Kramer et al. (1957), however, reported on two patients whose cricopharyngeus tired as quickly as their tongue and pharynx. Using cinefluorography, Donner and Siegel (1965) noted the marked fatigability of the tongue and pharyngeal musculature on repeated swallowing attempts. The pharyngeal walls showed prolonged barium coating with pharyngeal recess pooling and loss of tone. Repeated swallowing in some patients produced nasal regurgitation because the pharynx failed to rise adequately to seal the nasopharyngeal port.

The observation that patients with myasthenia have difficulty holding a bolus on the tongue suggests that patients may do better if they are given foods that do not fall apart easily during mastication. Such foods require more lingual effort and hasten fatigue.

Typically, patients with myasthenia are given anticholinesterase-producing drugs that, when administered in the proper doses, greatly facilitate muscle movement. It is important that these medications be coordinated with feeding times to facilitate swallowing. If possible, patients should be reminded to limit physical activity before a meal in an effort to maintain sufficient strength to complete it. Such activity can range from strenuous physical therapy to excessive talking. Conservation of energy in the early stages of dysphagia often makes the difference between oral or nasogastric feeding.

AMYOTROPHIC LATERAL SCLEROSIS

ALS, a progressive disease of the upper and lower motoneurons, is of unknown cause and is without known treatment. In a significant number of patients, bulbar muscles are involved and the patient experiences serious difficulties with swallowing. In other cases, the deterioration of ALS is confined to muscles supplied by the spinal cord, and dysphagia, if present, is related to the loss of respiratory muscle support.

Clinical findings in the ALS patient with bulbar involvement show a combination of spasticity and flaccidity. In the bulbar muscles specifically, the muscles of mastication (particularly the pterygoids) develop weakness that is experienced as chewing fatigue. The facial muscles (particularly the orbicularis oris) may become weak, and drooling is common. The lingual muscles are frequently the first bulbar muscles affected (Hillel and Miller 1989) and may look like a "bag of worms" because of muscle fasciculations (Blount et al.1979). As atrophy continues, the tongue weakens and may eventually be paralyzed. Palatal and pharyngeal weakness is common. Nasal regurgitation is possible when swallowing, but is not a common finding. The gag reflexes may range from hyperactive in one patient to absent in another. An intact gag can disappear during the course of the disease. The suprahyoid muscles that elevate the larynx may develop weakness, cramping, or both, and the cricopharyngeus may fail to open during swallowing. Impairment of vocal fold function is a frequent complication. Vocal cord adduction may be incomplete and the folds may appear bowed as they meet. More commonly, vocal cord abduction is impaired, causing restriction of breathing due to incomplete or even paradoxical movement (Hillel and Miller 1989). Progressive respiratory insufficiency and weakness of abdominal muscles lead to a poor protective cough. Loss of sensation is infrequently reported and most patients retain good cognitive function.

Since the dysphagia of ALS generally is progressive and the symptoms variable, establishing a baseline of function and following the patient throughout the course of the disease is recommended. The baseline data should include a thorough clinical examination for dysphagia (see Chapter 7) and a scaled assessment of bulbar and spinal muscle functions. The ALS Severity Scale is a reliable, easily administered ordinal instrument that can be used to measure speech, swallowing, and upper- and lower-extremity functions for staging the disease (Hillel et al. 1989; Yorkston et al. 1995). On follow-up examinations the clinician should obtain an accurate weight, a current diet and fluid intake record, a pulmonary vital capacity measure, and a functional staging of the disease. Some centers advocate following patients with a series of cineradiographic studies (Bosma and Brodie 1969). However, such studies are costly and not easily tolerated by patients with advanced disease. When dysphagia symptoms suggest the presence of concomitant disease (e.g., esophageal dysfunction) or the complaints are not consistent with motor neuron disease, fluoroscopic studies of swallowing should be considered.

Management of dysphagia should begin early in the course of the disease. The initial emphasis is on patient education and the prevention of complications associated with dysphagia and nutritional or fluid deficiencies. Patients need to be instructed to eat in an upright posture with the neck flexed (DeLisa et al. 1979). Foods that cause problems should be noted so that the consistency of the diet can be controlled. As expected, thin fluids are more easily aspirated than solids. Blenderized foods may act like liquid and fall apart in the mouth and pharynx. Soft, cohesive food boluses such as macaroni casseroles and custard tend to be tolerated well in early stages. Because abdominal muscles are weakened, constipation is a frequent complaint and high-fiber diets are recommended. As with other dysphagic patients, sticky food and dry, crumbly substances should be minimized in the diet. Optimal calorie and fluid intake requirements should be defined and the patient's progress toward these goals measured.

As the disease progresses, oral feeding may become unsafe and inefficient. In our experience, aspiration pneumonitis is not a common complication in ALS until the patient reaches end-stage disease. The progressive nature of the dysphagia and difficulties with self-feeding commonly result in a loss of enjoyment, fear, and even dread of eating. It is imperative to identify these feelings.

It is the dysphagia specialist's role to recommend procedures that may improve swallowing or alternative methods of providing nutrition. The alternative of choice for nutritional management is percutaneous endoscopic gastrostomy (PEG) performed under local anesthesia. This procedure does not interfere with swallowing functions and can be used either to supplement oral feedings or for primary nutritional intake. A nonsurgical feeding tube alternative that can be used when the patient's gag reflex permits is intermittent orogastric placement. A nasogastric tube may be used for patients in end-stage disease when other alternatives are not feasible.

Timing is very important when recommending surgical alternatives to swallowing. While many patients wish to maintain oral intake of food and liquid for as long as possible, those who quit eating and drinking for even short periods of time may become too weak to withstand surgical intervention. Others have severely compromised respiratory systems, predisposing them to surgical complications (Short and Hillel 1989). Even a PEG cannot be safely performed after pulmonary vital capacity falls below 1 L. Therefore, continuous monitoring of patients' ability and desire to eat and their nutrition and hydration status is necessary for optimal management.

Clinicians who offer symptomatic management for patients with progressive motoneuron disease should realize that the clinical course is highly variable and, so far, unpredictable. Although the primary symptoms cannot be arrested or prevented, the support offered by the dysphagia specialist may go far in preventing secondary complications of malnutrition, dehydration, aspiration, and improving the quality of the patient's remaining life (Strand et al. 1996).

HUNTINGTON'S CHOREA

Some of the feeding problems of patients with Huntington's chorea are unique to this disease; others are typical of patients with pseudobulbar dysphagia. The characteristic choreatic movements of Huntington's disease eventually severely compromise feeding and swallowing. At the time of diagnosis, feeding and swallowing disorders are infrequent. As the disease progresses, however, and the involuntary movements become more frequent and uncontrollable, dysphagia emerges as a significant problem. The constant movements burn a significant number of calories and patients frequently have appetites that are difficult to satisfy; their focus on food and eating becomes paramount. Difficulty with oral intake conflicts with their unsatisfied hunger and creates a significant feeding management problem. For some patients, their frustrations are compounded by documented changes in mental status that interfere with the ability to learn compensatory feeding and swallowing strategies. The majority are not cognizant of their swallowing deficits, but with treatment can learn to make necessary compensations (Kagel and Leopold 1992).

Typically, patients first lose the ability to manipulate utensils for self-feeding and require direct assistance in food transport. Once food and liquids are placed in the mouth they usually are managed without great difficulty. At this stage, some patients prefer to remain independent in feeding and therefore exercise the option of increasing the number of food items that can be consumed without utensils such as sandwiches, fruits, and selected vegetables.

As the choreatic movements intensify, there is marked involvement in the coordination of swallowing. In addition, unpredictable, sudden gulps of air during the inspiratory cycle open the glottis at irregular intervals, compromising protection of the airway. The head may suddenly be thrust back, exposing the airway. Because of the characteristic writhing tongue, lateralization and posterior transportation of food toward the pharynx are difficult. Forming the posterior bolus needed to trigger a swallowing reflex becomes an obstacle in completing a normal swallow (Kilman 1977). Foods and liquids reach the oropharynx with unpredictable speed. We can postulate that such irregular control may create abnormal timing sequences that invite laryngeal penetration and aspiration. Kagel and Leopold (1992) gathered diagnostic and treatment data on the behavioral and swallowing characteristics of 35 patients with Huntington's disease of a mean duration of 6.6 years. All but one had moderately advanced disease with dysphagia. Following videoradiographic and clinical evaluation, the patients fell into two categories: those with primary hyperkinetic features (30) and those with rigid and bradykinetic symptoms. Those with hyperkinetic features were not as liable to pharyngeal decompensation with aspiration as those with bradykinesia and rigidity. Interruption of normal esophageal peristalsis coincident with respiratory chorea resulting in distal-to-proximal bolus redirection was a finding in 14 patients with a hyperkinetic component and in none of those with bradykinesia.

Initial treatment for both groups (Kagel and Leopold 1992) focused on proper trunk and leg support, with below-the-waist food presentation to maintain neck flexion. The hyperkinetic group was trained in incentive spirometry to control respiratory patterns prior to attempts at oral feeding. Oral chorea was managed with precedent iced-lemon stimuli followed by a textured bolus with iced-lemon impregnation. For this group, crisp substances in textured foods enhanced mastication. For those with bradykinetic features, swallow was enhanced by lateral and dorsal tongue tapping, with training in a negative suck transfer focusing on labial closure. Iced-lemon stimuli were effective in clearing pharyngeal residue after each swallow. With a median re-evaluation period of 5 years, patients in both groups continued to eat by mouth. Some needed periodic treatment sessions to reinforce compensatory strategies.

Over a 5-year period, Groher had the opportunity to follow six patients with advanced Huntington's disease and swallowing complaints. All patients were hospitalized, nonambulatory, and could not meet most of their daily needs, including self-feeding. Four of the six had accompanying changes in mental status such as poor judgment, uncontrollable outbursts of temper, and disorientation. Their mean age was 47.6 years. All patients had had the disease for 12 years or more.

The patients were evaluated for their dysphagic complaints. At the time of the evaluation, all were receiving their nutrition orally; however, fluoroscopic evidence of increased laryngeal penetration suggested they should receive a complete dysphagia work-up. None had demonstrable aspiration pneumonia, although the nurses reported considerable choking, sputtering, and prolonged coughing at mealtimes. All six were eating puréed foods and not one was satisfied with this diet. The swallowing evaluation consistently revealed the following: (1) the nursing assistant who was feeding the patient had great difficulty placing the food in the patient's mouth due to marked choreatic movements of the head and trunk; (2) once the food was placed, the tongue often pushed the bolus anteriorly out of the mouth; (3) oral mastication was labored and the time between oral placement and a swallow reflex was not consistent, frequently being either too fast or delayed; (4) laryngeal elevation during swallowing was normal; (5) solids were managed better than liquids; (6) all had protective coughs; (7) all swallowed a soft mechanical diet without difficulty; and (8) all swallowed more efficiently when the environment was free of distraction (measured by less coughing and shorter total mealtime).

The evaluation revealed that the most crucial phase of swallowing management in patients with Huntington's disease took place in the preparatory stages of swallowing. For instance, two of six patients could not maintain a proper position for effective swallowing. This was managed as well as possible by providing head and trunk restraints during meals. Such restraints, of course, did not reduce the choreatic movements but did help patients to maintain upright posture. Spoon feeding was accomplished best when the feeder did not try to introduce the spoon at his or her will, but rather held the spoon in front of the patients waiting for them to take the food from it. Allowing the patient to take the food voluntarily resulted in fewer incidents of the tongue pushing the bolus out of the oral cavity. Finally, all patients were more motivated to eat because they received a diet that was more pleasing to their senses and equally as easy to swallow.

PARKINSON'S DISEASE

Another variant of pseudobulbar symptomatology is seen in patients with Parkinson's disease. The clinical features of tremor and rigidity may precipitate swallowing dysfunction. Like those with Huntington's chorea, patients with Parkinson's disease become progressively handicapped and are frequently not aware of their swallowing disability (Robbins et al. 1986; Bushmann et al. 1989). When rigidity is the prominent feature, dysphagia becomes a significant management problem (Lieberman et al. 1980).

Lieberman and associates (1980) contended that some degree of dysphagia may be present in 50% of cases, but it is rarely so severe as to require gastrostomy. Eadie and Tyrer (1965a) reported a similar figure, and our clinical experience suggests that most patients are able to take nutrition orally, even in the end stages of disease. Eadie and Tyrer (1965b) found no correlation between severity of disease and dysphagia. In 25% of these patients, dysphagic complaints began within 2 years of diagnosis. Their findings are supported by Lieberman and his colleagues (1980), who studied two cases with end-stage disease; one had adequate voice and tongue mobility but aspirated, and one had poor voice and tongue movement but did not aspirate. After studying six patients radiographically with varying stages of disease, Robbins and colleagues (1986) did not find correlative evidence between swallowing disability and disease stage, although the most severe did have the largest number of videoradiographic abnormalities.

The results of cineradiography are conflicting. Silbiger and associates (1967) found swallowing abnormalities in all 11 patients studied. Abnormalities were described as poor bolus formation, misdirected swallow, abnormal pharyngeal motility, pharyngeal stasis, and abnormal cricopharyngeal function. Eadie and Tyrer (1965a) questioned 107 patients and postulated that dysphagia existed secondary to faulty control of the pharyngeal constrictors. Palmer (1974) reported that the dysphagia associated with Parkinson's disease usually was due to hypopharyngeal dysfunction and recommended relief with posterior cricopharyngeal sphincterotomy. Calne and associates (1970) studied 20 patients and found no pharyngeal pathology. They attributed the differences between their studies and Silbiger's to the fact that the latter studied patients in the prone position rather than sitting upright. Calne et al. (1970) concluded that parkinsonism dysphagia was primarily related to oral or esophageal disorders or both, as they had noted lingual hesitancy and piecemeal deglutition in the oral stages. They presented fluoroscopic evidence of excessive mastication time, limited tongue and mandibular excursion, and poor posterior bolus formation. Once a swallow reflex was triggered, the larynx rose normally. Robbins et al. (1986) described both oral (most prominent) and pharyngeal stage abnormalities but did not find isolated impairment in the pharyngoesophageal segment. Of particular importance in their study was the prevalence of aspiration without cough in patients who had no dysphagic complaints, a finding supported by the work of Bushmann et al. (1989). Logemann et al. (1977) presented cineradiographic evidence showing that regardless of the stage of the disease, patients have slowed oral and esophageal transit times.

Other investigators have noted the presence of esophageal symptoms in patients with Parkinson's disease. Eadie and Tyrer (1965b) compared a group of 72 patients with parkinsonism with matched controls, finding a higher incidence of esophageal abnormalities in those with parkinsonism, including esophageal spasm, hiatal hernia, and gastroesophageal reflux. They speculated that some disorders of esophageal motility may be secondary to involvement of the dorsal vagal nucleus.

We can conclude from these investigations that swallowing disorders in parkinsonism may be present in varying degrees and combinations in the mouth, pharynx, and esophagus, and that the severity of the movement disorder probably does not correlate with the severity of the dysphagia.

Because of the excessive time taken for oral mastication, it is advantageous for patients to eat smaller portions more frequently, especially if feeding times are restricted. Changing the portions and increasing the length of mealtimes have two distinct psychologic advantages. First, patients feel they do not need to finish a large portion in a short time and therefore enjoy their meals more. Second, they are aware that they will not be left hungry if they do not finish one large meal in a fixed time segment. These facilitators are important motivators for swallowing.

In our experience, patients with Parkinson's disease generally do well with regular diets. In the end stages of disease, they find it easier to eat soft foods that require less effort to masticate. Teaching a more posterior spoon placement often helps reduce oral transit times, but patients must avoid bypassing sensory receptors that help trigger the swallow reflex.

The timing of dopaminergic medications should coincide with mealtimes so that their effect can facilitate oral and pharyngeal movements. Such an effect will vary from patient to patient depending on drug dosage and individual metabolic rates. Lieberman and associates (1980) pointed out that it is important to have patients swallow their medications because parenteral anticholinergics are not as effective as levodopa taken orally. However, ingestion of solid forms of medication may be problematic, retention of pills in the valleculae leading to irregular absorption and subsequent lack of a clinical response (Bushmann et al. 1989). Esophageal dismotility may compromise absorption further. In our experience, discontinuance of medications to manage parkinsonism to evaluate a clinical response to new drugs or dosage levels may put the patient at risk for aspiration. As the drug is withdrawn, patients should be monitored closely for signs of aspiration and changes in the physical and mental status examination that might predispose to decreased ability to protect the airway. The usefulness of levodopa in alleviating dysphagic symptoms remains controversial, however. Some patients have benefited, others have not (Cotzias et al. 1969; Calne et al. 1970; Lieberman et al. 1980). Bushmann et al. (1989) found general improvement in swallow for those patients on oral levadopa and carbidopa, but no improvement in swallow after increasing the dosage.

SUMMARY

This chapter contains some general treatment guidelines for patients who suffer from dysphagia secondary to neurologic impairments. Specific treatment and pretreatment considerations for this group are covered in the following chapter.

The clinician must remain cognizant of the fact that signs and symptoms of neurologic pathology may change over time. In addition, well-described disease entities and processes affect patients in differing ways. Therefore, we should not lose sight of the fact that dysphagia management with this group of patients is predicated on individualized plans.

REFERENCES

Barer DH. The natural history and functional consequences of dysphagia after hemispheric stroke. J Neurol Neurosurg Psychiatr 1989;52:236.

Bergman K. Dysphagia in the adult patient. Presented at conference on rehabilitation of dysphagia in adults. Detroit, Michigan, July 29 and 30, 1982.

Blount M, Bratton C, Luttrell N. Management of the patient with amyotrophic lateral sclerosis. Nurs Clin North Am 1979;14:157.

Bonanno PC. Swallowing dysfunction after tracheostomy. Ann Surg 1971;174:29.

Bosma JF, Brodie DR. Disabilities of the pharynx in ALS as demonstrated by cineradiography. Radiology 1969;92:97.

Bushmann M, Dobymeyer SM, Leeker L, et al. Swallowing abnormalities and their response to treatment in Parkinson's disease. Neurology 1989;39:1309.

Calne DB, Shaw DG, Spiers ASD, et al. Swallowing in parkinsonism. Br J Radiol 1970;43:456.

Campbell-Taylor I, Nadon GW, Schlacter AL, et al. Oro-esophageal tube feeding: an alternative to nasogastric or gastrostomy tubes. Dysphagia 1988;4:220.

Cotzias GC, Papavalilion PS, Gellene R. Modification of parkinsonism—chronic treatment with L-dopa. N Engl J Med 1969;280:337.

Crary M, Golasky A. Vocal fold immobility. In WS Brown, B Vinson, M Crary (eds), Organic Voice Disorders. San Diego: Singular Press, 1996.

Curran J, Groher ME. Development and dissemination of an aspiration risk reduction diet. Dysphagia 1990;5:6.

DeLisa JA, Mikulic MA, Miller RM, et al. Amyotrophic lateral sclerosis: comprehensive management. Am Fam Physician 1979;19:137.
Donner MW, Siegel CI. The evaluation of pharyngeal neuromuscular disorders by cinefluorography. Am J Roentgenol 1965;94:299.
Eadie MJ, Tyrer JH. Radiological abnormalities in the upper part of the alimentary tract in parkinsonism. Aust Ann Med 1965;14:23a.
Eadie MJ, Tyrer JH. Alimentary disorders in parkinsonism. Aust Ann Med 1965;14:13b.
English GM, Morfit HM, Ratzer ER. Cervical esophagostomy in head and neck cancer. Arch Otolaryngol 1970;92:335.
Groher ME. Bolus management and aspiration pneumonia in patients with pseudobulbar dysphagia. Dysphagia 1987;1:215.
Hargrove R. Feeding the severely involved patient. J Neurosurg Nurs 1980;12:102.
Hillel AD, Miller RM. Bulbar amyotrophic lateral sclerosis: patterns of progression and clinical management. Head Neck 1989;11:51.
Hillel AD, Miller RM, Yorkston K, et al. Amyotrophic lateral sclerosis severity scale. Neuroepidemiology 1989;8:142.
Isshiki N. Medialization of the Vocal Cord: Thyroplasty and Arytenoid Adduction. In CW Cummings, et al. (eds), Otolaryngology-Head and Neck Surgery. Update II. St. Louis: Mosby-Year Book, 1990;76.
Kagel MC, Leopold NA. Dysphagia in Huntington's disease: a 16-year retrospective. Dysphagia 1992;7:106.
Kilman WJ. Diseases of the pharynx and larynx. Curr Probl Diagn Radiol 1977;7:1.
Kramer P, Atkinson M, Wyman SM, et al. The dynamics of swallowing. II. Neuromuscular dysphagia of the pharynx. J Clin Invest 1957;36:589.
Krans DH, Ali MK, Ginsberg RJ, et al. Vocal cord medialization for unilateral paralysis associated with intrathoracic malignancies. J Thoracic Cardiovasc Surg 1996;111:336.
Larsen GL. Rehabilitating dysphagia: mechanica, paralytica, pseudobulbar. J Neurosurg Nurs 1976;8:14.
Lazzara GD, Lazarus C, Logemann JA. Impact of thermal stimulation on the triggering of the swallowing reflex. Dysphagia 1986;1:73.
Lieberman AM, Horowitz L, Redmond P, et al. Dysphagia in Parkinson's disease. Am J Gastroenterol 1980;74:157.
Lindeman RC. Diverting the paralyzed larynx: a reversible procedure for intractable aspiration. Laryngoscope 1975;85:157.
Logemann JA, Boshes B, Blonsky RE, et al. Speech and swallowing evaluation in the differential diagnosis of neurologic disease. Neurologica-Neurocirugia-Psiquiatria 1977;18:71.
Merritt HH. A Textbook of Neurology. Philadelphia: Lea & Febiger, 1967.
Miller RM, Groher ME. The evaluation and management of neuromuscular and mechanical swallowing disorders. Dysarthria Dysphonia Dysphagia 1982;1:50.
Montgomery WW. Surgery to prevent aspiration. Arch Otolaryngol 1975;101:679.
Murray JP. Deglutition in myasthenia gravis. Br J Radiol 1962;35:43.
Palmer ED. Dysphagia in parkinsonism. JAMA 1974;229:1349.
Robbins J, Levine RL. Swallowing after unilateral stroke of the cerebral cortex: preliminary experience. Dysphagia 1988;3:11.
Robbins JA, Logeman J, Kirshner A. Swallowing and speech in Parkinson's disease. Ann Neurol 1986;19:283.
Rosenbek JC, Robbins J, Fishback B, et al. Effect of thermal application on dysphagia after stroke. J Speech Hear Res 1991;34:1257.
Shin T, Tadatsugu M, Umezaki T, et al. Surgical Rehabilitation for Dysphagia Caused by Neuromuscular Disorders. In T Inouye, H Fukuda, T Sato et al. (eds), Recent Advances in Bronchoesophagology. Amsterdam: Excerpta Medica, 1990.
Short SO, Hillel AD. Palliative surgery in patients with bulbar amyotrophic lateral sclerosis. Head Neck 1989;11:364.

Silbiger ML, Pikielney R, Donner MW. Neuromuscular disorders affecting the pharynx: cineradiographic analysis. Invest Radiol 1967;2:442.
Smith AC, Spanling JM, Ardran G, et al. Laryngectomy in the management of severe dysphagia in nonmalignant conditions. Lancet 1965;2:1094.
Strand EA, Miller RM, Yorkston KM, Hillel AD. Management of oral-pharyngeal dysphagia symptoms in amyotrophic lateral sclerosis. Dysphagia 1996;11:129.
Yorkston KM, Miller RM, Strand EA. Management of Speech and Swallowing in Degenerative Disease. Tucson, AZ: Communication Skill Builders, 1995;81.

10

Management of Neurologic Disorders: The First Feeding Session

Wendy Avery-Smith

Evaluation of a patient with neurogenic dysphagia reveals whether the patient is alert enough for a feeding trial, what areas of oral and pharyngeal impairment may interfere with swallowing, and what risk factors may be associated with aspiration. Although a preliminary estimation of swallowing prognosis can be made based on clinical evaluation and radiographic studies, only implementation of a course of treatment will determine the patient's ultimate potential for safe eating. The goal for the patient with potential for dysphagia rehabilitation may range from independent consumption of a full oral diet to limited oral feeding with compensatory techniques and nonoral supplements.

Due to the changes in status that accompany many neurologic disorders, reevaluation is an inherent part of the initial feeding session and all subsequent ones. Patients with neurogenic dysphagia may have a safe but compensated swallow; decompensation caused by the natural course of disease may lead to an unsafe swallow (Buchholz et al. 1985). The clinician must keep in mind that changes in the care plan are an important and integral part of treatment.

This chapter begins with a program for prefeeding management to address the cognitive, perceptual, physical, and functional concerns that so often accompany dysphagia in the neurogenic dysphagia patient. Feeding training with emphasis on the initial feeding sessions is then presented.

PREFEEDING MANAGEMENT

Cognitive and Perceptual Status

Alertness and cooperation on the part of the patient are prerequisites for a safe feeding trial because lethargy and unwillingness to eat may increase the risk of aspiration. Mackay and Morgan (1992) observed that while head-injured patients at the Rancho Los Amigos Adult Levels of Cognitive Functioning Scale level 4, characterized by confusion and agitation, are ready to safely begin some oral intake, full oral intake did not occur until level 6, characterized by increasingly appropriate behaviors. For patients who are sleepy but easily roused, stimulation techniques may be used to improve the patient's level of arousal. Loud verbal and gentle physical stimulation, such as rubbing the patient's arm, may suffice. Occupational or physical therapy may have a beneficial effect on attention span, postural control, and swallowing skills; it may be therapeutic to schedule feeding sessions after other rehabilitative procedures. The room should be well lit and the patient positioned properly, as these factors have a stimulating effect on the central nervous system. Feeding sessions for patients who need intensive stimulation to pay attention for even brief periods should be deferred until the patient demonstrates a sufficient level of arousal.

Various strategies are helpful in working with the cognitively impaired or aphasic patient. Because eating is such a familiar and overlearned behavior, minimal orientation to the activity may be necessary. Even a very confused and distracted patient may demonstrate the attention span to eat, especially if he or she is hungry. Mere presentation of a serving of food provides a strong cue as to the activity at hand. Providing foods that are normally eaten at the time of day they are presented, such as oatmeal at breakfast, has an orienting effect on the patient. A quiet room with a minimum of distractions helps to direct the patient's attention to the food. Self-feeding helps to direct attention as well. For patients with unilateral inattention, a colorful "anchor," such as a piece of red construction paper, helps to draw the attention to the neglected side of the meal tray. Reducing the complexity of the visual array on the tray by presenting only one or two foods at a time may be helpful for these patients and for those with visual-perceptual dysfunction. Feeding sessions should not occur when a patient is fatigued, such as after test procedures. If a patient's overall endurance is reduced, time spent out of bed should be during mealtime. Because continuous drip and bolus tube feedings may suppress appetite and thus reduce motivation to eat, arrangements should be made to halt or delay these for several hours prior to the feeding session.

Apraxia

Apraxia is defined as the inability to plan and execute a skilled movement in the absence of sensory and motor deficits. The apraxic patient is not able to demonstrate a movement on verbal request. Oral and limb apraxias are frequently encountered in the dysphagic patient. Thus, the patient with oral apraxia is unable to smile when asked. Similarly the patient with limb apraxia is unable to demonstrate how to bring a spoon to the mouth. In treatment, the apraxic patient benefits from a natural setting, with food as the focus of activity. Demonstrating movements in addition to giving verbal cues enhances the patient's ability to execute oral movements. The patient may be able to self-feed in the context of the actual activity, even though demonstration of self-feeding out of context was impossible. If the patient is unable to initiate or follow through with movements, tactile cuing or guiding helps to organize available movements into self-feeding (Affolter 1987). Figure 10.1 demonstrates the sequence of movements as the therapist gently guides the patient during self-feeding. Often, guiding is necessary at the beginning of a session, but after several mouthfuls the patient can continue independently. Oral movements that were not elicited with verbal cues and demonstration may be observed during eating.

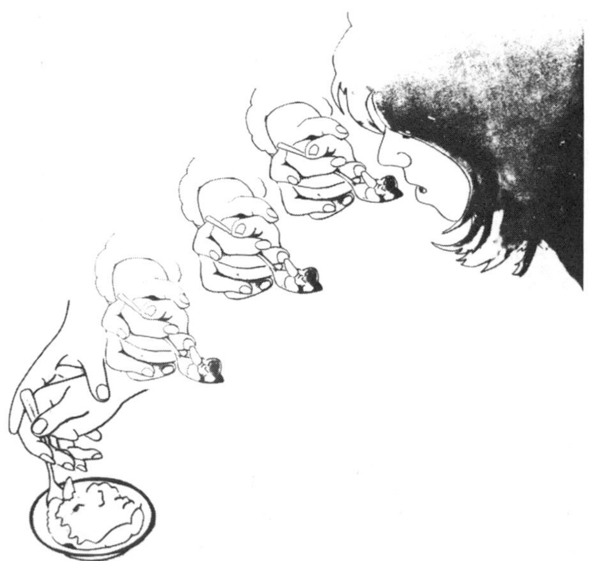

Figure 10.1 Tactile cueing or guiding to help the apraxic patient self-feed.

Sensory Impairment

When oral or facial sensation is impaired, the patient or caregiver must be educated as to the type and extent of impairment. Safety techniques for alterations in sensation may be done by the patient who is intellectually capable of remembering and carrying out techniques or by the caregiver. Such precautions must be emphasized to prevent injury from hot foods, biting, or other sources. Abnormal sensation may result from sensory loss or from heightened sensation.

In patients with severe hyposensitivity, food should be placed initially in the most sensitive area of the mouth, both to protect the patient and to provide maximal sensory stimulation. Taste, temperature, texture, shape, weight, and size define the sensory qualities of a bolus (Coster and Schwarz 1987). These characteristics stimulate swallowing, and the therapist may wish to experiment with these components to find the best bolus type for the patient. If there is food retention in sensory-impaired areas, the use of verbal cues, a mirror, and frequent observation of the oral cavity is helpful. As the patient progresses, food should be placed at midline to encourage sensory retraining and normal oral patterns. As skills improve, compensatory techniques may be gradually withdrawn.

Hypersensitivity to touch may be noted in brain-injured patients. This may take the form of aversive reactions such as grimacing or backing away from sensory stimuli. To treat this, Farber (1982) recommends applying continuous pressure with a finger to the perioral area across the maxilla between the nose and the upper lip. Once this is tolerated, pressure to the lips and the dorsum of the anterior third of the tongue may be maintained with a tongue blade and lip

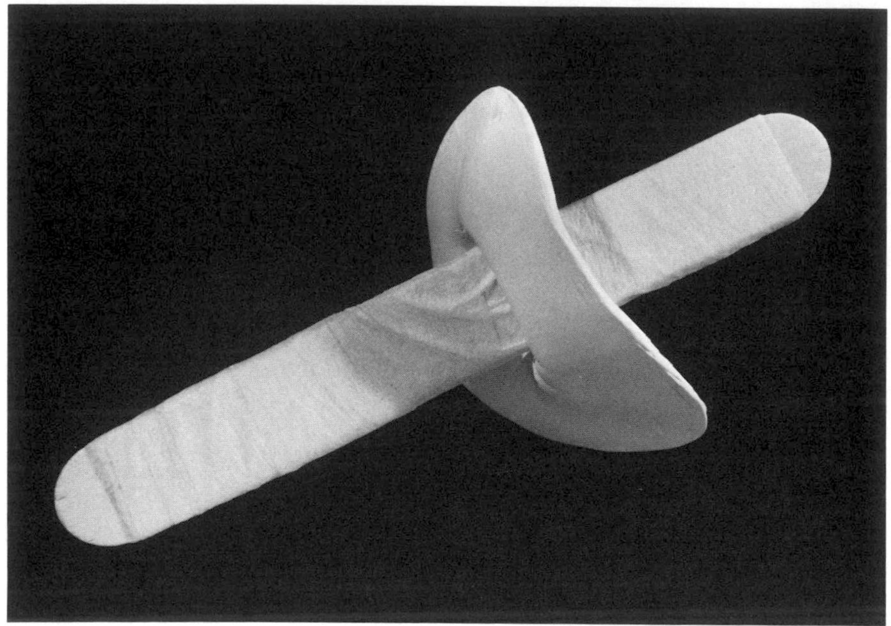

Figure 10.2 A modified tongue depressor can be used to apply pressure to the tongue dorsum to inhibit hypersensitivity.

mold (Figure 10.2). This device is fabricated by molding lip-shaped thermoplastic splinting material around a padded tongue blade. The patient may then progress to a graded program of application of sensory stimuli. Firm touch with a hard object is more easily tolerated, so the program starts with harder objects, such as eating utensils, and then progresses to softer objects, such as toothbrushes and moistened swabs. Touch is gradually reduced in pressure. The patient may be better able to tolerate self-application of stimuli (O'Sullivan 1990). For patients in whom the fear of eating or choking causes or exacerbates hypersensitivity to touch, muscle relaxation techniques may be useful in reducing anxiety and heightened oral muscle tone (Brown et al. 1992).

Oral Hygiene and Prosthetic Considerations

Extra care must be taken in providing oral hygiene to dysphagic patients. Because of diminished sensation, the patient may not feel residual food particles in the oral cavity. Mouth breathing may cause additional drying of oral structures, secretions, and residual food. Dried food and secretions further inhibit sensation and promote growth of bacteria. Oral care should be provided after each feeding session and may need to be done before feeding. Lemon glycerine swabs or a swab dipped in diluted mouthwash may be used to clean around the teeth and gums. Synthetic salivas, originally developed for the cancer patient with xerostomia, may be useful with this population as well. Secretions that are thick or hardened in the oral cavity should be moistened and removed with a damp washcloth. If the patient has the oral control and airway protection to do so, he or she should brush the teeth and rinse the mouth, with assistance and supervision as needed.

Dentures and partial plates should be worn. If muscle tone has been affected by neurologic illness, oral prostheses may be loose or fall out. It may be difficult for the patient to insert dentures due to reduced intraoral pressure. This can be remediated by use of a dental adhesive. The wearing of oral prostheses lends contour to the mouth and supports oral structures, permitting more normal movement. Indeed, specialized modifications to dentures may assist with dysphagia rehabilitation. A "palatal training appliance" is a wire loop that attaches to the back of the upper denture and serves to elevate the soft palate, possibly providing sensory stimulation to the area and preventing posterior tongue humping (Selley et al. 1995). Lower dentures may be lengthened on the affected side to prevent pocketing of food (Selley et al. 1995). If dentures or partial plates are loose or cause pain or lacerations, they should be removed and their fit checked by a dentist.

Muscle Tone

Patients with upper motoneuron disease may demonstrate abnormalities in muscle tone proximally in the body and distally in the head, neck, and extremities. Both proximal and distal tone abnormalities may interfere with the movements needed for eating and swallowing. Muscle tone may be increased or spastic, or decreased or flaccid. A combination of spasticity and flaccidity is often seen, and compensatory or substitution movements are observed as the patient tries to move. Pathologic reflexes also may be seen. Mood, stress, discomfort, and effortful activities all influence muscle tone. Various techniques are useful in eliciting more normal tone and movement. Treatment techniques that reduce spasticity are termed "inhibitory"; techniques that increase muscle tone or movement are "facilitory." The treatment techniques outlined here are used with both acutely and chronically impaired neurologic patients. These techniques should be applied by trained occupational, physical, and speech therapists because of their complexity in application as well as their consequences to overall movement and function. Treatments should be part of an integrated multidisciplinary program of rehabilitation.

Treatment should begin proximally in the trunk because establishing improved proximal control facilitates improved distal control (Bobath 1990; Nelson et al. 1994). Appropriate positioning provides a stable postural base which then serves as a basis for trunk and limb movement. Postural stability and mobility are a basis for the "synchrony" of oral movements, swallowing and breathing of the ingestion process (Oetter et al. 1995). Hulme and colleagues (1987) have shown that in a pediatric population, efforts to correct trunk pos-

NAME: ______________________

THE NEW YORK HOSPITAL
DEPARTMENT OF REHABILITATION MEDICINE

Positioning Guidelines for Sitting

1. Have patient sit straight, not tilted.
2. Head in midline with neutral chin position.
3. Support both arms on tabletop where patient can see them.

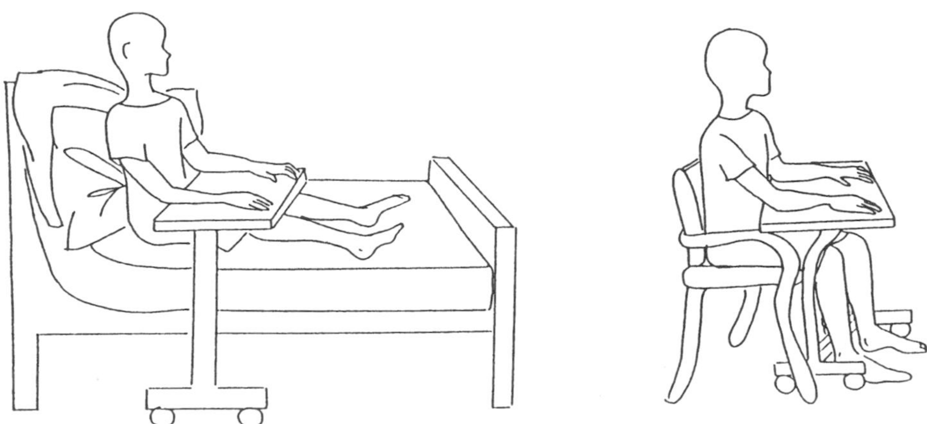

Figure 10.3 Proper sitting position. (Reprinted by permission of the Department of Rehabilitation Medicine, The New York Hospital-Cornell Medical Center.)

ture resulted in improved oral motor performance and the ability to safely swallow a wider variety of textures. Treatment may begin with mobilization techniques to loosen soft-tissue structures and increase range of motion in specific areas of the trunk and limbs that have become tight because of abnormal tone or posture. This may be followed by inhibitory techniques to reduce abnormal or compensatory movements and facilitory techniques to allow normal movement. For example, in a stroke patient, mobilization techniques may be required to increase anterior tilt of the pelvis, reduce abnormal weight shift due to muscle imbalances in the thoracolumbar areas, and permit increased extension in the cervical-thoracic area. This may be followed by facilitating active selective thoracic extension while inhibiting extension at the hips. As a result, the patient presents with more symmetric posture, as illustrated in Figure 10.3, with upper trunk extension available for respiratory effort and upper extremity use for self-feeding, and control of the neck available for swallowing as well as compensatory swallowing techniques.

Enhancement of distal control then proceeds to the neck area. Facilitation of a neutral neck position (see Figure 10.3) allows more symmetric oral motor function. The ability to use neck movements for compensatory swallowing techniques should be preceded by a range-of-motion assessment and mobilization, inhibition, and facilitation as needed. Achieving chin tuck or capital flexion at the atlanto-occipital joint is important to emphasize because this movement is critical for airway protection and as a compensatory swallowing technique. Mobility in the cervical spine is a prerequisite for swallowing techniques such as lateral flexion or rotation at the neck.

Self-feeding plays a role in coordinated swallowing. The dominant hand should be used for eating if at all possible. For hemiplegic or brain-injured patients in whom the dominant upper extremity is affected, severe hypo- or hypertonicity may prevent self-feeding. In these cases, the nondominant upper extremity should be used. Adaptive equipment, discussed later in this chapter, helps to make this less awkward for the patient. For those with emerging dominant upper extremity movement, occupational therapy treatments to facilitate muscle tone and coordinated movement may enhance the ability to self-feed with normal movement patterns prior to the meal. It may be easier to begin with finger foods than with utensils. Eating with the affected elbow supported on a high table may facilitate distal hand control over a utensil. Wrist cockup splints alleviate "wrist drop" and may be useful if adequate elbow and shoulder movements are intact. A utensil may be attached to the splint if grasp is not present. Hand-over-hand guiding and adaptive equipment also may be useful with these patients. Efforts should also be made to facilitate nondominant upper extremity function during eating. The ability to hold and use the napkin or stabilize the rim of the plate with the nondominant hand should be addressed. Fatigue should be avoided in the affected upper extremity as this may contribute to abnormal compensatory movements.

Since oral movements are the beginning of the continuum of coordinated oral-pharyngeal movements during swallow, it may be desirable to practice them to enhance movement, either before eating or even before oral intake begins. A variety of inhibition and facilitation techniques may be applied to specific muscles to improve oral and pharyngeal movements (Silverman and Elfant 1979; Farber 1982; Davies 1982; Langley 1987; O'Sullivan 1990). Sustained pressure, slow stretch, slow rocking, and prolonged icing are inhibitory; quick touch, quick pressure, quick stretch, and quick icing are facilitory (Farber 1982). Excessive spasticity in the cheek can be relieved by stretching it slowly from inside with the back of a spoon or a gloved finger. Vibration is facilitory; an electric toothbrush can be used to activate tone in the cheeks and stimulate lip closure (Davies 1985). A quick touch with ice to the lips or cheek in the direction of the desired movement may help to stimulate that movement. Stimuli should be applied unilaterally if the movement deficits are unilateral. Gustatory stimuli can be used to stimulate movement. Flavored water may be applied on the tongue with a cotton swab or an eyedropper if the patient is not yet able to manage a bolus.

For patients whose oral movement is intact but slow or poorly coordinated, treatment focuses on developing coordination between opposing muscle groups and on developing speed. This is done through direct exercises that focus on speed and timing or by using games such as blowing bubbles or blow darts.

Lip, tongue, cheek, and jaw movements may be retrained using "retrievable boluses" such as Life-Savers on a string, or food wrapped in gauze.

Oral and Pharyngeal Reflexes

Reflexes may be categorized as abnormal, such as bite and root, or normal, such as cough and gag. Treatment focuses on inhibiting abnormal reflexes and facilitating normal ones. Proper positioning is critical in both reducing abnormal reflexes and in promoting normal movement. While not true reflexes, the sensory and motor events that promote swallowing may be used therapeutically to elicit a swallow reflex.

Abnormal Reflexes

Abnormal reflexes include the bite reflex, rooting, mouth opening, tongue thrust, sucking, and hyperactive gag. A distinction is made between reflexes that are abnormal at any age, such as the bite reflex, and those that are seen early in development, such as rooting. Developmental reflexes may not interfere with swallowing as much as pathologic reflexes. Diminution of all abnormal reflexes may be a goal in feeding training.

Abnormal reflexes may be indirectly inhibited by avoiding the stimuli that elicit them (Silverman and Elfant 1979). Not touching the teeth, gums, or cheeks minimizes occurrence of the bite reflex. If the bite reflex is elicited, the therapist should wait until it relaxes and not force the jaw open, as this further elicits the reflex. Applying direct pressure at the temporomandibular joint may inhibit this reflex. Avoiding tactile stimulation of the lips and cheeks prevents accidental triggering of the rooting reflex. The mouth opening reflex is elicited by the visual stimulus of food on a utensil coming toward the mouth and may be used to overcome a tonic bite reflex. Asking the patient to open the mouth before visual presentation of food may help to control this reflex at the cortical level. These reflexes often diminish as neurologic recovery occurs.

Tongue thrust is reduced by facilitating tongue retraction (Silverman and Elfant 1979; Farber 1982). Retraction of the tongue occurs simultaneous to chin tuck or capital (head) flexion. Thus, capital flexion may be useful in conjunction with other maneuvers to stimulate tongue retraction. Retraction may be facilitated by applying manual vibration on either side of the frenulum under the tongue to the muscles of tongue retraction, or by quick stretch to the tongue in the direction opposite the desired movement (Farber 1982). Sucking activities reduce tongue thrust by promoting stabilization of the tongue in a retracted position, an important skill that permits movement of the posterior portion of the tongue during swallowing.

Sucking is considered a primitive reflex if the patient is unable to control it, or it may depend on the presence of a stimulus on the tongue, lips, or both, such as a straw or lollipop. Reflexive sucking may be observed as part of a suck-swallow sequence. The sucking reflex may be used to elicit a reflexive swallow when a volitional swallow is absent. Both reflexive (Farber 1982) and volitional

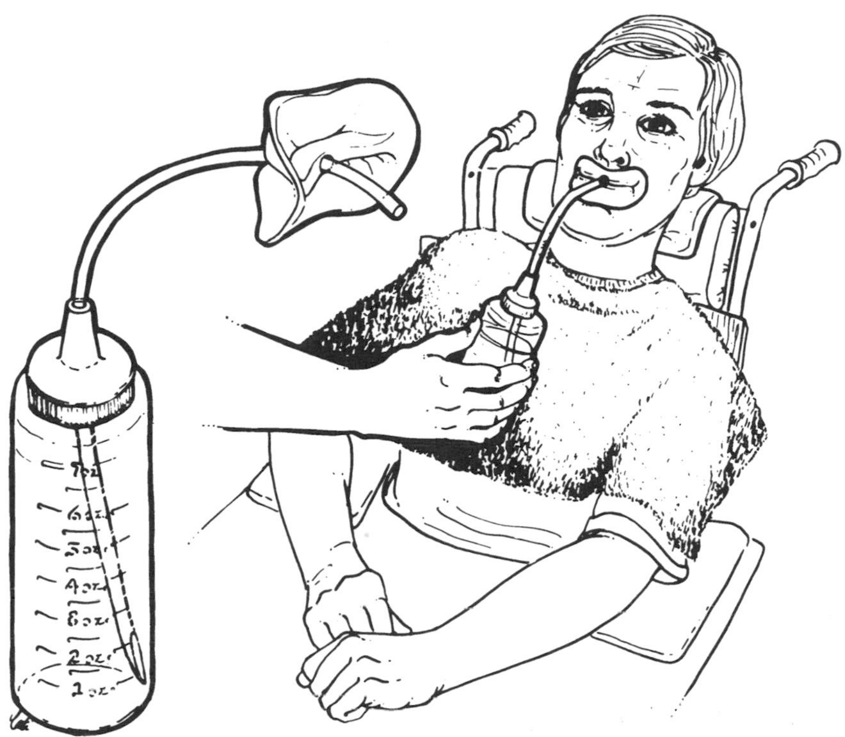

Figure 10.4 A plastic squeeze bottle, fish tank hose, and thermoplastic material can be used to promote swallowing behavior. (Reprinted with permission from SD Farber. Neurorehabilitation: A Multisensory Approach. Philadelphia: Saunders, 1982.)

sucking (Ramsey 1986) have been used therapeutically to elicit a swallow for nutritional purposes. Farber (1982) recommends a simple device to promote swallowing that can be constructed from a plastic squeeze bottle, fish tank tubing, and thermoplastic material (Figure 10.4). The mouthpiece and tube extending into the mouth provide pressure over the tongue and lips, which stimulates the reflex. The fish tank tubing must be bonded to the mouthpiece with a heat gun, and optimally the mouthpiece is molded on the individual patient, with a "shelf" between the lips.

An abnormal hyperactive gag reflex may be seen in the brain-injured adult. To inhibit the gag reflex, pressure is applied on the dorsum of the tongue using a padded tongue depressor, maintaining pressure for several seconds and then gradually moving back (Farber 1982).

Normal Reflexes

Normal reflexes include the gag, palatal, and cough reflexes. Silverman and Elfant (1979) advocate stroking the posterior tongue, uvula, and anterior and posterior faucial arches to elicit a depressed or absent gag reflex. The palatal reflex may be stimulated by stroking the soft palate with a cotton swab followed by attempts to phonate (Sullivan et al. 1982; Davies 1985). Activities that encourage palatal movement through nasopharyngeal closure, such as sucking through a straw, also may be done provided a Valsalva maneuver is not contraindicated. Both volitional and reflexive cough are important for airway protection during swallowing. Volitional cough may be strengthened by performing deep breathing exercises and vocal cord adduction, followed by active attempts at coughing and by applying manual pressure to the abdominal musculature while trying to cough (Kisner and Colby 1985). A "tracheal tickle," which is done by pressing posteriorly toward the trachea at the sternal notch with a circular movement, helps to stimulate a reflexive cough (Frownfelter 1987; Kisner and Colby 1985).

The swallowing reflex can be facilitated if the dry swallow is observed to be weak or absent. Swallowing is facilitated by stroking the anterior faucial arches with a cold stimulus, such as an iced laryngeal mirror, followed by active attempts at swallowing (Logemann 1983; Helfrich-Miller et al. 1986; Lazzara et al. 1986). Silverman and Elfant (1979) describe the use of other maneuvers, including icing the sternal notch for several seconds during attempts to swallow, upward stroking under the chin, and manual vibration under the chin and lateral to the larynx. Activities aimed at improving oral skills also improve swallowing. As consecutive dry swallows are difficult to achieve, these techniques may be more successful using ice slush, a few drops of fruit juice or a retrievable bolus such as a lollipop. Because of the many sensory and motor stimuli that facilitate swallowing, each patient should be evaluated individually to determine the success of the maneuvers attempted.

Weakness

Patients with weakness caused by lower motoneuron involvement require a treatment program that focuses on strengthening weakened structures. Strengthening activities may be contraindicated in some diagnoses, such as amyotrophic lateral sclerosis, in which exercise produces further weakness. A complete muscle test helps the clinician develop an exercise program for specific muscles or muscle groups. Compensatory movements are often seen as stronger muscles attempt to compensate for weakened muscles. Prefeeding treatment may involve reducing the activity of these muscles before proceeding with exercises and strengthening activities. The facilitory techniques described in the section on muscle tone are useful with those with lower motoneuron impairment (Sullivan et al. 1982). Movement in weakened cheek and lip musculature due to a peripheral facial nerve palsy may be facilitated with quick icing and quick stretch, followed by active smiling and sucking exercises. Once active movement is possible, resistive exercises such as sucking or blowing on a pinched straw should begin. To improve strength, the appropriate amount of resistance must be supplied (Farber 1982). It is important not to overfatigue weak muscles, especially before a meal.

FEEDING TRAINING

When the patient is alert and has been deemed a candidate for attempts at eating, feeding training may begin. Feeding training is differentiated from nutritional feeding; if the patient cannot swallow safely, the training session is rehabilitative, and the patient receives complete nutrition through an alternative route (Logemann 1983). During feeding the patient should be observed for signs and symptoms of aspiration, which may include changes in respiratory or heart rate, color, voice quality, or coughing. It is also helpful to auscultate with a stethoscope at the neck, to assess whether audible pooling develops in the upper airway. Auscultation of the lungs before and after swallowing helps to assess pulmonary integrity. During initial feeding sessions, suctioning equipment should be available in the circumstance of suspected aspiration, but every effort should be made to avoid aspiration.

Positioning and Environment

Appropriate positioning is critical for safe and maximally independent eating and swallowing. The upright position allows optimal functioning of oral and pharyngeal structures (Farber 1982; Oetter et al. 1995). The patient in an upright position is better able to keep the airway clear by coughing (Frownfelter 1987). A flexed position is physiologically associated with swallowing success (Farber 1982) and prevents mass extension through the trunk and limbs that may be seen in the neurologically impaired patient. The seated position illustrated in Figure 10.3 incorporates flexion at the hips, knees, and shoulders; the arms are supported on the table and flex toward the body as the patient self-feeds. The head should be neither flexed nor extended, but in a neutral position with a slight chin tuck. Positioning aides such as special cushions and lumbar supports should be provided. This position minimizes the possibility of food entering the airway. For patients who have difficulty maintaining position, repositioning may be necessary during the feeding session. Patients should remain upright for 15–30 minutes following eating, longer if there is an accompanying esophageal disorder.

The first feeding sessions should be conducted in a quiet room that allows the patient to concentrate on eating activity. If possible, the therapist should sit directly in front of the patient, as this promotes postural symmetry. If the patient has cognitive or perceptual problems, the therapist may wish to present one food item at a time. Conversation should be kept to a minimum to discourage simultaneous eating and talking, although brief conversation between swallows may help the therapist to assess changes in the patient's voice quality that may indicate compromise to the airway.

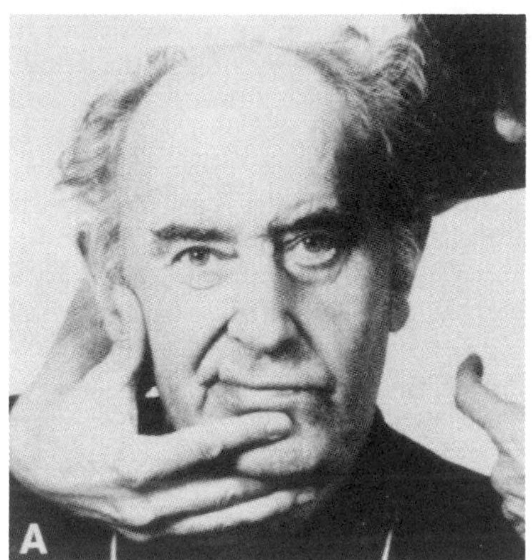

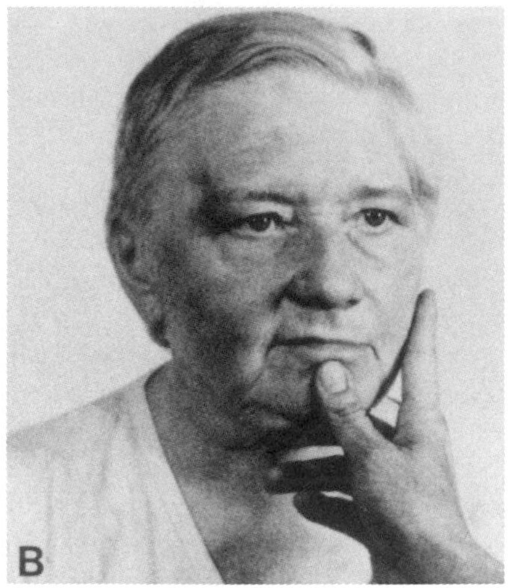

Figure 10.5 Hand placement to facilitate oral-pharyngeal movement during swallowing. A. Facilitation for the patient with poor head and neck control. B. Facilitation for the patient with primarily oral-pharyngeal control problems. (Reprinted with permission from PM Davies. Steps to Follow: A Guide to Treatment of Adult Hemiplegia. Berlin: Springer-Verlag, 1985.)

Food Selection and Administration

Patients with neurogenic dysphagia should first be evaluated with a soft, semiformed bolus that requires a minimum of oral manipulation, such as applesauce or gelatin. Sour boluses have been found to enhance both oral and pharyngeal aspects of swallowing (Logemann et al. 1995). Increased bolus viscosity (pudding vs. liquid) and volume (5 ml liquid vs. 1 ml liquid) have been found to reduce a delay in pharyngeal timing in patients who have had strokes (Bisch et al. 1994). While cold boluses have not been found to alter pharyngeal function in stroke patients and normal subjects (Bisch et al. 1994), they may be stimulating to oral functioning and may facilitate sucking (Farber 1982). Liquids should be avoided initially as they can be easily aspirated, although they may be easier to manage for tracheostomized patients or those with cricopharyngeal dysfunction. Crumbly or solid textures are difficult because they require more oral preparation, dropping prematurely into an unprepared pharynx.

The therapist may use two positions, illustrated in Figure 10.5, to facilitate eating and swallowing (Davies 1985). In Figure 10.5A, the therapist stands at the patient's side and uses his or her arm to maintain the correct head position by reinforcing a neutral position of the neck with a gentle upward force. The head should never be pushed forward from behind (Farber 1982), because this triggers an extension response. The position depicted in Figure 10.5B is used when the patient has adequate head control. In both positions the therapist's hand is used to monitor tone and control and to facilitate movement in the lips, cheeks, and tongue. To administer food, the therapist should bring the utensil toward the mouth, allowing the patient to see and smell it. Presenting the spoon from below the level of the mouth helps maintain head position. If the patient is being fed, the spoon should be placed firmly on the tongue to stimulate removal of food from the spoon by the oral structures. The bolus should be placed at midline on the tongue. If the patient is unable to mobilize it from this position, it may initially be placed toward the stronger or more sensitive side of the mouth. The first few spoonfuls should be considered test swallows and the patient monitored for signs and symptoms of aspiration. The mouth should be inspected and residual food removed if the patient is unable to clear it. For patients at high risk for aspiration, initial attempts at feeding should be done under videofluoroscopy to assess whether prefeeding treatment with an alternative nutritional route is necessary.

To avoid confusing patients with cortical lesions, verbal cues, if needed at all, should be short and simple. Some patients, because of reduced safety judgment and attention, may not be safe when eating and may require supervision, assistance, or both at mealtime indefinitely. Patients who need to use more complex swallowing maneuvers, as described in the following section, must be able to follow directions and remember to use such techniques.

Once test swallows have been successful, several ounces of a trial food should be attempted. Different soft foods should be tried because tolerance of subtle changes in texture may vary; for instance, some patients may tolerate pudding but not applesauce. Once the patient tolerates soft foods, other textures should be attempted. A frequently used continuum of foods is soft chewables (canned fruit, well-cooked vegetables), thick liquids (fruit nectars), thin liquids (fruit juice and water), chewables (raw vegetables and cooked meat), foods that require biting (rolls), and finally mixed textures (pills and water). Progression through this continuum is individualized and may take from days to months. Some patients may never be able to safely manage certain textures, particularly thin liquids, chewables, and mixed textures. Individual food preferences as well as cultural attitudes toward types of foods and eating habits should be taken into consideration.

Special swallowing techniques may be appropriate for the patient with neurogenic dysphagia. Chin tuck has been shown to change the dimensions of the pharynx in such a way as to afford greater airway protection (Welch et al. 1993). Logemann et al. (1989) noted that head rotation during swallowing in patients with unilateral pharyngeal weakness facilitated bolus propulsion by the pharyngeal musculature on the stronger side and enhanced relaxation of the cricopharyngeus muscle. While a true supraglottic swallow may be difficult for neurogenic dysphagia patients, a swallow, throat clear, reswallow maneuver may be useful in the presence of a wet-sounding voice after swallowing certain textures. Voluntarily prolonging the rise of the larynx by prolonging tongue contraction, ("Mendelsohn's maneuver") may help improve opening of the pharyngoesophageal segment (Kahrilas et al. 1991). Compensatory swallowing

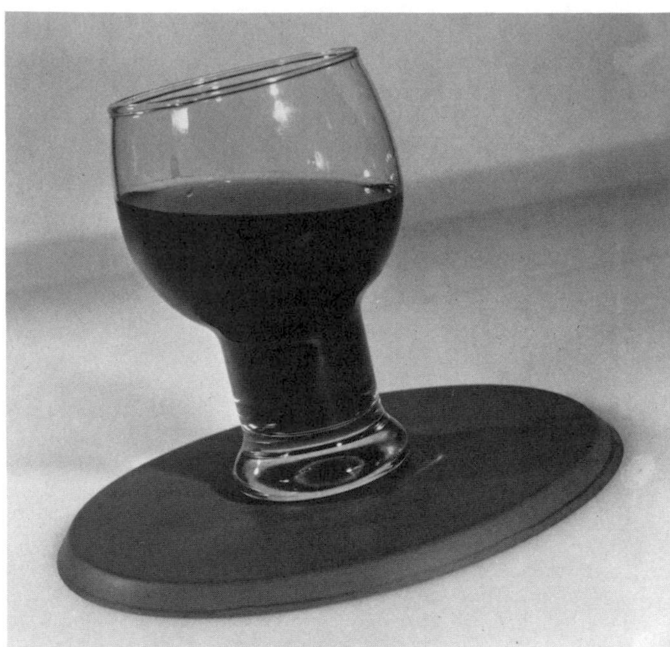

Figure 10.6 Use of a nonslip rubberized disk for holding eating utensils in place to prevent sliding. (Reprinted by permission of Maddak, Inc., Pequannock, NJ.)

maneuvers should be verified radiographically with the use of relevant food textures to assess their usefulness for the individual patient (Linden 1989).

Biofeedback technology is increasingly available (Crary 1995). It may be useful for nondirect treatment of facial nerve palsy that can interfere with the oral stage of eating. Perlman (1993) discusses the use of electroglottography biofeedback during direct treatment to help a patient with multiple sclerosis perform a more effective Mendelsohn maneuver. The essence of biofeedback is to heighten awareness; Logemann and Kahrilas (1990) use the term *indirect biofeedback* to refer to verbal cuing in a direct treatment context for swallowing retraining.

Adaptive Equipment

Adaptive feeding equipment may be useful in increasing eating independence and safety. A wide range of equipment is available. Such equipment should be chosen with care by the occupational therapist, who can assess patient needs and skills and train the patient or caregiver in its use. Nonskid pads (Figure 10.6) or a wet cloth under a dish prevents slipping. A high-rimmed plate allows the patient to load food onto the utensil more easily (Figure 10.7). A cup with a nose cutout helps to prevent atlanto-axial and neck extension during drinking (Figure 10.8). For patients with distal upper extremity weakness, a universal cuff fitted with a utensil allows increased independence in eating (Figure

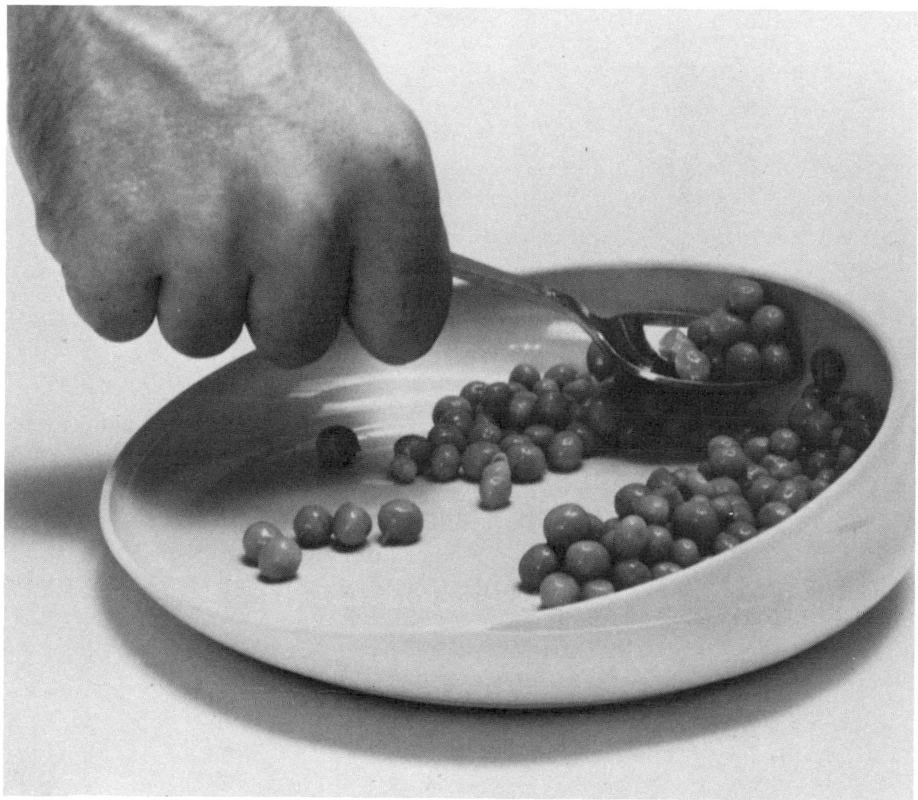

Figure 10.7 Example of a high-rimmed dish that assists the patient in loading the utensil for self-feeding. (Reprinted by permission of Fred Sammons, Inc.)

10.9). Many types of equipment are available for patients with proximal weakness, such as ball-bearing feeders (Figure 10.10) and overhead slings (Figure 10.11). More complex electronic and computerized feeding devices for the more disabled patient are under development and will be more readily available in the future (Hartmann and Cerna 1992).

SUMMARY

This chapter provides the swallowing clinician with a prefeeding and feeding program for use with the neurogenically dysphagic patient following diagnostic evaluation. Intervention that addresses the patient's cognitive, perceptual, physical, and functional abilities will maximize safe and independent eating and swallowing. Some patients require intervention in these areas as well as indirect dysphagia treatment before oral intake may safely begin. Both indirect dysphagia treatment techniques, including sensory stimulation and exercises, and direct

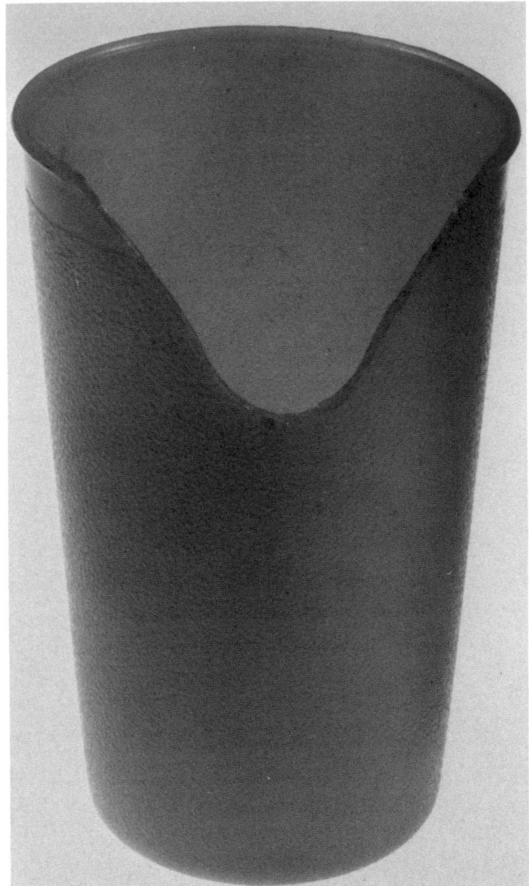

Figure 10.8 Example of a nose cutout cup to avoid neck extension while drinking. (Reprinted by permission of Fred Sammons, Inc.)

treatment techniques, including techniques for use during swallowing, have been shown to be effective (Neumann 1995). Promising studies are also emerging regarding treatment for patients with chronic neurogenic dysphagia (Crary 1995; Helfrich-Miller et al. 1986). Treatment should be designed for the individual patient, and the effectiveness of treatment strategies should be reevaluated frequently.

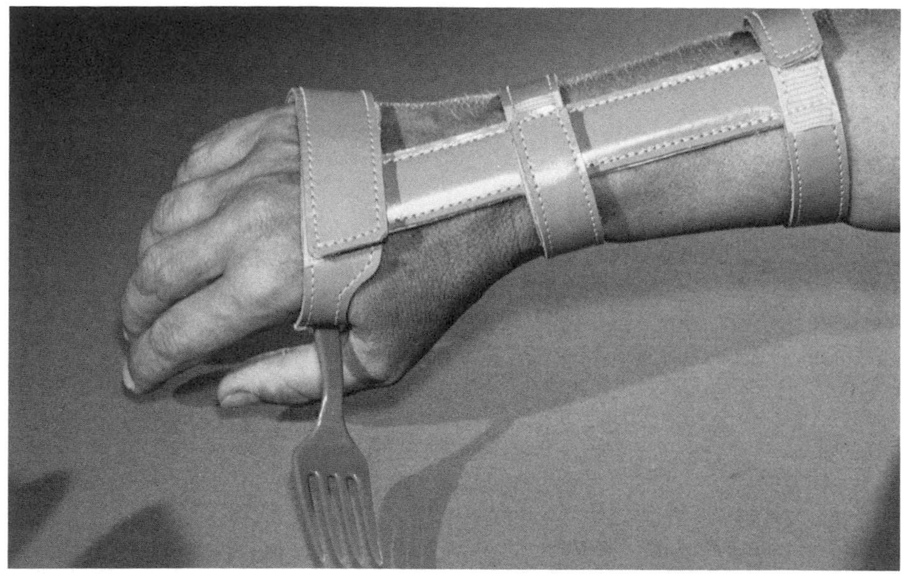

Figure 10.9 The universal cuff fits over the hand, pictured here with a wrist support splint; it requires only arm motion for feeding. (Reprinted by permission of Fred Sammons, Inc.)

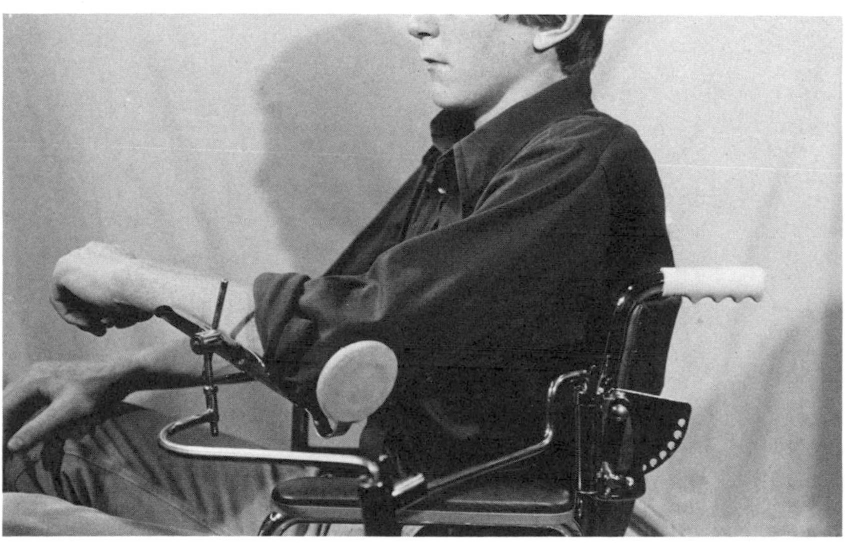

Figure 10.10 The Michigan ball-bearing feeder is useful for patients with large-muscle or proximal weakness. (Reprinted with permission from CA Trombly. Occupational Therapy for Physical Dysfunction. Baltimore: Williams & Wilkins, copyright 1989. Photographer, Judith LaDrew.)

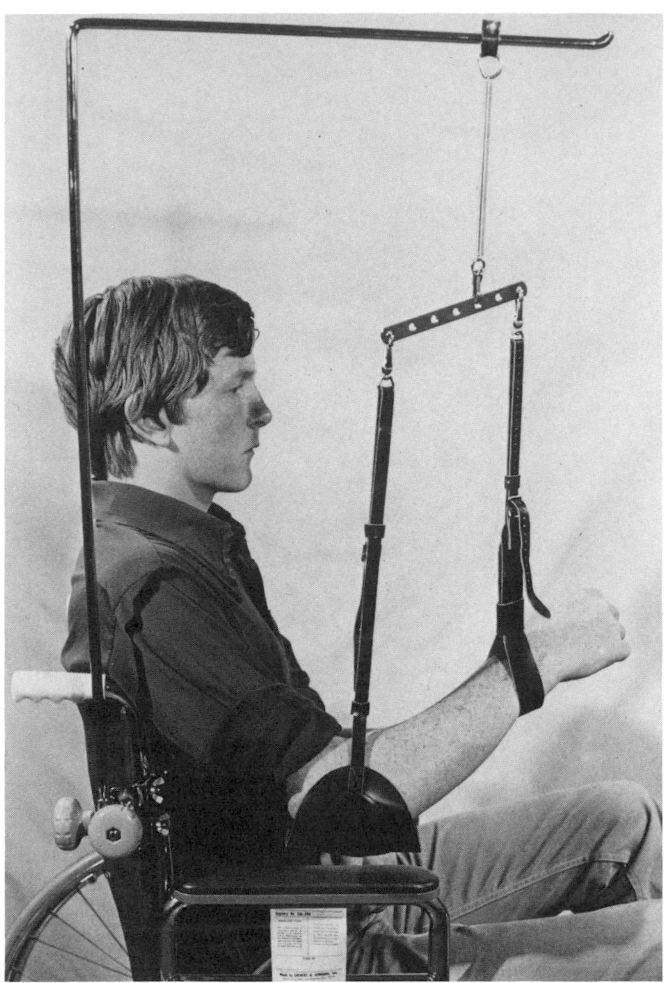

Figure 10.11 Use of the suspension sling can aid patients in self-feeding. (Reprinted with permission from CA Trombly. Occupational Therapy for Physical Dysfunction. Baltimore: Williams & Wilkins, copyright 1989. Photographer, Judith LaDrew.)

REFERENCES

Affolter FD. Perception, Interaction, and Language. Berlin: Springer-Verlag, 1987.

Bisch EM, Logemann JA, Rademaker AW, et al. Pharyngeal effects of bolus volume, viscosity, and temperature in patients with dysphagia resulting from neurologic impairment and normal subjects. J Speech Hear Res 1994;37:1041.

Bobath B. Adult hemiplegia: evaluation and treatment. Oxford, England: Heinemann Medical Books, 1990.

Brown GE, Nordloh S, Donowitz AJ. Systematic desensitization of oral hypersensitivity in a patient with a closed head injury. Dysphagia 1992;7:138.

Buchholz DW, Bosma JF, Donner MW. Adaptation, compensation, and decompensation of the pharyngeal swallow. Gastrointest Radiol 1985;10:235.

Coster ST, Schwarz WH. Rheology and the swallow-safe bolus. Dysphagia 1987;1:113.

Crary MA. A direct intervention program for chronic neurogenic dysphagia secondary to brainstem stroke. Dysphagia 1995;10:6.

Davies PM. Steps to Follow: A Guide to Treatment of Adult Hemiplegia. Berlin: Springer-Verlag, 1985.
Farber SD. Neurorehabilitation: A Multisensory Approach. Philadelphia: Saunders, 1982.
Frownfelter D. Chest Physical Therapy and Pulmonary Rehabilitation: An Interdisciplinary Approach. Chicago: Year Book, 1987.
Hartmann KD, Cerna R. Present and future prospects for a robot as an assistant in feeding. Occup Ther Prac 1992;3:75.
Helfrich-Miller KR, Rector KL, Straka JA. Dysphagia: its treatment in the profoundly retarded population with cerebral palsy. Arch Phys Med Rehabil 1986;67:520.
Hulme JB, Shaver J, Acher S. Effects of adaptive seating devices on the eating and drinking of children with multiple handicaps. Am J Occup Ther 1987;41:81.
Kahrilas P, Logemann J, Krugler C, et al. Volitional augmentation of upper esophageal sphincter opening during swallowing. Am J Phys: Gastro Liv Phys 1991;G450.
Kisner C, Colby LA. Therapeutic Exercise: Foundations and Techniques. Philadelphia: FA Davis, 1985.
Langley, J. Working with Swallowing Disorders. Bicester, Oxon, England: Winslow Press, 1987.
Lazzara GD, Lazarus C, Logemann JA. Impact of thermal stimulation on the triggering of the swallow reflex. Dysphagia 1986;1:73.
Linden P. Videofluoroscopy in the rehabilitation of swallowing dysfunction. Dysphagia 1989;3:189.
Logemann JA. Diagnosis and Treatment of Swallowing Disorders. San Diego: College-Hill Press, 1983.
Logemann JA, Kahrilas PJ. Relearning to swallow after stroke—application of maneuvers and indirect biofeedback: a case study. Neurology 1990;40:1136.
Logemann JA, Kahrilas PJ, Kobara M, et al. The benefit of head rotation on pharyngo-esophageal dysphagia. Arch Phys Med Rehabil 1989;70:767.
Logemann JA, Pauloski BR, Colangelo L, et al. Effects of a sour bolus on oropharyngeal swallowing measures in patients with neurogenic dysphagia. J Speech Hear Res 1995;38:556.
Mackay L, Morgan AS. Early swallowing disorders with severe head injuries: relationships between the RLA and the progression of oral intake. Departments of Rehabilitation Medicine and Surgery, St. Francis Hospital, Hartford, CT. Abstract from the Fourth Multidisciplinary Symposium on Dysphagia, 1992, The Johns Hopkins Swallowing Center, Baltimore, MD.
Nelson CA, Meek MM, Moore JC. Head-Neck Treatment Issues as a Base for Oral-Motor Function. Albuquerque: Clinician's View, 1994.
Neumann S. Swallowing therapy of neurologic patients: correlation of outcome with pretreatment variables and therapeutic methods. Dysphagia 1995;10:1.
Oetter P, Richter RW, Frick SM. M.O.R.E.: Integrating the Mouth with Sensory and Postural Functions (2nd ed). Hugo, MN: PDP Press, 1995.
O'Sullivan N. Dysphagia Care: Team Approach with Acute and Long Term Patients. Los Angeles: Cottage Square, 1990.
Perlman AL. The successful treatment of challenging cases. Clin Comm Disord 1993;3;37.
Ramsey WO. Suckle facilitation of feeding in selected dysphagia patients. Dysphagia 1986;1:7.
Selley WG, Roche MT, Pearce VR, et al. Dysphagia following strokes: clinical observations of swallowing rehabilitation employing palatal training appliances. Dysphagia 1995;10:32.
Silverman EH, Elfant IL. Dysphagia: an evaluation and treatment program for the adult. Am J Occup Ther 1979;33:382.
Sullivan PE, Markos PD, Minor MAD. An Integrated Approach to Therapeutic Exercise. Reston, VA: Reston Publishing, 1982.
Welch MV, Logemann JA, Rademaker AW, et al. Changes in pharyngeal dimensions effected by chin tuck. Arch Phys Med Rehab 1993;74:178.

11

Treatment of Mechanical Swallowing Disorders

Susan M. Fleming

Although deglutition has been studied for many years, it has been only in the last two decades that there has been significant interest in the subject, particularly in approaches to treatment (Kasprisin et al. 1989). Most clinicians and researchers appreciate the range of intrasubject and intersubject variability in the normal swallow (Christrup 1964; Ekberg and Nylander 1982; Hamlet 1989). At some point on this continuum of deglutition variability, the normal swallow becomes decompensated, with resultant dysphagic symptomatology. Dysphagia itself is also on a continuum, with the extent of abnormal variability influencing the degree of severity.

This chapter begins with clarification of problems associated with dysphagia to establish a clearer concept of subsequent management suggestions. This description of disorders is followed by suggestions for treating postsurgical patients with difficulties of bolus transport during the oral and pharyngeal stages of swallowing. Esophageal performance also may be influenced by some of these suggestions (e.g., upright versus supine positioning). The astute clinician will want to remember that although, by convention, we often speak in terms of the three stages of swallowing, the normal swallow is a rapid, synchronous process that exceeds the sum of its representative parts.

DESCRIPTION OF DISORDERS

When dysphagia is present, swallowed contents do not traverse the normal route of deglutition in a timely fashion. Rather, one or more of the following events occurs: drooling, nasoregurgitation, aspiration, esophageal regurgitation or reflux, or swallowed contents remaining as residual. These contents may eventually follow four alternative routes: anteriorly past the lips, into the nasal cavity, into the airway, or from the esophagus or stomach into the mouth or pharynx. Dysphagia, therefore, is not a disease, but a sign or symptom of another underlying disease or disorder that may be debilitating or life-threatening.

Forces of swallowed materials such as increased viscosity may impair bolus flow. When this occurs, a mechanical dysphagia becomes more apparent. The problems associated with mechanical dysphagia are multifaceted and allow an array of management possibilities. Consequently, determining the optimal plan can be challenging.

Aspiration is of greatest concern since it is life-threatening (Weiss 1988). At one time or another, most people have aspirated food or liquid into their airway. In healthy persons this results in a cough to expel the substance. Dysphagic patients, whose overall physical status may have deteriorated, may tolerate aspiration poorly (Kirsch and Sanders 1988).

Aspiration may be caused by unilateral incompetence of the hypoglossal nerve. When this occurs the process of swallowing is out of control; the tongue is no longer able to regulate the passage of the bolus. The pharynx receives the bolus prematurely, threatening the unprotected airway. Considering also that the laryngeal elevators may be impaired with hypoglossal nerve dysfunction, care must be taken in assessing potential risk of aspiration. In other words, disruption of tongue control is not the only factor in hypoglossal nerve dysfunction.

Involvement of the soft palate alone does not result in aspiration. In many neurologic disorders, however, problems of the soft palate accompany problems of the pharynx because they have common innervation by the vagus and glossopharyngeal nerves. If peristalsis is disrupted, aspiration is possible since swallowing is such a rapid, synchronous process. Bolus stasis in the pharynx indicates that once the structures assume an at-rest or nonswallowing position, food may enter the unprotected airway. Further down the alimentary tract, a stricture of the cricopharyngeus or upper esophagus could result in reflux of swallowed substance that might then be spilled into the unprotected airway. Aspiration of this refluxed material, particularly if it contains hydrochloric acid, a normal constituent of gastric juice, may further compromise pulmonary status.

Problems of bolus transport can occur anywhere along the feeding route. For example, a person with unilateral involvement of the hypoglossal nerve with resection of portions of the tongue would have difficulty lateralizing a bolus for mastication and transport into the oropharynx to initiate the second stage of swallowing. Resection or paralysis of the soft palate may result in nasal regurgitation of the bolus, especially if the bolus is liquid (Kilman and Goyal 1976). Pharyngeal involvement results in disrupted peristaltic activity of the pharyngeal constrictors. Stenosis or narrowing of the alimentary tract at the level of the cricopharyngeus may prevent a food bolus from moving beyond that point. Esophageal transit may be disrupted in a similar manner.

Before deciding which mechanical devices to use in aiding bolus transport, the clinician must have medicolegal clearance to work with the dysphagic patient. Presuming legal consent such as clinical privileges and medical clearance has been obtained, the clinician must completely review the patient's chart as a beginning to a thorough assessment. If the patient appears to be at risk for aspiration (e.g., frequently coughs, has a "wet-sounding" voice, or is unable to clear secretions well), the clinician must discuss this with the attending physician. Assuming that the patient is not at significant risk of aspiration, mechanical devices can be considered to enable the patient to eat more easily and more conveniently, and most importantly, to maintain nutrition and hydration.

SCINTIGRAPHY

Used with the appropriate procedures and instrumentation, scintigraphy can be extremely helpful in managing dysphagic patients, especially those who have persistent dysphagia (generally >4 months) that is not showing progressive deterioration. Experience has shown that in about 4 months' time, these dysphagic patients acquire compensatory strategies and the dysphagia severity plateaus. It is not uncommon to see atypical videofluoroscopic studies in these patients (those with dysphagia not showing progressive deterioration), yet they frequently show no signs of aspiration pneumonia. Thus, scintigraphy may be initiated to quantify any pulmonary aspiration. Although considered diagnostic in nature, scintigraphy is useful for management because it is the only method that (1) can quantify the amount of material ingested, (2) can quantify the amount of oropharyngeal residue, (3) measures bolus transit time, and (4) most significantly, quantifies pulmonary aspiration of boluses containing radionuclides (Humpreys et al. 1987; Hamlet et al. 1989; Muz et al. 1990; Hamlet et al. 1992; Hamlet et al. 1996). This gives the attending physician and dysphagia team members a powerful tool for patient management.

The use of scintigraphy may improve the patient's quality of life. Following scintigraphic assessment, feeding tubes have, with a high degree of confidence, been removed (Fleming et al. 1990) and tracheostoma cuffs, on ventilator-dependent patients, have safely been deflated, enhancing swallowing as well as speaking (Tippett and Siebens 1991). Clinically, decisions can be made on a more timely basis, reducing delays for management intervention. The author has seen inpatient lengths of stay reduced and unnecessary procedures avoided because of the timely and reliable information given by scintigraphic assessment.

Although other sources are much more comprehensive, we provide a brief description of scintigraphic assessment.

Scintigraphic assessment uses a radionuclide, usually technetium-99m sulfur colloid, which may be mixed with a liquid or more viscous substance. For clinical studies we frequently use 10 ml of a carrier substance such as apple juice or applesauce, preferably of known viscosity, to which 2.5 mCi technetium-99m sulfur colloid has been added. Another 2.5 mCi technetium-99m sulfur colloid is added to 110 ml of the same carrier substance. Thus, only one texture is evaluated at a time. The 10-ml volume is given initially for the transit study while the additional 110 ml is given to the patient to determine what percentage is aspirated. Glottal-level aspiration does not necessarily mean that the patient will be unable to clear the trachea or bronchi of the aspirated material. Patients often clear the aspirate before it reaches the bronchi. Furthermore, if aspirated materials do make it to the lung or lungs, pneumonia is not a requisite consequence. A major challenge is to correlate clinical data (e.g., pulmonary function, mobility, immunosuppressive status, etc.) with percentages of lung aspirate as determined scintigraphically. For the clinical test, the patient is given a total of 120 ml of the liquid, purée, or solid carrier. This is approximately 4 oz, which is more representative of quantities the patient would take if he or she were to ingest normally.

With videofluoroscopy, radiation is emitted from the instruments. With scintigraphy, the radiation comes only from radionuclide that the patient ingests. Although radiation doses are low, generally less than that given fluoroscopically, extreme care is exercised. A scintillation camera and computer are used to determine radiation counts within specified anatomic areas. Unlike with videofluoroscopy, discrete anatomic structures are not visible. To better identify important landmarks for analysis, cobalt markers are taped to the right angle of the mandible and to the anterior neck at the level of the cricoid cartilage.

Patient positioning for the scintigraphic study is important. For the clinical study, the patient is typically positioned for the transit study in a right anterior oblique manner, close to the scintillation camera so that as much as possible of the oral-to-stomach areas may be "viewed." Figure 11.1 shows a patient positioned for a right anterior oblique view. For the aspiration quantification phase the view is anterior-posterior.

For quantification, the scintillation camera displays an image and the computer enhances it (Figure 11.2) and "counts" the radionuclide particles in any area of interest. These areas may include, for example, the oral, pharyngeal, and esophageal areas, or a lung such as that shown in Figure 11.3. With the computer, any combination of areas may be viewed for quantifying scintigraphic activity.

Clinical and research needs determine specific protocols. It is imperative, however, that the radiation physicist be consulted for matters such as the half-life of the radionuclide needed (and the implications of this half-life), differing attenuation of body tissues that affect scintigraphic counts, and issues related to safety and policy.

The decision about whether to use scintigraphy is made case by case. As stated earlier, the best candidates for scintigraphic assessment are those who have had dysphagia for more than 4 months and are not showing progressive deterioration, such as those with nonsevere, nonrecurring strokes and some persons who have undergone head and neck surgery. Additional good candidates would be those who have been considered "dysphagic" but who have not shown clinical signs of aspiration pneumonia. Patients who are relatively mobile but have dysphagia are possible scintigraphy candidates since their activity appears to help contribute to clearing in the event of aspiration. Finally, scintigraphy should be considered when the patient or significant others insist on oral feedings. When patients and others have been told that aspiration may result in pulmonary complications and pneumonia and the findings are quantitatively validated, acceptance is better and patient management progresses.

The cost of scintigraphic assessment varies with the institution and region. The amount appears to be close to that of videofluoroscopy. We have found the cost to be justified and accepted if the patient has improved outcome or if the test's findings conserve health care resources. Scintigraphy is not intended to supplant other standard and recognized procedures. Instead, it is presented as a valuable means of quantifying aspiration and perhaps aspiration tolerance for optimal patient management.

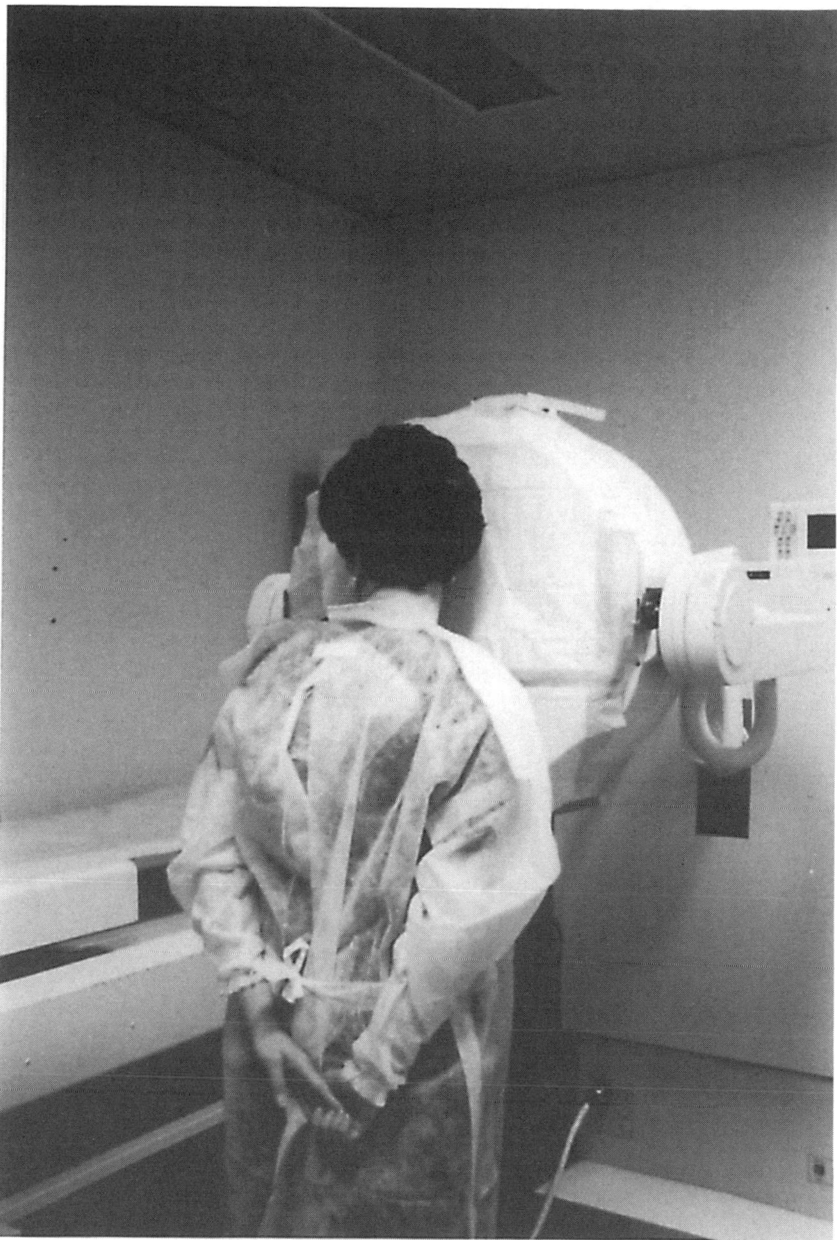

Figure 11.1 The patient is positioned in the right anterior oblique view. Note that the scintillation camera has been covered in the event of accidental coughing or spillage of the radionuclide material.

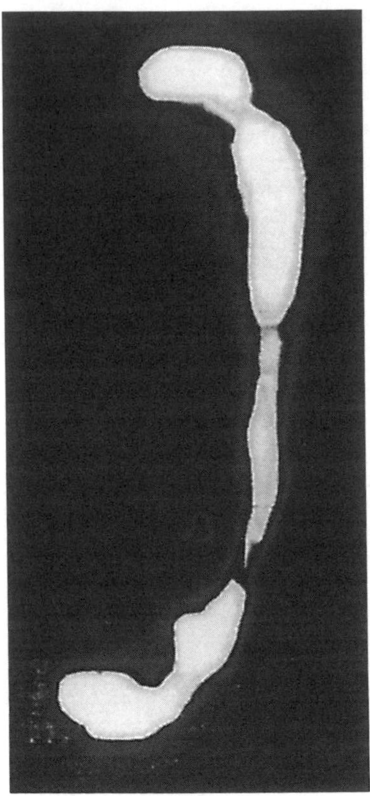

Figure 11.2 A computer-enhanced display of scintigraphic activity in the oral, pharyngeal (top), esophageal, and stomach areas (middle to bottom). The computer enhances the display for ease of viewing, but the radionuclide counts are not altered in the process.

POSITIONING

The position taken while eating affects bolus transport. If the head is lowered and there is incomplete lip closure, drooling may occur. In patients with insufficient velopharyngeal closure, lowering the head, as when drinking from a water fountain, may result in nasoregurgitation. With some esophageal disorders, reflux is greater in the supine than the upright position. Depending on the manifestation of the swallowing disorder, aspiration secondary to pharyngeal incompetence may be reduced by turning the head to the involved side (Logemann et al. 1989). Turning the head toward the involved side eliminates that side of the pharynx from its participation in bolus transit, allowing the non-impaired side to propel the bolus. This is demonstrated both clinically and radiographically. Flexing the neck so that the head tilts forward improves protection of the laryngeal vestibule (Ekberg 1986). This chin-tuck maneuver is frequently seen as a compensation made by patients in the absence of any deglutition training. Apparently, experience has taught these patients that this compensatory technique improves their swallow efficiency.

The size of the bolus ingested is related to positioning. Tracy et al. (1989) found that as bolus volume increased, the oral transit time of the bolus head

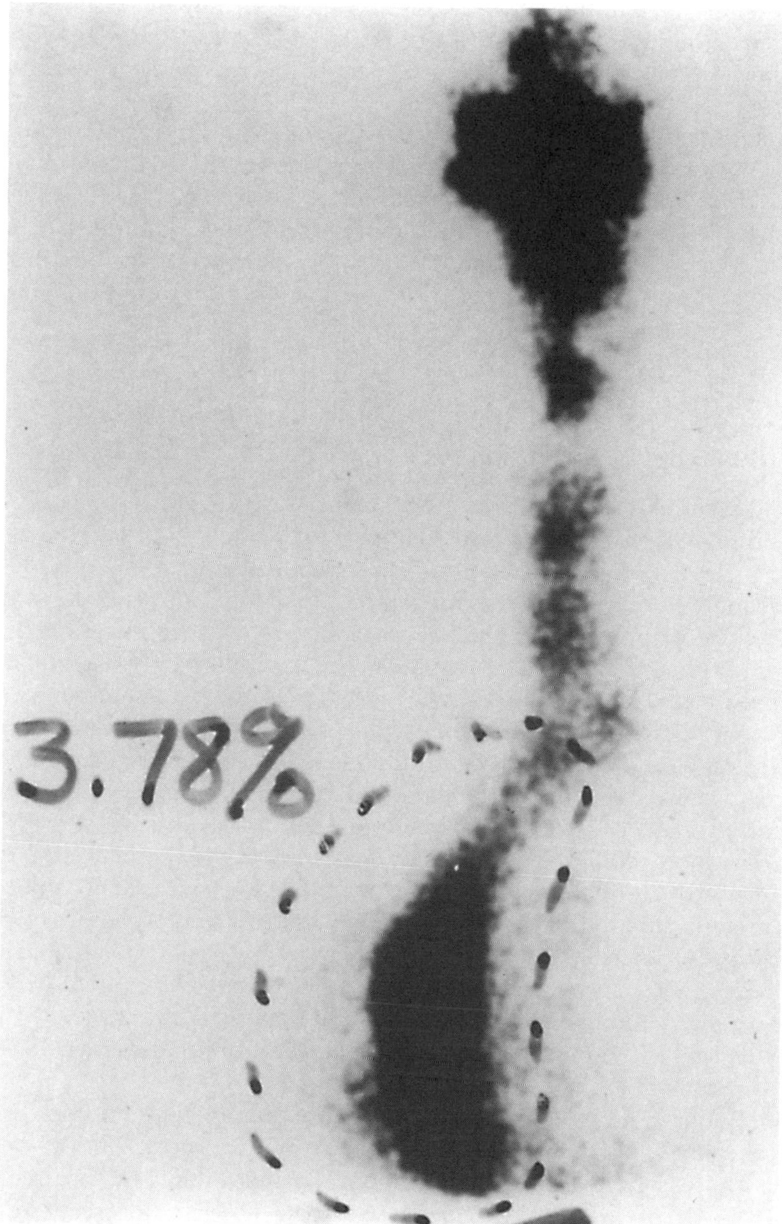

Figure 11.3 Scintigraphic display showing 3.78% of the radionuclide substance in the area enclosed by the dotted lines. This display indicates that 3.78 of the total amount ingested was misdirected into the right lung field. Note that without the computer to count the radionuclide particles, with visual inspection alone one might expect a much higher percentage of aspiration. (Courtesy of Dr. Sandra Hamlet.)

decreased and the duration of the cricopharyngeal opening increased. Significant changes in swallow coordination were reported by Castell et al. (1990) when comparing the factors of upright versus supine, wet versus dry swallows, and varying textures.

Collectively, many factors alter patterns of deglutition in both normal individuals and those with swallowing impairment. Variations in performance suggest that there are no equations or recipes for resolving dysphagic complications, even for those who present with what appear to be similar problems. One must integrate what is known in the laboratory about the normal swallow with one's clinical experience in managing the disordered mechanism to formulate the most appropriate treatment program.

FEEDING DEVICES

Glossectomy Feeding Spoons

Glossectomy feeding spoons are a means of transporting the bolus of food to the oropharynx. Not all patients with a partial or total glossectomy are candidates for the device. There are two criteria for use of the spoon. First, the patient should not be at high risk for aspiration. Significant resection of the base of the tongue or problems at the pharyngeal stage of swallowing might render the larynx vulnerable to the oncoming bolus. In addition, swallowing may be compromised severely in patients with resection of the hyomandibular complex (Summers 1971). Second, the patient can use the glossectomy feeding spoon with greatest ease if at least 50% of the tongue has been resected. The presence of more tongue actually interferes with placement of the device.

Puréed (blenderized) or finely chopped food is placed in the bowl of the spoon. The food should be ground to a consistency that eliminates the need for mastication. If lubrication is a problem, gravies, juices, and the like can be mixed in with the food. Holding the spoon level to keep the bolus from falling off, the bowl is placed as far back into the oral cavity as possible (avoid eliciting a gag reflex). Placement should be on the side where the patient has greater tongue mass remaining or better sensation. Sliding the triggering mechanism on the handle causes the push plate on the bowl of the spoon to move and deposit the food onto the base of the tongue.

The glossectomy feeding spoon is useful because it gives patients an opportunity to enjoy something besides liquids that are transported by way of other devices. It is also more esthetically acceptable than a tube since it closely resembles commonly used flatware. At least two types of metal glossectomy feeding spoons available today (Figure 11.4). The one shown on the bottom of the figure is available through Maddock, Inc. Developed at the VA Medical Center, Allen Park, Michigan, the device has been used by several patients and found quite acceptable. Shown in the middle of Figure 11.4 is a measuring spoon used for cooking. It is included here only to show what should not be used for feeding patients; other than being somewhat unwieldy, it is risky to use because the

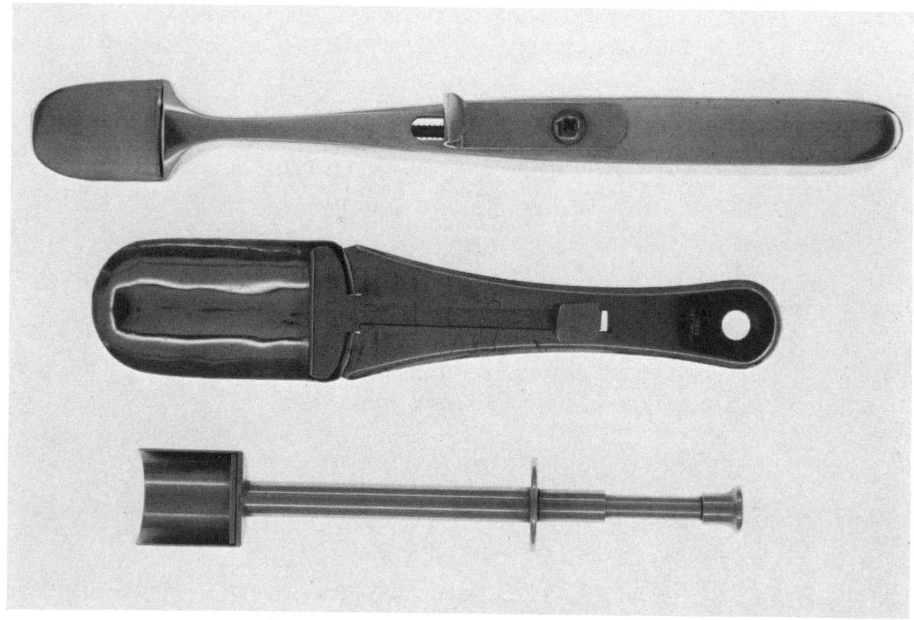

Figure 11.4 Top: Commercially available glossectomy feeding spoon. Middle: Cooking measuring spoon that should not be used for feeding. Bottom: Glossectomy feeding spoon originally available for eligible military veterans, but now commercially available.

push plate easily slides out from the spoon's handle and may be inadvertently deposited into the patient's oropharynx.

If funding is not available to purchase the commercially available spoon, the clinician can readily construct a glossectomy feeding spoon (Fleming and Weaver 1983). It may not be as esthetically pleasing or as easy to use (particularly if trismus is present) as the one described, but it is economical and based on the same principles. It is made from a 20-cc plastic syringe (Figure 11.5). Using a medium-fine hacksaw blade, a horizontal cut is made to one side of the protruding tip at the distal end of the syringe. A second cut is made perpendicular to the first cut so that the larger portion of the distal tip may be removed and discarded. A beveled 45-degree third cut is made on the cylinder wall about 3 cm from the distal end of the cylinder. This cut should continue only to the midpoint of the cylinder. Finally, two parallel cuts are made into the cylinder from the distal end toward the proximal end, intercepting the third cut. The portion of the cylinder that is sectioned by the third and fourth cuts is discarded. The inner portion of the cylinder is then ground down enough so that the piston can move freely. Fine sandpaper is used to remove bits of plastic and to smooth rough edges. The entire process takes less than 10 minutes. At the top of Figure 11.6 is a glossectomy feeding device made from a plastic syringe in the manner described.

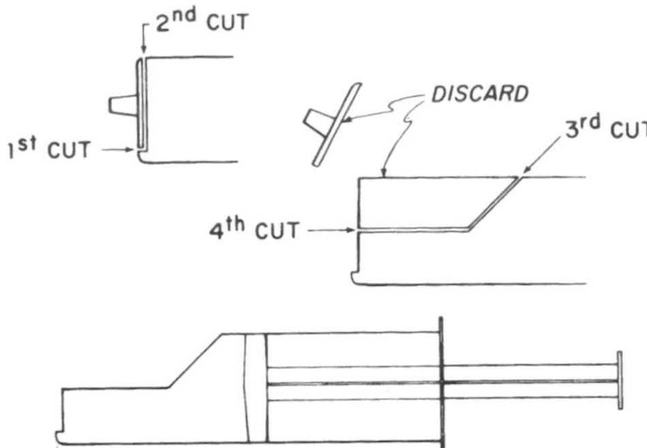

Figure 11.5 Steps used in making a glossectomy feeding spoon from a 20-ml plastic syringe. See the top of Figure 11.6 for the finished product.

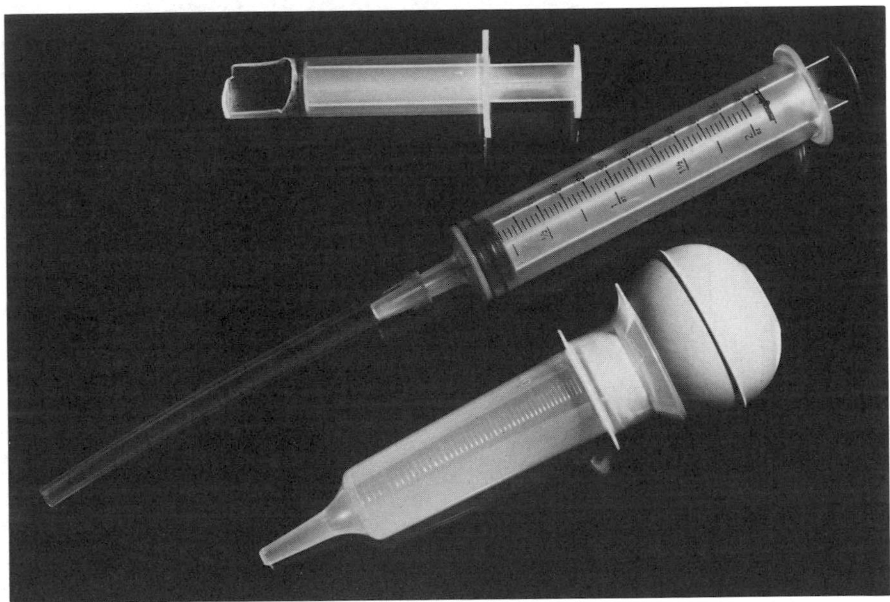

Figure 11.6 Top: Glossectomy feeding spoon made from a 20-ml plastic syringe. Middle: Catheter-tipped 60-ml syringe with tubular extension device for feeding. Bottom: Bulb type syringe sometimes used for feeding.

Patients whose treatment has included resection of bone or muscle tissue may need a maxillofacial prosthesis (Hurst 1988). Depending on the size of the prosthesis, its location, and patient tolerance, it may be necessary to desensitize the patient to the prosthesis. Usually this is most successful when started with the least noxious stimulus (e.g., the clinician placing a clean, soft, nonbreakable object such as a pliable spatula to the area where the prosthesis is to be placed), and ultimately placing the prosthesis itself for more extended periods of time. This desensitization requires a well-motivated patient and a supportive clinician. Fortunately, however, not many patients require such a level of intervention.

Syringes

Patients with lingual paresis or those having less than 50% tongue resection also may have trouble transporting an oral bolus. For these patients, use of the glossectomy feeding spoon is impractical because of the presence of tongue mass. A 50- or 60-ml catheter-tipped syringe (Bakamjian and Cramer 1960) with a 15-cm extension of pliable connecting tubing can be used in these cases (see Figure 11.6, middle). The syringes are available in glass but they are more expensive (approximately $40 each) and more easily broken than the plastic ones. They do have advantages, however, in that they are easy to clean and the pistons slide easily within them. Plastic syringes are more difficult to keep clean and the washerlike tip at the distal end of the piston demonstrates wear by sticking, particularly if very warm foods are used. The major advantages of the plastic syringes are that they cost about one-twentieth as much as glass syringes and they are unbreakable. Individual circumstances suggest which type of syringe to use, but in most settings it is probably better to start with a plastic model and progress to a glass one when the patient can manage the device handily.

Before issuing a catheter-tipped syringe with a tubular extension, the risk of aspiration must be considered. Again, it is incumbent upon the clinician to obtain medical clearance before attempting to use the device with a patient. In addition, the clinician must consider the patient's overall ability to handle the syringe. For example, although only a few patients manage syringe feedings with only one hand, the majority of patients require use of both hands (one to support the device and the other to regulate the piston). The bottom of Figure 11.6 shows a bulb-type syringe. Most patients find this difficult to control, complaining that it squirts food into their mouths, resulting in a startle or recoil response.

The patient must fill the catheter-tipped syringe by slowly withdrawing the piston as the distal tip of the tubular extension is submerged into a liquid or thin purée. The object is to fill the syringe with food without pockets of air. Practice enables most patients to acquire this skill within the first session. To make the task easier, the purée should be strained and not too thick. Once the syringe is filled with food, the patient places the distal tip of the tubular extension at the place in the mouth where there is greatest sensation and ability to move the bolus with the tongue. For patients with surgical excision, that is usually on the back of the unresected portion of tongue. For those who have had a cerebrovascular accident or other neuromuscular problem, the distal tip should be placed where the bolus can be most easily handled.

Connecting tubing is the most convenient tubular extension to use since it is available in most settings and its large diameter (approximately 6 mm or 18 French) allows puréed foods to pass. Smaller-diameter tubing (e.g., 3 mm or 10 French) may have at least two applications. First, it allows more precise placement, which is beneficial in stimulation exercises. Second, some patients, such as those with severe trismus, may be unable to open their mouths wide enough for even the 6-mm connecting tube extension. For them a narrower tube may be more easily tolerated.

Finally, there are patients who, through trauma or elective surgery, must have their teeth wired to prevent jaw opening. For them the problem is usually only a mechanical one—getting liquid food into the oral cavity. A small-gauge feeding tube can be threaded behind the third molar into the oral cavity. Feeding may then proceed with syringe or gavage (feeding) bag, the pliable plastic container used to hold the tube feeding. The attending physician must be informed of the intended method of feeding and be assured that the patient can handle the feedings without aspiration.

The optimal position for feeding dysphagic patients is upright, with head support if necessary (Buckley et al. 1976). The head should not be tilted back; such a posture only increases the chances of aspiration. The one exception to the upright position is when the patient has a problem transporting an oral bolus compounded by drooling and intraoral pooling, but does not have significant risk of aspiration. Eating may be easier if these patients assume a semireclining position (e.g., 50 degrees), but with the head and body on the same plane. The goal is to decrease aspiration (the head remains on same plane with the body, not tilted) while increasing oral transport of the bolus (gravity helps the patient move the bolus to the oropharynx).

The patient with a supraglottic laryngectomy should not extend the head posteriorly in an effort to swallow. There is no reason to extend the head in this way since oral transport of the bolus is not a problem. Extending the head posteriorly only increases aspiration because the laryngeal inlet becomes more accessible to the oncoming bolus.

Sometimes it is necessary to remind or train these patients to learn the supraglottic swallow. This technique, also known as the "controlled" or "safe" swallow, can be applied to many patient populations. It is just an extension of what one normally does when swallowing—i.e., masticate the food, assemble it as a collecting mass bolus, position it on the tongue, inhale, hold the breath, swallow, exhale, swallow again, and exhale again. This sequence of events is almost normal and should be reinforced since it serves to protect the airway and to clear pooled food from the laryngeal aditus. Two points deserve emphasis when teaching this normal sequence. First, exhalation, not inhalation, must follow the swallow. If one were to inhale immediately following a swallow, aspiration would probably occur. Second, the swallow must occur at the beginning, not the end, of the exhalation phase of respiration. This allows an adequate amount of pulmonary air to help clear the laryngeal aditus. Another swallow must follow to clear any materials pooled in the pharyngeal recesses.

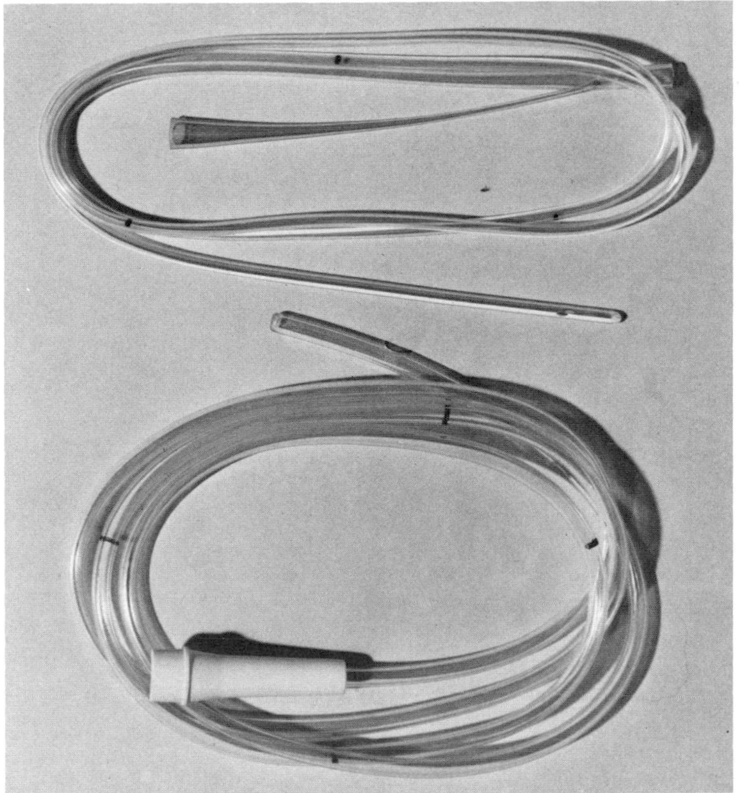

Figure 11.7 Top: Small (10 French) nasogastric feeding tube. Bottom: Large (16 French) nasogastric feeding tube.

Nasogastric Tubes

Unfortunately, in spite of efforts to rehabilitate dysphagic patients, adequate oral nutrition and hydration are sometimes impossible. Although problems associated with patients handling their own secretions persist, problems associated with aspiration of food and fluids can be circumvented through other means. Surgically, an altered feeding route, such as a feeding gastrostoma, jejunostoma, percutaneous endoscopic gastrostoma, or esophagostoma, can be created. These procedures are reserved for patients whose eating problems are considered long term (see Chapter 14). Parenteral feeding is one method of supplying nutrition (Hegedus and Pelham 1975) (see Chapter 13). Another option is to use a nasogastric (NG) feeding tube (Figure 11.7). Although feeding tubes come with a variety of features, perhaps the most important is their diameter. From the standpoint of patient comfort and fewer complications, the smaller size (10 French) is preferred; it also achieves a slower rate of feeding. Patients with larger feeding tubes (16–18 French) tend to feed themselves too rapidly,

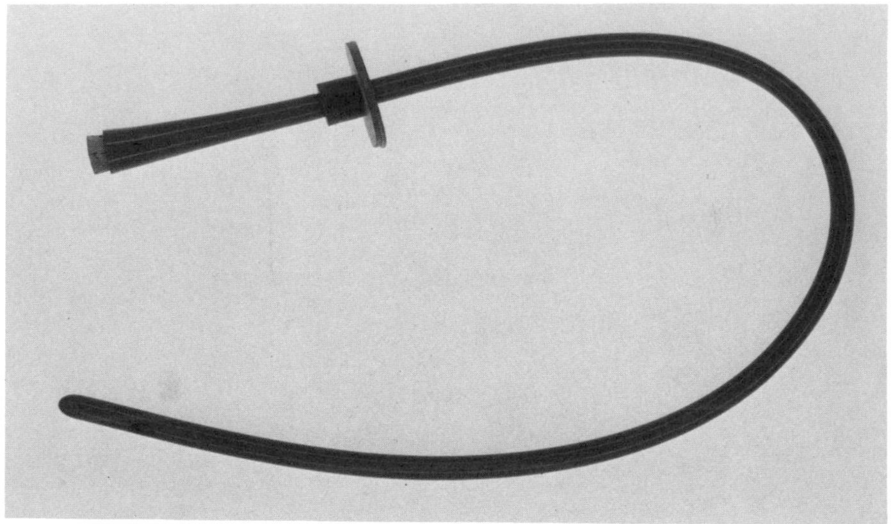

Figure 11.8 Nasoesophageal feeding tube with safety retention flange.

which causes gastric distress (Cataldo and Smith 1980). Also, esophageal ulceration increases with larger tubes, especially if they are used for an extended period. The only advantages of larger feeding tubes are that they are easier to insert and do not clog as easily as the smaller ones. (See Chapter 13 for additional discussion of NG tubes.) These are staff conveniences that do not necessarily improve the patient's comfort and tolerance.

For patients who abhor the thought of being seen outside the hospital setting with a nasogastric feeding tube in place, there is an alternative. They can be taught to carefully insert a shorter feeding tube, take the feeding, withdraw the tube, and clean it properly after use (Donaldson et al. 1968) (Figure 11.8). If they so desire, they can become accustomed to the procedure. The obvious risk is, of course, incorrect insertion of the tube. The objective is to place the distal tip of the reusable tube into the upper esophagus so that it bypasses the level of the pharynx where food might be aspirated into the larynx. The decision to use this device rests with the physician and dysphagia team members and is based on their perception of how adequately the patient can adapt to the method.

TRACHEOSTOMA TUBES

Many patients with mechanical dysphagia have a tracheostoma tube in place, especially in the acute stage of their illness. While tracheostoma tubes assure an airway, they do interfere with swallowing (Feldman et al. 1966; Nash 1988). In a retrospective study, Arms et al. (1974) demonstrated increased risk of aspiration with their presence. Normally, when one swallows, the larynx is lifted in an anterosuperior direction to protect the laryngeal inlet from the

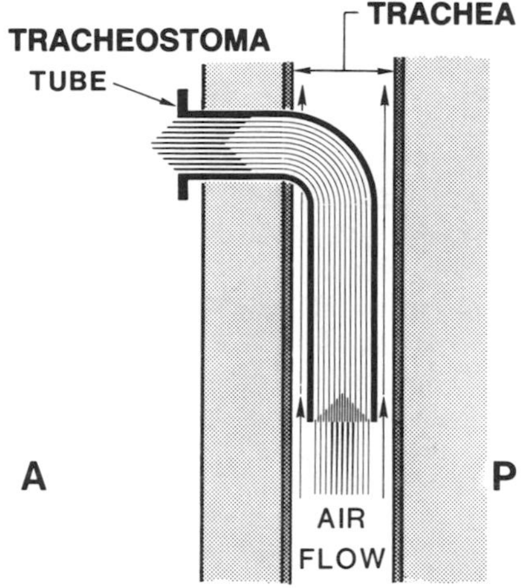

Figure 11.9 The large arrow within the tracheostoma tube indicates a significant proportion of air shunted out of the tracheostoma tube. Smaller arrows show a relatively small proportion of pulmonary air available for clearing the laryngeal aditus.

oncoming bolus. The presence of a tracheostoma tube may anchor the larynx and make it more accessible to the bolus (Bonanno 1971). Another problem concerns pulmonary air, which cannot be used to clear the larynx if obstructions impede the flow of air. Normally, immediately following a swallow we exhale to clear the laryngeal aditus of foreign substance. With a tracheostoma tube, pulmonary air is shunted out via the tube. Evidence, including scintigraphic data, indicates that aspiration usually increases when a tracheostomy tube is not occluded (Fleming et al. 1989; Muz et al. 1989). Figure 11.9 illustrates how most of the pulmonary air is shunted out of the tracheostoma tube when the outer cannula takes up such a large portion of the inner diameter of the trachea. The usual manner of clearing the larynx is not available. Nothing can be done about the presence of the tracheostoma tube limiting anterosuperior laryngeal elevation, but there are some things to consider about improving the flow of pulmonary air through the larynx.

The most practical way to effect passage of air through the larynx instead of out the tracheostoma tube itself is to plug or cover the opening of the tube. The patient can do this with the index finger, which is effective for the immediate purpose, but it is not convenient since it necessitates the continued use of one hand. Full closure plugs (Figure 11.10) can be used to occlude the port. These (Pilling Co.) are tapered and fitted by size so that there is no danger of their being drawn into the trachea. Another means of closing the opening of the tracheostoma tube is by use of a one-way Kistner valve (Figure 11.11). The Kistner valve opens on inhalation and closes when the user exhales. Exhaled air passes upward through the larynx. It should be noted that if a tracheostoma tube diameter is so large that it occludes much of the inner tracheal diameter, no amount of plugging at the open end of the tube will allow pulmonary air to reach the larynx; this mechanical blockage must be dealt with. The simplest solution is to

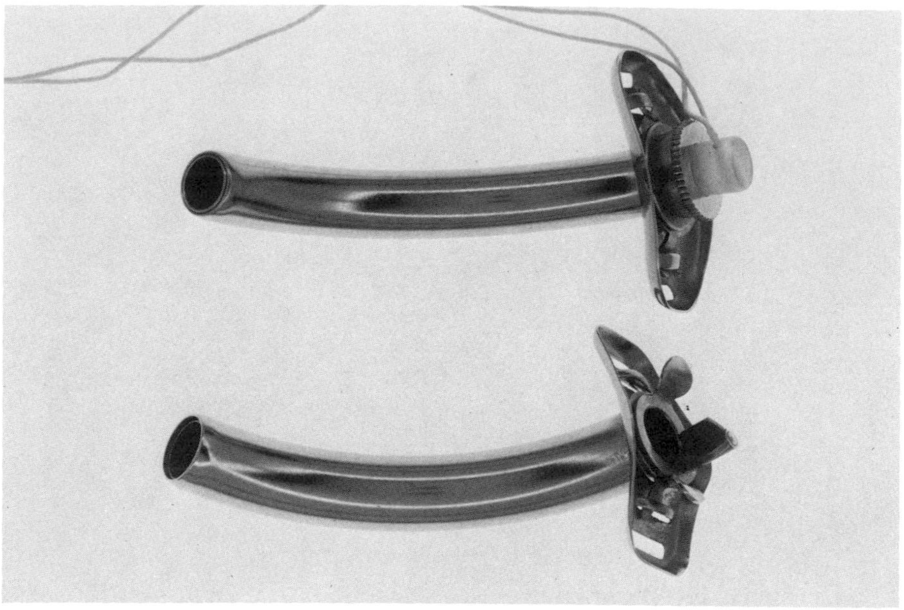

Figure 11.10 Top: Full-closure plugs can be used to occlude the tracheostoma. Bottom: Unplugged tracheostoma tube.

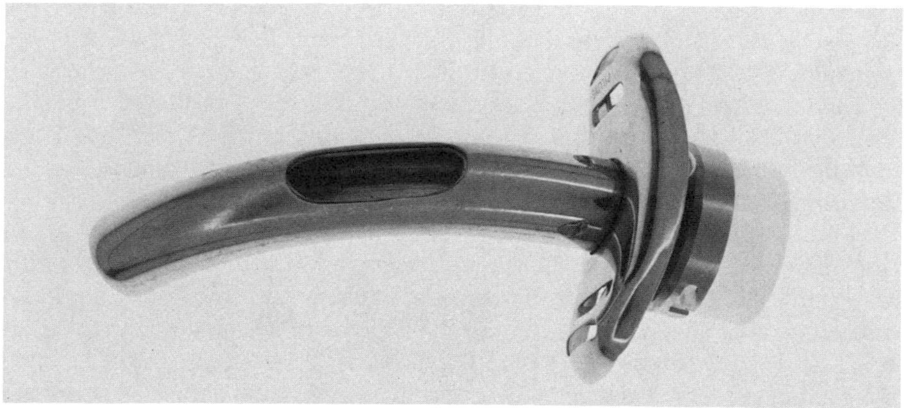

Figure 11.11 A one-way valved tracheostoma tube.

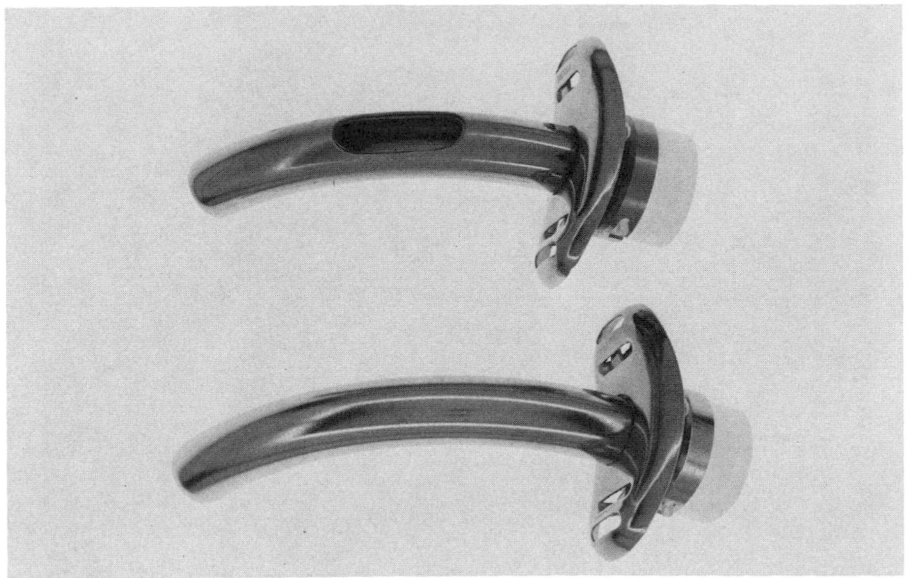

Figure 11.12 Top: Fenestrated and one-way valved tracheostoma tube. Bottom: Unfenestrated and one-way valved tracheostoma tube.

reduce the tracheostoma tube by two sizes. For example, if a patient with a number 8 tube cannot get adequate air to the larynx for phonation or coughing when the tracheostoma opening is plugged, a number 6 tube should be used.

Another way to get pulmonary air to pass upward into the larynx is by use of a fenestrated tracheostoma tube (Figure 11.12, top). Some of these have a valve for the fenestration. These work well unless the patient has copious secretions that could impede the functioning of the fenestration and its valve. Their use may be limited because of problems associated with irritation of the tracheal wall. To eliminate this irritation no part of the fenestration should be adjacent to the tracheal wall. Verification of fenestration location may be done radiographically.

Cuffed tracheostoma tubes present problems such as infection, tracheal stenosis, esophageal erosion, and innominate artery fistualization (Cooper and Grillo 1969; Sasaki 1980). Aspiration cannot always be prevented by a cuffed tracheostoma tube (Cameron et al. 1973; Bone et al. 1974; Pavlin et al. 1974; Bernhard et al. 1979; Petring et al. 1986; Nash 1988). A cuffed tracheostoma tube may well give a false sense of security to the patient and caregivers. The cuff is inflated in an attempt to keep food, liquid, and secretions from getting into the lungs. The top of Figure 11.13 shows a cuff that is inflated; the cuff in the bottom of the figure is not inflated. The cuff should be inflated to the specifications of the physician (Nahum and Harris 1981).

There are, however, three reasons for not feeding patients orally while their tracheostoma cuffs are inflated. First, if a patient's medical condition is so

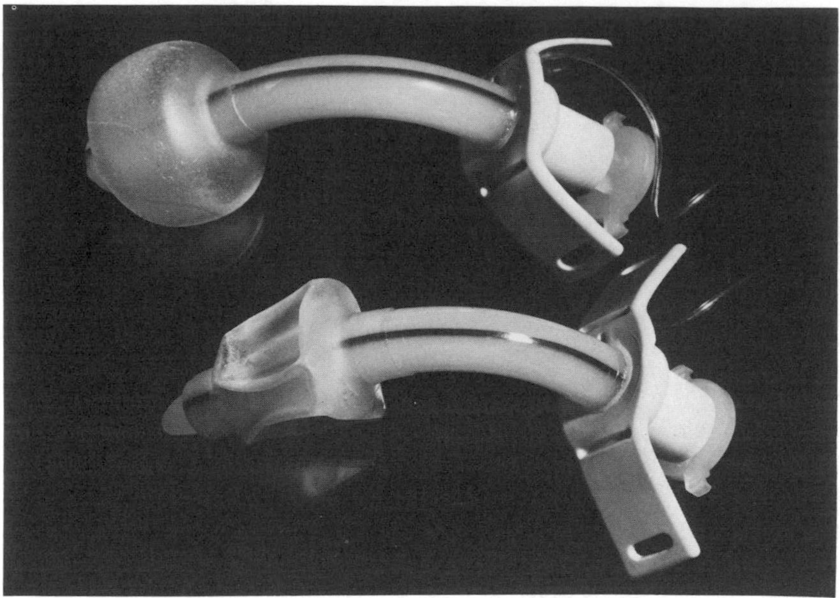

Figure 11.13 Top: Cuffed tracheostoma tube with cuff inflated. Bottom: Cuffed tracheostoma tube with cuff somewhat deflated.

precarious that a cuffed tracheostoma tube is warranted, perhaps oral feeding is premature. It has been demonstrated radiographically that a liquid bolus may get past the cuff and enter the lower trachea. Second, the presence of an inflated cuff prevents pulmonary air from clearing the larynx; this mechanical blockage is not desirable. Third, if a patient is aspirating the food bolus it is vital to know when it occurs so that suctioning can be done immediately. With an inflated cuff that knowledge is delayed.

For tracheotomized ventilator-dependent patients the problems become even more complex. The first consideration is the mode of mechanical ventilation. The mode selected by the physician depends on the patient's ability to independently initiate and maintain aspiration. Rate and volume vary with the patient's condition. As the patient's physical status improves, the weaning process begins. Although there is a good tracheostoma speaking valve for ventilator-dependent patients (Passy-Muir), it is preferred that, whenever possible, cuffs be deflated to enhance deglutition. Tippett and Siebens (1991) reported good clinical outcomes in five ventilator-dependent patients when cuffs could be deflated. These were five selected and well-managed patients with varying medical conditions, but the success nonetheless underscored the need to consider alternative management approaches.

There are guidelines for working with these patients. Once medical clearance has been obtained, the tracheostoma should be suctioned, the cuff deflated, and suctioning repeated. Then the patients may be fed. Adding blue food coloring to the food will help verify aspiration. Once the patients have been fed they should be suctioned again and the cuff inflated to the physician's specifications.

SYNTHETIC SALIVA

Patients taking certain medications, those who have salivary gland dysfunction, and those who are receiving irradiation to the oral or pharyngeal areas will experience xerostomia or dry mouth (Shedd 1976; Dreizen et al. 1977; Sobol et al. 1979; Caruso et al. 1989). In addition to physical discomfort, this causes at least two other problems. First is the loss of saliva that normally serves to cleanse and protect the teeth. Without the protection provided by saliva, dental caries increase (Trowbridge and Carl 1975). Second, decreased saliva reduces the ability to moisten food and facilitate mastication and deglutition (Mansson and Sandberg 1975). This leads to weight loss in many patients.

Although saliva cannot be replaced, artificial saliva is available to provide lubrication. Presently, several synthetic saliva products are commercially available. They are not alike, however. They differ in terms of viscosity, preference, and performance. Ideally, the synthetic saliva should lubricate both hard and soft oral tissues (Aguirre et al. 1989). Usually patients are directed to take the synthetic saliva as needed. Most rinse with a spoonful of the synthetic saliva just prior to eating. Some of these products contain fluoride to deter caries (Dudgeon et al. 1980). Unfortunately, some may have a drying effect (Daeffler 1981), so their use must be assessed on an individual basis.

Lemon-glycerin swabs are available for the patient to cleanse and freshen the mouth. Although for many patients these special swabs provide relief, others find that they add to oral dryness with long-term use. Patient preference will help determine the amount and frequency of use of lemon-glycerin swabs.

In addition to synthetic saliva, a surface anesthetic applied just prior to eating may help reduce the pain associated with deglutition. Surface anesthesia should be used carefully in patients at high risk for aspiration, since the swallowing mechanism should not be further compromised by reduced sensation.

FOOD BLENDERS

Perhaps the most a clinician can do for the patient is to provide the food consistency that the patient tolerates best. Unfortunately, most people assume that liquid consistency is best. This is not necessarily so. Many patients with mechanical disorders leading to dysphagia do better with food of purée consistency (Ardran and Kemp 1952; Summers 1971; Edwards 1973; Paavolainen 1977; Silverman and Elfant 1979). Puréed material is less mobile than liquid, and for those with an impaired oropharyngeal mechanism it is important to minimize aspiration. This is especially true of the patient who has undergone a supraglottic laryngectomy. Evidence that puréed material is preferable for some patients is supported by our clinical experience and radiographic observations.

Fluids are more easily tolerated by patients who demonstrate an organic stenosis (Hellemans et al. 1981).

Dentition status influences masticatory performance. Additionally, patient perceptions about actual texture acceptability affect anxiety associated with chewing and swallowing performance (Garcia et al. 1989). Consequently, offering easy-to-chew foods or foods that have been blenderized to a patient's optimal texture may facilitate deglutition (von Branchitsch and May 1968).

Although aspiration is not possible in patients who have undergone a total laryngectomy (unless, of course, there is an unplanned fistula), this patient population frequently experience difficulty swallowing (Schobinger 1958; Kaplan 1984; McConnel et al. 1988). When comparing total laryngectomees to normal healthy controls, Hamlet et al. (1992) reported that there is an increased role for tongue propulsions in laryngectomee swallows. Clinically, laryngectomized patients report more effort swallowing solids, the tongue seems to "pump" the food into the esophagus, and food texture needs to be altered. Thus, a food blender can be helpful to the patient with a total laryngectomy. Laryngectomized patients also report that alternating a food bolus with a liquid bolus is helpful. Apparently the liquid helps to "flush" the bolus through the stenotic area.

Food consistency is of such importance that some facilities make food blenders available to patients. An added benefit of blenders is that the cost of purchasing specially prepared products can be reduced as patients are able to purée items consumed by the rest of the family (Farrior and Kelly 1979).

Just as food blenders are available for altering the rheologic characteristics of solid foods, there are commercially available food thickeners to modify the viscosity of liquids. Significant concerns for the dysphagic patient are not only calories and nutrition but also hydration. For the patient who is quite compromised with liquids, the use of food thickeners may well determine whether a feeding tube (nasogastric or surgical) is necessary. Caution dictates, however, that in patients who are severely dysphagic, the use of food thickeners still may not be sufficient. Some patients who have been taking artificially thickened fluids on a long-term basis complain that they fail to quench their thirst. As with many treatment and management techniques, the problem may be ameliorated but not eliminated.

SUMMARY

Mechanical swallowing disorders in the mouth, pharynx, and esophagus usually result from a combination of structure loss and rearrangement and potential peripheral nerve involvement secondary to removal of cancerous lesions. Such lesions in the mouth and pharynx may require glossectomy, partial pharyngectomy, and partial laryngectomy, resulting in difficulty transporting and channeling a bolus. Decisions concerning the appropriate mechanical device and diet needed to obviate mechanical disorders are based on the type and amount of resection, concomitant medical complications, and patient acceptance and cooperation. Alternatives to regular dietary intake via nasogastric tube feeding, surgically created feeding routes, and blenderized textures need to be considered.

REFERENCES

Aguirre A, Mendoza B, Reddy MS, et al. Lubrication of selected salivary molecules and artificial salivas. Dysphagia 1989;4:95.

Ardran GM, Kemp FH. The protection of the laryngeal airway during swallowing. Br J Radiol 1952;23:406.

Arms RA, Dines DE, Tinstman TC. Aspiration pneumonia. Chest 1974;65:136.

Bakamjian V, Cramer L. Surgical management of advanced cancer of the tongue. Ann Surg 1960;152:1058.

Bernhard WN, Cottrell JE, Sivakumaran C, et al. Adjustment of intracuff pressure to prevent aspiration. Anesthesiology 1979;50:363.

Bonanno PC. Swallowing dysfunction after tracheostomy. Ann Surg 1971;174:29.

Bone DK, Davis JL, Zuidema GD, et al. Aspiration pneumonia. Prevention of aspiration in patients with tracheostomies. Ann Thorac Surg 1974;174:30.

Buckley JE, Addicks CL, Maniglia J. Feeding patients with dysphagia. Nurs Forum 1976;15:69.

Cameron JL, Reynolds J, Zuidema CD. Aspiration in patients with tracheostomies. Surg Gyn Obstet 1973;136:68.

Caruso AJ, Sonies BC, Atkinson JC, et al. Objective measures of swallowing in patients with primary Sjögren's syndrome. Dysphagia 1989;4:101.

Castell J, Dalton C, Castell D. Effects of body position and bolus consistency on the manometric parameters and coordination of the upper esophageal sphincter and pharynx. Dysphagia 1990;5:179.

Cataldo CB, Smith L. Tube Feedings: Clinical Applications. Columbus, Ohio: Ross Laboratories, 1980.

Christup J. Normal swallowing of foodstuffs of pasty consistency. Dan Med Bull 1964;11:79.

Cooper JD, Grillo HC. The evolution of tracheal injury due to ventilatory assistance through cuffed tubes: a pathologic study. Ann Surg 1969;169:334.

Daeffler R. Oral hygiene measures for patients with cancer. Cancer Nurs 1981;4:29.

Donaldson RC, Skelly M, Paletta FX. Total glossectomy for cancer. Am J Surg 1968;116:585.

Dreizen S, Daly TE, Drane JB, et al. Oral complications of cancer radiotherapy. Postgrad Med 1977;61:85.

Dudgeon BJ, DeLisa JA, Miller RM. Head and neck cancer, a rehabilitation approach. Am J Occup Ther 1980;34:243.

Edwards H. Neurological disease of the pharynx and larynx. Practitioner 1973;211:729.

Ekberg O. Posture of the head and pharyngeal swallowing. Acta Radiologica Diag 1986;27:691.

Ekberg O, Nylander G. Cineradiography of the pharyngeal stage of deglutition in 150 individuals without dysphagia. Br J Radiol 1982;55:253.

Farrior JB III, Kelly MT. Home nutrition for patients with head and neck tumors. Ear Nose Throat J 1979;58:84.

Feldman SA, Deal CW, Urquhart W. Disturbance of swallowing after tracheostomy. Lancet 1966;1:954.

Fleming S, Muz J, Hamlet S. Practical scintigraphic application for the dysphagic patient. ASHA 1990;32:72.

Fleming S, Nelson R, Muz J, et al. Scintigraphy in the dysphagic patient. Presented at National Conference, American Speech-Language-Hearing Association, St. Louis, November 1989.

Fleming SM, Weaver AW. Glossectomy feeding device readily adapted from a plastic syringe. Arch Phys Med Rehabil 1983;64:183.
Garcia RI, Perlmutter LC, Chauncey HH. Effects of dentition status and personality on masticatory performance and food acceptability. Dysphagia 1989;4:136.
Hamlet S. Dynamic aspects of lingual propulsive activity in swallowing. Dysphagia 1989;4:136.
Hamlet S, Choi J, Zormeier M, et al. Normal adult swallowing of liquid and viscous material: scintigraphic data on bolus transit and oropharyngeal residues. Dysphagia 1996;11:41.
Hamlet SL, Muz J, Farris R, et al. Scintigraphic quantification of pharyngeal retention following deglutition. Dysphagia 1992;7:12.
Hamlet SL, Muz J, Patterson R, et al. Pharyngeal transit time: assessment with videofluoroscopic and scintigraphic techniques. Dysphagia 1989;4:4.
Hamlet SL, Patterson RL, Fleming SM, et al. Sounds of swallowing following total laryngectomy. Dysphagia 1992;7:160.
Hegedus S, Pelham M. Dietetics in a cancer hospital. J Am Diet Assoc 1975;67:235.
Hellemans J, Pelemans W, Vantrappen G. Pharyngoesophageal swallowing disorders and the pharyngo-esophageal sphincter. Med Clin North Am 1981;65:1149.
Humphreys B, Mathog R, Rosen R, et al. Videofluoroscopic and scintigraphic analysis of dysphagia in the head and neck cancer patient. Laryngoscope 1987;97:25.
Hurst PS. The role of the prosthodontist in the correction of swallowing disorders. Otol Clin North Am 1988;21:771.
Kaplin JN. The incidence of hypopharyngeal stenosis after surgery for laryngeal cancer. Otol Clin North Am 1984;89:656.
Kasprisin A, Clumeck H, Nino-Murcia M. The efficacy of rehabilitative management of dysphagia. Dysphagia 1989;4:48.
Kilman WJ, Goyal RK. Disorders of pharyngeal and upper esophageal sphincter motor function. Arch Intern Med 1976;136:592.
Kirsch CM, Sanders A. Aspiration pneumonia: medical management. Otolaryngol Clin North Am 1988;21:677.
Logemann J, Kahrilas P, Kobara M, et al. The benefit of head rotation on pharyngoesophageal dysphagia. Arch Phys Med 1989;70:767.
Mansson I, Sandberg N. Salivary stimulus and swallowing reflex in man. Acta Otolaryngol 1975;79:445.
McConnel F, Cereuko D, Mendelsohn M. Dysphagia after total laryngectomy. Otol Clin North Am 1988;21:721.
Muz J, Fleming S, Hamlet S. Bolus consistency and aspiration: quantification with scintigraphy. Presented at The Johns Hopkins Third Symposium on Dysphagia, Baltimore, MD, March 22–23, 1990.
Muz J, Mathog RH, Nelson R, et al. Aspiration in patients with head and neck cancer and tracheostomy. Am J Otolaryngol 1989;10:282.
Nahum AM, Harris JP, Davidson TM. The patient who aspirates—diagnosis and management. J Otolaryngol 1981;10:10.
Nash M. Swallowing problems in the tracheotomized patient. Otolaryngol Clin North Am 1988;21:701.
Paavolainen M. Rehabilitation of eating after supraglottic laryngectomy. Minerva Otorhinolaryngol 1977;27:91.
Palvin EG, Van Nimwegan D, Hornbein TF. Failure of a high-compliance low-pressure cuff to prevent aspiration. Anesthesiology 1974;42:216.
Petring OU, Adelhoj B, Jensen BN, et al. Prevention of silent aspiration due to leaks around cuffs of endotracheal tubes. Anesth Analg 1986;65:777.
Sasaki CT. Paralysis of the larynx and pharynx. Surg Clin North Am 1980;60:1079.
Schobinger R. Spasm of the cricopharyngeal muscle as a cause of dysphagia after total laryngectomy. Arch Otolaryngol 1958;67:271.

Shedd DP. Rehabilitation problems of head and neck cancer patients. J Surg Oncol 1976;8:11.

Silverman EH, Elfant IL. Dysphagia: an evaluation and treatment program for the adult. Am J Occup Ther 1979;33:382.

Sobol SM, Conoyer JM, Sessions DG. Enteral and parenteral nutrition in patients with head and neck cancer. Ann Otolaryngol 1979;88:495.

Summers GW. Physiologic problems following ablative surgery of the head and neck. Otolaryngol Clin North Am 1971;7:217.

Tippett DC, Siebens AA. Using ventilators for speaking and swallowing. Dysphagia 1991;6:94.

Tracy J, Logemann J, Kahrilas P, et al. Preliminary observations on the effects of age on oropharyngeal deglutition. Dysphagia 1989;4:90.

Trowbridge JE, Carl W. Oral care of the patient having head and neck irradiation. Am J Nurs 1975;75:2146.

von Branchitsch H, May W. Deaths from aspiration and asphyxiation in a mental hospital. Arch Gen Psychiatry 1968;18:129.

Weiss MH. Dysphagia in infants and children. Otolaryngol Clin North Am 1988;21:727.

12

Nutritional Considerations in Dysphagia

Jean E. Curran

The importance of early recognition of patients at risk for developing protein-calorie malnutrition in both acute and chronic care settings, and subsequently providing appropriate therapy and nutritional support, has only recently begun to receive the attention it deserves. The distressing prevalence of malnourishment in hospitalized patients and the deleterious effect of malnutrition on clinical outcome have been the major causes of health professionals' increasing concern about the need for timely nutrition intervention in a manner comparable to that provided with other medical or surgical treatment (Bistrian et al. 1976). The assessment of nutritional status, implementation of a care plan, and continuous monitoring and evaluation of individual patients to determine the effectiveness and appropriateness of the nutritional care plan must give greater precedence to correcting nutrient imbalances, restoring nutritional well-being, and maintaining quality of life.

Patients presenting with dysphagia and the inability to take adequate food and fluid by mouth, whether as a result of neurologic disease or surgical resections involving any part of the alimentary tract, should be considered at high nutritional risk. Over the past few decades there has been heightened awareness of the adverse events caused by inadequate intake in this population; optimal patient care depends on adequate nutritional support (Jones and Altschuler 1987). The consequence of untreated dysphagia is protein-calorie malnutrition (Hynak-Hankinson 1984), which may lead to life-threatening nutrition-associated complications (Detsky et al. 1984) including increased susceptibility to infection due to compromise of the immune system, respiratory failure, poor wound healing, skin breakdown (Detsky et al. 1984) in both the bed-bound and the wheelchair-bound, and death.

ASSESSMENT OF NUTRITIONAL STATUS

The registered dietitian in a clinical setting is the primary health professional responsible for ensuring that all patients are adequately nourished, either by providing nutrients appropriate in both quality and quantity to individual needs, or by counseling patients, their families, or both in their own food choices (Zeman 1983). Dietitians are uniquely trained not only in biochemistry, anatomy and physiology, food science, and diet therapy, but also in behavioral sciences, counseling skills, and institutional management. They are therefore qualified to assume the role of nutrition specialist and are instrumental in preventing problems associated with malnutrition by identifying patients with predisposing factors, planning and implementing the appropriate route and mode of nutrient delivery, and monitoring and evaluating the whole process (Kamel 1990).

The initial step in preventing complications of malnutrition is being able to identify patients with predisposing factors who are at risk and likely to benefit from nutritional support. Malnutrition generally results from factors that affect ingestion or digestion and impair absorption or utilization of nutrients (Lang and Cashman 1989). Table 12.1 lists the variety of physiologic, psychological, and psychosocial factors that suggest a patient might be at nutritional risk. Acute care facilities should use such a list to help dietitians identify patients at risk by noting the number and severity of risk factors in each patient. The routine screening process normally includes recording the initial diagnosis, medical and surgical history, height and weight, dental status, medication orders, and serum albumin concentration. The use of individual objective (laboratory) measures such as serum albumin, which may be affected by hydration status, stress, and other comorbid disease processes (hepatic disease, protein-losing enteropathies), may be inadequate when evaluating the effects of nutritional repletion due to albumin's prolonged half-life. Use of laboratory measures can also be slow because there is often a wait for the return of laboratory data (Detsky et al. 1984).

The presence of protein-calorie malnutrition is not easily determined by an individual lab test or diagnostic procedure. Objective data collection such as diagnosis and history, anthropometric measurements, prescribed medications, and serum albumin concentration is routinely used to perform a nutrition assessment, historically viewed as a means of diagnosing protein-calorie malnutrition (Baker et al. 1982). Unfortunately, a single test or lab value continues to be of little value in determining whether a patient is malnourished (Blackburn et al. 1977). In addition, clinical examination, when used as part of a nutrition assessment, has not been critically analyzed or tested for validity and reproducibility (Baker et al. 1982). Therefore, there are no definitive tests for diagnosing protein-calorie malnutrition and no universally accepted criterion for malnourishment. However, there is clearly a consistent relationship between poor nutritional status and the risk of developing these nutrition-related complications (Detsky et al. 1987a).

The benefits of nutritional status assessment for surgical patients have been confirmed in studies on the relationship between poor nutritional status and increased risk postoperative complications using a more prognostic than diagnostic instrument, Subjective Global Assessment (SGA) (Detsky et al. 1987a). The use of SGA relies heavily on the clinical assessment—that is, the result of the routine history and physical examination. Patients are classified as either well nourished, moderately malnourished, or severely malnourished (Figure 12.1).

Table 12.1 Factors Suggesting Nutritional Risk

Diagnosis indicative of nutritional risk
Alcoholism and/or drug abuse
Acquired immunodeficiency syndrome
Cancer
Coronary heart disease
Dehydration
Diabetes
Gastrointestinal tract disease
Liver disease
Lung disease
Malnutrition
Neurologic disorders
Obesity
Infection, trauma, burns
Psychiatric illness
Physical findings indicative of nutritional risk
Cachexia
Involuntary weight loss
Poor dentition, ill-fitting dentures
Inability to feed self
Anorexia from illness, drugs, therapy
Dysphagia
Losses from diarrhea, draining wounds, and fistulas
Hospital treatment indicative of nutritional risk
Chemotherapy
Radiation therapy
Surgical resections of head and neck or gastrointestinal tract
Dental
Drug-nutrient interactions
Chronic use of medications that affect digestion, absorption, or utilization
Prolonged use of inadequate diets (i.e., clear liquids)
Nothing by mouth for >3 days
Psychosocial factors
Fear, anxiety, depression about illness
Isolation, inability to shop or cook for self
Dislike of hospital food and/or therapeutic diet
Food idiosyncrasies or concern about the side effects or after effects of eating specific foods (i.e., milk)

It is important to note that studies (Detsky et al. 1987a) concluded that SGA is a useful and accurate nutritional assessment technique and that this method performed better in determining patients most likely to develop nutrition-related complications than single objective measures such as percentage ideal body weight on admission and serum albumin level. Although these studies were performed to predict postoperative complications in surgical patients, SGA

History

1. Weight change
   Overall loss in past 6 months:
   Amount = _____ kg; ____%
   Change in past 2 weeks: ______ increase
   ______ no change
   ______ decrease
2. Dietary intake change (relative to normal)
   ____ no change
   ____ change ____ duration = _____weeks
   ____ type _____ suboptimal solid diet
   _____ full liquid diet
   _____ hypocaloric liquids
   _____ starvation
3. Gastrointestinal symptoms (that have persisted for >2 weeks)
   _____ none
   _____ nausea
   _____ vomiting
   _____ diarrhea
   _____ anorexia
4. Functional capacity
   _____ no dysfunction (e.g., full capacity)
   _____ dysfunction _____ duration = _____ weeks
   _____ type: _____ working suboptimally
   _____ ambulatory
   _____ bedridden

Physical

For each trait specify:
0 = normal
1+ = mild
2+ = moderate
3+ = severe
_____ loss of subcutaneous fat (triceps, chest)
_____ muscle wasting (quadriceps, deltoids)
_____ ankle edema
_____ ascites

Rating

_____ A = well nourished
_____ B = moderately (or suspected of being) malnourished
_____ C = severely malnourished

Figure 12.1 Subjective Global Assessment. (Adapted from AS Detsky, JR McLaughlin, JP Baker, et al. What is subjective global assessment of nutritional status? J Parenter Enteral Nutri 1987;11:8.)

Class A
<5% weight loss
>5% total weight loss but with recent gain and improvement in appetite
Class B
5–10% weight loss without recent stabilization or gain
Poor dietary intake
Mild (1+) loss of subcutaneous tissue
Class C
Ongoing weight loss of >10%
Severe subcutaneous tissue loss and muscle wasting, often with edema

Figure 12.1 (*continued*)

is likely to be a useful tool on chronic medical wards. Patients in these wards are also at risk for developing skin breakdown and infections such as pneumonia, potentially increasing complications and costs, slowing recovery, and increasing lengths of hospital stay (Smith et al. 1989).

Another assessment technique, the prognostic nutritional index, combines a variety of objective measurements to derive a specific index from statistics. SGA is less sensitive and more specific, meaning that very few well-nourished patients will receive a false-positive diagnosis, though some mildly depleted patients may be missed (Detsky et al. 1994). Good clinical judgment in interpreting the SGA data based on their overall relationship to the patient's medical or surgical status will allow the clinician to formulate a feasible, appropriate nutritional care plan.

Classification or "rating" of patients into A, B, or C levels is based on subjectively combining features of the history and physical examination. Particular importance is given to the history of weight loss expressed as a proportionate loss from a patient's usual body weight (net loss of more than 10%, which is considered a serious loss), inadequate nutrient intake, muscle wasting, and loss of subcutaneous fat.

Case 1

An ambulatory head-and-neck-cancer patient presented with a laryngeal mass and a history of severe odynophagia and dysphagia over a 4-week period. His subsequent intake was restricted to thin, hypocaloric liquids (broth, gelatin, juice, soda). He had an ongoing weight loss of more than 5% and normal to mild (1+; see Figure 12.1) subcutaneous fat loss. During a preoperative nutritional assessment, this patient was ranked as class B, moderately malnourished.

Case 2

On transfer to an intermediate care ward pending discharge with home health care assistance, a class A (well-nourished) status was assigned to a normal-weight 75-year-old man with Parkinson's disease accompanied by solid food dysphagia over a 2-year period. Recently widowed, the patient was unable to procure his own food and unable to prepare meals; previously, his wife had prepared his food according to the outpatient dietitian's diet instruction. The patient had a weight loss of 12% of usual body weight over a 3-month period at home, mild (1+) loss of subcutaneous fat, and acute onset of thin-liquid aspiration due to mental status changes resulting from changes in medication. The patient was referred by family members to a local medical center, who contacted the dysphagia team for a consultation. Admitted to an acute ward, the patient was rehydrated with intravenous solutions. Because of the degenerative, progressive, and irreversible nature of the disease, a percutaneous endoscopic gastrostomy tube was placed for future use. The patient's appetite increased as his mental status improved. His weight loss stabilized and a subsequent 6% weight gain followed over the next month (so net weight loss was 6% for the entire period) as the patient continued to tolerate a dysphagia diet with feeding assistance on intermediate care pending discharge home.

Case 3

A robust, physically fit 65-year-old diabetic male was admitted with an acute stroke. The patient was initially kept on a non-oral diet, receiving only intravenous fluid for hydration and medication. Subsequently, he received inadequate nasogastric feedings due to large gastric residuals secondary to diabetic gastroparesis. A follow-up demonstrated gross evidence of protein-calorie malnutrition via muscle and fat wasting and development of skin breakdown with the formation of decubitus ulcers. Despite the presence of lower-extremity edema due to hypoalbuminemia and its accompanying loss of fluid from the intravascular to extravascular space, his weight clearly followed a pattern of ongoing weight loss. Despite overall good health, this patient would be classified as severely malnourished on a routine reassessment using SGA.

Successful management depends on accurate and timely assessment of nutritional status. With the recent birth and ongoing evolution of managed care systems, the use of SGA may be of great importance to a variety of health care professionals in prioritizing patients who require immediate referral to the clinical dietitian. The SGA can be performed by one of the first clinicians assigned to interview or examine the patient, eliminating the need to wait for laboratory results. Those who are or are likely to become malnourished can thus receive more aggressive nutritional support before nutrition-associated complications can set in. In this way, SGA may indirectly facilitate faster recovery from illness, preventing extended lengths of stay in health care facilities.

The registered dietitian in a clinical setting is the primary health professional responsible for ensuring that all patients are adequately nourished, but a variety of clinicians, including nurses, physicians, and medical students, should be able to apply the method. A good level of inter-rater reproducibility agreement on SGA ratings has been documented (Detsky et al. 1987a). Registered dietitians may lead training in the use of SGA, beginning with a group in-service approach. Subsequently, to test clinical reproducibility, students collect data on a series of patients independently and then compare their rankings (Detsky et al. 1994).

PATIENT IDENTIFICATION: THE DIETITIAN'S ROLE

Dietitians can play an important role in identifying patients with swallowing problems and can be instrumental in initiating referrals to the swallowing team. Dietetic clinicians working specifically with populations at risk for swallowing disorders should be familiar with the principal causes of dysphagia, such as neurologic disease, cerebrovascular disease, demyelinating disorders, end-stage dementia, comatose state, late-stage Parkinson's disease (Ciocon 1990), impairment from surgical resections of the head and neck (glossectomy, hemilaryngectomy, supraglottic laryngectomy), acute inflammatory processes (pharyngitis, tonsillitis, thrush), and the potential side effects of radiation therapy that influence normal deglutition (Fleming et al. 1977). The medical and surgical history should be reviewed, taking into account the problems mentioned above and any history of aspiration pneumonia, lung disease, or esophageal disorders. The dietitian's involvement with identifying and preventing potential drug-nutrient interactions has expanded greatly in recent years (Murray and Healy 1991), and a review of the patient's current medication orders may identify the use of drugs that frequently cause xerostomia (Table 12.2) and subsequent problems with chewing or swallowing. Familiarity with the symptoms of dysphagia, such as reduced attention, distractibility, abnormal head and body position, drooling of liquid bolus, pocketing, coughing, choking, changes in vocal quality, slow eating, and observed patient inability to feed independently and use eating utensils, can alert the dietitian that a patient may have a problem. "Meal rounds," observation of patients at mealtime that are usually done on a routine basis, are an invaluable way to obtain firsthand information on any problems in chewing, swallowing, self-feeding ability, or overall food intake.

Finally, the dietitian's expertise in eliciting subjective information about usual eating habits may be a key factor in identifying a patient in need of a thorough swallowing evaluation. In patients with swallowing disorders secondary to altered mental status or impaired speech, however, obtaining information from patients themselves may be difficult or impossible (Miller 1992). The patient, caregiver, or both may initially deny problems with swallowing, but further investigation may reveal a diet history suggestive of avoidance of solid or liquid food items, food preparation methods such as mashing, chopping, or blenderizing, reliance on nutritional supplements, or the use of commercial baby food.

Table 12.2 Classes of Drugs with Xerostomic Side Effects

Analgesic mixtures
Anticonvulsants
Antiemetics
Antihistamines
Antihypertensives
Antinauseants
Antiparkinsonism agents
Antipruritics
Antispasmodics
Appetite suppressants
Cold medications
Decongestants
Diuretics
Expectorants
Muscle relaxants
Psychotropic drugs
Central nervous system depressants
Benzodiazepine derivatives
Monoamine oxidase inhibitors
Phenothiazine derivatives
Tranquilizers, major and minor
Sedatives

Source: Reprinted with permission from SL Bahn. Drug-related dental destruction. Oral Surg 1972;33:50.

Alternative Nutrition: Options and Issues

In most circumstances, relatively healthy, well-nourished hospitalized patients can withstand the effects of about 1 week of starvation and stress secondary to surgery, trauma, or illness (Blackburn 1988). However, based on the American Society of Enteral and Parenteral Nutrition (ASPEN) Guidelines for Enteral Feeding (ASPEN 1987), the following necessitate use of enteral nutrition support:

- Protein-calorie malnutrition (>10% loss of usual weight or serum albumin levels of <3.5 g/dl) with inadequate intake of nutrients for the previous 5 days
- Normal nutritional status with less than 50% of required nutrient intake orally for the previous 7–10 days
- Severe dysphagia
- Major full-thickness burns
- Small-bowel resection in combination with administration of total parenteral nutrition (TPN)

As nutritional repletion improves muscle strength, swallowing function (Vreudge 1994), the ability to concentrate and interpret instructions (Beadle et al. 1995), and overall quality of life, dysphagic patients in a weakened and debilitated state due to poor intake require enteral feeding as part of routine care to improve nutritional status before dysphagia therapy can be initiated successfully. Malnutrition in this population may also compound the already-present depression, apathy, and feelings of weakness that are often misinterpreted as loss of the will to eat (Beadle et al. 1995). For patients with severe neurologic impairments that compromise the mechanism and cognitive integrity needed to protect the airway during swallow, an oral diet is contraindicated due to the high risk of aspiration and its life-threatening consequences. Enteral feeding is also initiated for patients who have undergone surgical procedures for head and neck cancer.

When developing initial dysphagia treatment strategies, the "when, how, and what to feed" question is a most distressing one, often provoking uncertainty and biased opinions. The risk of developing pneumonia in a patient already weak and debilitated, together with the patient's potential inability to maintain successful oral nutrition and hydration, poses crucial questions to those involved in the care of dysphagic patients (Scott and Heughan 1993).

It is generally agreed that using nasogastric tube feeding for alimentation purposes over an extended period has undesirable consequences, particularly for dysphagic, elderly, bedridden, and comatose individuals. Dramatic increases in the volume of oropharyngeal secretions, greater difficulty in swallowing saliva, regurgitation of stomach contents, pooling of pharyngeal secretions around the tube, inability to clear pulmonary secretions effectively, and suppression of the cough reflex due to the tube's constant presence (Scott and Austin 1994) all contribute to the risk of aspiration. Other complications include tube dislodgement, often by self-extubation, frequent interruption of feeding with concomitant weight loss while awaiting tube replacement, discomfort from frequent reintubation, social or cosmetic unacceptableness, nasal and skin irritation from the tube and the tape used to secure it in place, routine clogging, and difficulty passing medications due to their narrow bore.

The associated costs of replacement tubes—the extra nursing time required to monitor patients for proper upright positioning in bed, gastric residual checks, more frequent suctioning, and long-term nutritional support—are also an issue. Although the gastrostomy tube, particularly the percutaneous endoscopic gastrostomy tube (PEG), can produce both insertion and management complications, including infection and aspiration (Park et al. 1992), it has gained widespread acceptance as a means of providing long-term nutrition. Despite lack of data supporting the view that the risk of aspiration pneumonia is lower with a gastrostomy tube than a nasogastric tube, a history of aspiration pneumonia was found to be the only risk factor associated with future episodes during gastrostomy tube feedings (Cogen and Weinryb 1989). This study found that the only gastrostomy tube patients who developed pneumonia were those who had a prior episode of aspiration pneumonia (in other words, they seemed to have a compromised respiratory system to begin with).

Many patients who are candidates for swallowing rehabilitation ultimately require non-oral feeding for more than 4–6 weeks, so PEG feeding is a major advance in helping to restore or maintain nutritional status while enhancing quality of life and rehabilitation potential (Raha 1993). The basic decision about whether to feed becomes an issue in the period after the patient has been identified, when consultations are being conducted and before management options are implemented. Nasogastric tube feeding continues to be used routinely as a temporary means of providing nutrition during this time, although some researchers no longer consider it an option in acute stroke (Hussain and Cox 1993).

The use of TPN, administration of a hypertonic nutrient solution directly into a central vein, has been suggested for use in dysphagic patients (Sitzman 1990). Historically, TPN has been reserved for patients with nonfunctioning gastrointestinal tracts or extremely high nutrient requirements. When considering this option, the possibility of aspiration in a dysphagic patient must be weighed against the risk of multiple technical and metabolic complications, including infection, sepsis, and gut atrophy if TPN continues over an extended period. Although this feeding method bypasses the gastrointestinal tract completely, patients who cannot swallow their own saliva are still at risk for developing aspiration pneumonia. The inability of a peripheral vein to tolerate hypertonic nutrient solutions makes peripheral parenteral nutrition appropriate for mildly to moderately malnourished patients and those with normal to slightly elevated metabolic rates (Mahan and Arlin 1992). This method is deemed appropriate for administering up to 1,800 calories per day for short-term use, where enteral or oral feeding is expected to resume within 5–7 days (Mahan and Arlin 1992). As most acutely ill hospitalized patients have peripheral intravenous lines placed for hydration and administration of intravenous medication, this form of nutrition support may be valuable in patients awaiting PEG placement during the time period generally required before short- and long-term feeding strategies can be determined in patients who have had cerebrovascular accidents (Hussain and Cox 1993). The use of enteral and parenteral nutrition therefore plays an extremely important role in managing dysphagia patients but does not always meet the patient's psychological and physical needs.

Videofluoroscopy may enable clinicians to visualize an uncoordinated swallow, pooling of liquid in the vallecula, frank aspiration, or a normal to near-normal pattern of deglutition. This diagnostic tool has revolutionized management in a population on which there was limited empiric information, and it often provides extremely valuable objective data that helps determine whether a patient should be fed by mouth or placed on nonoral feeding status. A range of issues that affect the benefits and burdens of different management options must also be considered. These may include the patient's degree of malnutrition and his or her expectations of outcome once provided with nutrients; denial of a progressive disease, which may influence attempts to educate the patient or caregiver on alternative feeding before a crisis situation; and religious beliefs and the right to refuse or accept artificial nutrition if death is imminent (Scott and Heughan 1993).

Behavioral and cognitive factors, such as alertness, judgment, orientation to time and place, memory and sequencing skills, attention span, recognition of food, and oral sensation all influence the appropriateness of oral feeding, even in a patient with a physiologically normal swallow (Logemann 1990). If any of these factors has been impaired by disease and the volume of food and fluid consumed is inadequate, life-threatening situations may ultimately arise.

The majority of health care institutions have organized dysphagia teams, which identify these patients and optimize expedient, appropriate care (Logemann 1990). The team's ultimate ethical obligation is to the patient (Russell and Hill 1992). Continuing education, team meetings and rounds to review cases and management options, frequent and ongoing contact and communication with patients and their loved ones, and, above all, the experience that comes with evaluating outcomes of specific treatments in different as well as similar individuals all facilitate discussing both the advantages and disadvantages of feeding options among team and family members. These interactions help to alleviate patient concerns and foster informed decisions (Mahon and Arlin 1992), enabling patients and their families to make the best possible decision, one that satisfies the body's need for nutrients while maintaining an optimal quality of life.

ENTERAL FEEDING

Formula Selection

Among the wide assortment of enteral feeding formulas available for nutrition support, two basic varieties exist. Elemental, or monomeric formulas, contain predigested nutrients and are appropriate for patients with maldigestion or malabsorption. Polymeric formulas contain intact nutrients and thus require normal digestive and absorptive ability (Heanue 1994). They generally provide 1.0–1.2 cal/ml and are able to satisfy all known micronutrient needs in 1.0–2.5 liters of formula. Since most patients who are not acutely ill require 30 kcal/kg actual body weight and 0.8–1.0 g of protein/kg/day, standard polymeric formulas are generally the first choice when initiating enteral feedings. Disease-specific formulas containing altered levels of macronutrients are also available (Pasulka and Crockett 1994). The use of a high-nitrogen formula may be appropriate for a patient with a decubitus ulcer. The decreased production of carbon dioxide associated with low carbohydrate feedings may be beneficial in patients with compromised respiratory status. Fiber-containing formulas have been shown to improve bowel function in those on long-term enteral feeding regimens.

Administration

Continuous-drip feedings are recommended for patients at risk for aspiration. The use of an enteral pump assures an accurate flow rate and is preferred over gravity drip. There is no reason to dilute isotonic formulas as the gastrointestinal tract generally adapts as the volume of formula is gradually increased in a continuous feeding (Mahan and Arlin 1992). Full-strength feedings should be started at 10 ml/hour and advanced every 12–24 hours until nutrient needs are met (Heanue 1994).

Case Study

The patient is a 67-year-old male S/P with cerebrovascular accident and severe dysphagia, S/P PEG placement. His weight is 64.5 kg. His calorie needs resting comfortably in bed are 1,936 kcal/day or 30 cal/kg. His fluid needs are 1,936 ml/day or 1 ml/kcal. The formula used is the "house" formula, isotonic 1.08 cal/ml. The amount needed to meet the patient's needs is 1,793 ml/day.

Day	Time	Rate of formula (over 24 hrs)	Calories provided
1	6 AM	10 ml/hr	259
	6 PM	20 ml/hr	518
2	6 AM	30 ml/hr	778
	6 PM	40 ml/hr	1,037
3	6 AM	50 ml/hr	1,296
	6 PM	60 ml/hr	1,555
4	6 AM	75 ml/hr	1,944

By day 4, the patient is tolerating the volume of formula to meet his needs. Standard 1.0–1.2 kcal/ml formulas are 80–85% free water (Mahan and Arlin 1992). Therefore, the patient is receiving 1,555 ml of free water from formula. To meet fluid needs, the tube needs to be flushed with an additional 50 ml water every 3 hours. His intravenous is discontinued by day 4 as the patient is tolerating the volume of formula and free water to meet his needs via enteral tube.

As dysphagia improves with therapy and initiation of oral feedings is recommended, "cyclic" enteral feedings, those given over a specific time period, also are begun. As continuous feedings cause elevated circulating insulin levels, which in turn can depress appetite (Heanue 1994), it is appropriate to "cycle" tube feedings overnight to optimize oral intake during the day. Due to decreased "cyclic" time (e.g., 6 PM to 6 AM, or 12 hours), the feeding rate generally needs to be increased to provide adequate volume to meet needs. As this is often intolerable to the patient and inappropriate if at risk for aspiration, the formula may need to be changed to a calorically dense product.

Transition Feeding

Once oral feedings are initiated, all intake should be recorded. Calorie counts should include food and fluid taken from the meal tray, medication cart, and items brought in by visitors. An ongoing evaluation of daytime intake is necessary to determine the decrease in nocturnal cycling time for enteral feedings. A steady improvement in oral intake facilitates decreasing the tube feeding from 12 hours on day 1, to 10 hours on day 2, to 8 hours on day 3. When calorie counts establish that a patient is consuming two-thirds to three-fourths of daily requirements for calories and protein over a 3-day period, the enteral feeding can be discontinued (Trujillo and Queen 1994). In some cases, patients who are gradually able to advance to a semisolid dysphagia diet but who remain intolerant to liquids, require continued use of the gastrostomy tube to meet fluid needs while enjoying their food tray during meal service.

Problems and Possible Solutions

Routine flushing of the tube with 20 ml of warm water helps keep it patent and prevents clogging, particularly before and after medications are administered. If the feeding tube does clog, often as the result of protein coagulation, an enzyme called papain can be ordered from the pharmacy. In a 2.5% solution, papain hydrolyzes the components of protein (Thibault 1994). Cola soft drinks have been shown to be as effective as warm water, and both are more effective than cranberry juice in clearing a clogged feeding tube (Metheny et al. 1988). Liquid medications or very finely crushed pills must not be mixed into the feeding formula as this may cause the formula to clump. Syrups high in alcohol (Thibault 1994), dyazides, ibuprofen, magnesium oxide, psyllium, potassium chloride, and theophylline also tend to clog tubes. Enteric-coated and time-released medications, liquid-filled capsules, and sublingual tablets should never be administered by feeding tube. Serum drug levels of medications such as dilantin and theophylline should be closely monitored when given enterally, as interaction with the feeding formula may necessitate an adjustment in dosage.

The aspiration of gastric contents in patients fed intragastrically is a serious, life-threatening complication, particularly in a compromised individual. Delayed gastric emptying may be the result of infection, fever, hyperglycemia, diabetic gastroparesis, high fat intake, or a variety of drugs (Thomas 1994). Patients generally benefit from a standard 1.0–1.2 cal/ml feeding formula because these products generally do not provide excessive amounts of fat. Since body position can increase gastric emptying, the patient should lie on his or her right side with the head of the bed elevated.

Monitoring the volume of gastric residuals is critical. Stomach contents should be aspirated every 4 hours and if residual volume is greater than twice the tube feeding rate, or a maximum of 100–150 ml, the feeding rate should be reduced. Gastric contents should be returned to the stomach before initiating feeding again. If the patient is consuming an oral diet with daytime enteral feedings, the timing of residual checks should be considered to prevent a clogged tube due to the inadvertent aspiration of solid food particles back through the tube.

If high gastric residuals remain a consistent problem, medications that increase gastric emptying should be initiated. Metoclopramide, 10 mg four times a day, is commonly used for this purpose. Recurrent high gastric residuals and episodes of aspiration may necessitate the PEG being converted to a percutaneous endoscopic gastrostomy-jejunostomy (Thomas 1994).

It is not unusual for those directly involved in patient care to be troubled by both sanitation concerns and patient comfort in enterally fed patients with diarrhea. Classified as more than 300 ml liquid stool/day or greater than four loose bowel movements per day (Pasulka and Crockett 1994), diarrhea is the most frequent gastrointestinal complication associated with tube feeding. Except in patients who have not had oral feedings for an extended period as a result of gut atrophy secondary to disuse, choice of feeding formula is rarely the cause. Before treating the diarrhea, its etiology must be determined. In the presence of a normally healthy gastrointestinal tract, the following are most often related to diarrhea (Thomas 1994):

- Medications
  - Failure to discontinue laxatives
  - Metoclopramide
  - Erythromycin
  - Quinidine
  - Medications in sorbitol suspensions
  - Magnesium-containing antacids
  - Antibiotic therapy
- Formula
  - Lactose containing
  - Inadequate fiber content
  - Hyperosmolar
  - Bacterial contamination of formula
- Nutritional status
  - Hypoalbuminemia
  - Prolonged nonoral feeding

Clostridium difficile (bacteria related to antibiotic use), if present in stool samples, should be treated with vancomycin. Appropriate alternatives for diarrhea-inducing medications should be initiated and, when applicable, given intravenously. A change to formula that is lactose-free, contains fiber, or, if continuous intolerance occurs, to an elemental diet, may provide relief. If all attempts to control diarrhea fail to disclose its etiology, and if diarrhea persists, hypomotility agents such as Lomotil, paregoric, or tincture of opium may be administered. Ultimately, the patient may require bowel rest, necessitating parenteral nutrition so as not to further compromise nutritional status.

DIETARY MANIPULATION

When the primary physician, in consultation with the speech-language pathologist, considers the patient able to safely ingest an oral diet, the choice of the appropriate food and fluid consistency becomes a critical factor in subsequent management. A dysphagia evaluation tray, provided by the department of nutrition services and containing a variety of food and fluid textures, can be used during a bedside evaluation to determine what foods and fluid consistencies the patient tolerates best. A systematic way to prepare and deliver these foods and fluids from kitchen to bedside should be developed and implemented, taking into account the kitchen and food production and service schedule, the availability of certain food items at specific times during the day, and the available manpower needed to deliver food trays and pick them up after evaluation. Based on the results of the food texture evaluation and, if necessary, the modified barium swallow, the speech-language pathologist and dietitian must coordinate efforts to determine the oral diet most suitable for the patient.

Liquid or puréed food is often the only consistency safely tolerated by patients with mechanical disorders leading to dysphagia or with the oral mucosa changes that frequently accompany other concurrent treatment modes such as radiation or chemotherapy (Fleming et al. 1977). However, for patients with suspected oropharyngeal pathologic conditions that would put them at risk for aspiration of food and fluid, thin puréed and liquid diets are often contraindicated (Groher 1987). Such patients have more difficulty with fluids and thinned (puréed) foods because the disordered mechanism cannot respond in time with sufficient control to protect the airway. Studies have demonstrated that, in general, substances that are easy to chew (puréed consistency) are not always easy to swallow, especially for those with neurogenic oropharyngeal pathologic conditions (Groher 1987). Semisolid consistencies that do not easily disperse in the mouth and can be swallowed as a single bolus are more palatable and better tolerated than thin puréed foods. Unlike runny purées, textured soft foods with high moisture content and flavor can help trigger a weak reflex (Table 12.3).

Many institutions offer a dysphagia diet in stages or levels. The diet may be advanced to the next level based on overall progress with swallowing rehabilitation and individual patient tolerance. An example is presented in Table 12.4.

Further modifications may be necessary on each diet level based on individual tolerances. For instance, many patients find it difficult to tolerate the thick, ropy texture that oropharyngeal secretions take on with the ingestion of dairy products, requesting they be eliminated from the meal tray. Staff who care for postsurgical head and neck cancer patients find that bread may pose a threat to the airway. Acidic foods such as citrus and tomato products are generally irritating to patients with mucosal burns following radiation to the oral cavity or chemotherapy. Finally, many institutional kitchens do not always obtain specific food items due to availability, season, and vender contracts. Therefore, if administration is not sure that bread slices procured will always be coarse-textured rather than doughy, that grapefruit sections will always be supplied without membranes, or that canned fruit is always pitless, these items should be excluded from the dysphagia menu cycle.

An advanced dysphagia diet, or level 4, is often confused with a "mechanical soft" regimen. It is important to distinguish one from the other because tiny, bite-sized food items with a hard texture and those that easily fall apart in the oral cavity or pharynx (Table 12.5) are easy to chew for most individuals but pose safety issues in dysphagics. Omission of these food items reduces the risk of small pieces of food entering the airway, which would increase the risk of respiratory compromise.

Table 12.3 Food and Fluid Selection Tailored to the Suspected Dysphagic Condition

Slow/weak/uncoordinated swallow
Highly seasoned foods
Very warm or very cold food
Highly textured foods (diced, chopped)
Semisolids that form a cohesive bolus
Small frequent meals; minimize fatigue, optimize food intake
Weakened/poor oral-muscular control
Semisolids that form a cohesive bolus
Avoid slippery, sticky foods
Small frequent meals
Reduced oral sensation
Food positioned in most sensitive area of oral cavity
Avoid foods with two or more textures
Very cold foods
Highly seasoned foods
Cricopharyngeal dysfunction
Liquid or thin puréed texture
Decreased laryngeal elevation
Soft solids with medium and spoon-thick liquids
Avoid sticky and bulky foods and foods that fall apart
Decreased vocal cord closure
Avoid foods that fall apart
No thin liquids

The importance of serving a diet to the dysphagic patient that provides contrasting color, flavor, texture, size, shape, and temperature cannot be overemphasized. However, recent studies have shown that a high percentage of elderly residents in nursing homes receive puréed or blenderized food. Puréed food is ordered most often for behavioral feeding problems such as a patient's reluctance to eat, confusion and lack of cooperation during mealtime, and inability to self-feed (Cluskey 1989). The widespread use of food processors, thickening agents, and attractive serving dishes (Mayes 1985) has finally brought us to an era where puréed foods are now finished products with eye as well as taste appeal. Table 12.6 lists main dish entrees that combine taste and visual appeal as well as mastication ease.

Commercial thickeners that thicken both hot and cold liquids without cooking are now available for institutional use (Table 12.7). Fluids can generally be thickened to the consistency levels noted above, depending on the amount of thickener used. During the process of digestion, starch-based thickeners, as opposed to vegetable gum thickeners, release the fluid back into the gastrointestinal tract, where 98% of the liquid is directly absorbed for hydration (Vartan 1989). Although they are easy to use and readily available, issues such as cost, patient acceptance, and personnel responsible for preparing the thickened

Table 12.4 Progressive Diet Levels for Dysphagic Patients

Dysphagia Diet Level 1

Characteristics: Based on the puréed diet, food is blenderized and has a mashed potato–like consistency. Food is smooth but should not be thin and runny. Bread and thin liquids, including water, are excluded. Does not require chewing. The diet is nutritionally adequate.

Food category	*Suggestions*
Breads and cereals	Farina, Cream of Wheat, Cream of Rice
Eggs	Soft poached, soft boiled eggs, baked custard
Dairy	Plain yogurt, thickened milk
Soups	Blenderized and creamed soups, strained; thicken as needed to pudding consistency
Meats/entrees	Thick puréed meat with gravy; puréed casseroles or puréed mixed dishes
Vegetables	Thick puréed vegetables (strain before thickening as needed)
Fruit	Thick puréed fruit (strain before thickening as needed)
Dessert	Pudding, ice cream, sherbet, double-strength gelatin
Beverages	Cold and thickened

Dysphagia Diet Level 2

Characteristics: A puréed consistency with some textured foods. Thin liquids are not included; thick/thickened liquids should be cold. All foods served on level 1 are included in level 2 with the addition of the following.

Food category	*Suggestions*
Breads and cereals	Thinned oatmeal (strained), pancakes with extra syrup
Eggs	Soft scrambled eggs with gravy or melted cheese
Dairy	No additions
Soups	No additions
Meats/entrees	Soft noodles or macaroni with sauce (e.g., cheese)
Vegetables	Moist mashed white or sweet potatoes with extra gravy
Fruit	Ripe, mashed bananas
Desserts	No additions
Beverages	Very thick juice and milk, all other cold and thickened beverages

Dysphagia Diet Level 3

Characteristics: Moist and well-lubricated semisolids that are easy to masticate. Foods served should be cohesive and swallowed as a single bolus. Although puréed-consistency foods from the previous levels can be served on this diet, it is important from a motivational and psychological standpoint to present food that resembles regular soft foods.

Table 12.4 *(continued)*

Food category	*Suggestions*
Breads and cereals	Biscuits and grits with gravy, cooked and cold cereals in milk, waffles with extra syrup, moist bread dressing with gravy
Eggs	Soft fried eggs
Dairy	Whipped, soft cream cheese or smooth cheese spreads
Soups	Mixed textures as long as ingredients are well cooked and in tolerable pieces
Meat/entrees	Diced or ground with gravy, soft casseroles, omelets
Vegetables	Canned or well-cooked asparagus tips, cooked carrots or green beans, fresh tomato without skin or seeds or stewed tomatoes
Fruits	Canned or fresh (overripe) without seeds or skins, baked apple without peel, stewed fruit (no pits), jellied cranberry sauce
Desserts	Custard and cream pies, plain, soft cake, doughnuts softened in milk, moist cheese cake with sauce, cobblers with softened crust
Beverages	All beverages, thickened as needed

Source: Adapted from AW Martin. Dietary management of swallowing disorders. Dysphagia 1991;6:129.

Table 12.5 Problem Foods

Dry muffins
Pound cake
Plain rice
Peas or dried beans
Corn, mixed vegetables, lima beans
Any soup with loose floating contents
Chili con carne
Coconut, nuts, seeds
Fruit cocktail
Items containing celery, nuts, or raisins
Dried fruit
Coconut cake or coconut pie
White bread
Toasted bread
Crackers
Hard boiled or hard fried eggs
Hard cheese (uncooked)
Cheeses that crumble easily
Bacon, sausage, hot dogs
Peanut butter
Baked potato with skin

Table 12.6 Dysphagia Main Dishes and Entrees*

Corned beef hash
Omelets or quiche
Moist, boneless fish, baked or broiled with sauce
Sliced, tender meat or poultry with gravy
Small curd cottage cheese and soft cheese
Macaroni and cheese
Meatloaf or salmon loaf with sauce or gravy
Stew made with diced or chopped ingredients
Chopped tuna, egg, or potato salad made without celery or onion pieces
Cheese blintzes
Soufflés or aspics
Tender Salisbury steak
Chopped beef burgundy
Shepherd's pie made with diced or chopped meat
Swedish meatballs with gravy
Ground beef and noodle or macaroni casserole
Noodles Alfredo
À la kings
Tuna noodle casserole
Turkey tetrazzini
Lasagna, ravioli, or spaghetti casseroles

*Patients who are unable to tolerate thin liquids are at increased risk for aspiration and dehydration. Liquids can be classified into four consistencies based on their viscosity (see Table 12.7).

liquids need to be addressed. Therefore, modified cornstarch and maltodextrin-based commercial thickeners are recommended. Rice, tapioca, instant or mashed potatoes, unflavored gelatin, or baby cereal can be used for thickening purposes, especially for patients discharged home (Table 12.8), but these media may mask or alter food flavor or texture.

Often, the most difficult challenge for dysphagic patients is consuming adequate quantities of thickened liquids to meet fluid needs. According to a survey of 40 rehabilitation dietitians, the primary problem in persons with dysphagia was low tolerance to thick liquids (Schmitz 1990). Incorporating high–fluid content foods such as puréed fruit, custards, gelatin desserts, and frozen juice helps increase the overall fluid content of the diet. Also, the addition of extra margarine, cream, Half-and-Half, powdered or evaporated milk, and whipped topping to recipes can add extra calories to the diet without substantially increasing the volume of food the patient is required to consume to meet caloric needs.

Commercial nutritional supplements served with meals or as between-meal nourishment are generally available in most institutions for patients who are unable to meet nutrient needs. These may be given for those with poor appetites, difficulty swallowing, increased requirements secondary to illness, or excessive fatigue during the feeding process, rendering them unable to complete

Table 12.7 A Classification System for Liquid Consistencies

Thin: Low viscosity
- Water
- Fruit juice (except prune)
- Broth
- Nutritional supplements
- Milk
- Coffee and tea
- Cocoa
- Carbonated beverages
- Liquor, wine, beer, cordials

Medium thick: "naturally" of medium viscosity
- Buttermilk
- Tomato and vegetable juice
- Nectar
- Prune juice
- Thick milkshakes, eggnog
- Blenderized soup

Medium thick plus: "honey" consistency
- All liquids brought to a "honey" consistency with use of a commercial thickener.

Spoon thick: High viscosity, pudding consistency. Liquids that "mound" or are "plopable" at room temperature. Too thick for a straw; generally require spoon for feeding or eating.
- Frozen shakes or extra-thick shakes
- Thick juice with pureed fruit added
- Custard and pudding
- Yogurt
- Whipped gelatin
- All liquids thickened to this consistency with a commercial thickener

Source: Adapted from P Womack. The dysphagia challenge. Techniques for the individual. Bellevue: WA: Womack, 1993.

meals. Multivitamin and mineral preparations, including calcium supplements, also can be ordered by physicians, especially for patients who exclude a food group from their diets due to intolerance or personal preference (e.g., dairy, vegetables, red meat).

As most texture-modified diets contain low levels of fiber, constipation often becomes problematic, especially for elderly bedridden residents who are unable or unwilling to take adequate amounts of fluid. The addition of bran to hot cereals, soup, mashed potatoes, casseroles, and dishes such as meatloaf or meatballs helps increase the fiber content of the diet. Prune juice can be invaluable for preventing or treating constipation and serves as a thicker liquid for dysphagic patients who cannot manage thin liquids.

Patient food preferences must be taken into account. Modified ethnic or cultural foods should be incorporated into the dysphagic diet as frequently as

Table 12.8 Food-Thickening Preparations*

Hot liquids
Milk-based liquids: add rice cereal (baby product) or plain gelatin
Other liquids: add potato flakes, mashed potatoes, or flaked baby cereal
Cold liquids: add plain gelatin or Jell-O, puréed fruits, banana flakes
Pureed fruits: add flaked rice cereal (baby product), gelatin or Jell-O, cooked cream of rice or wheat cereal
Puréed vegetables: add mashed white or sweet potatoes, potato flakes, plain sauces
Puréed soups: add potato flakes, mashed potatoes, thick sauces or gravies, or canned puréed or strained baby meat (e.g., chicken noodle soup, puréed and thickened with strained baby meat)

*Specific measurements for thickening are not given due to the variety of thicknesses desired.
Source: Reprinted with permission from B Dereiko, PM Stout. Swallowing Safely, Swallowing Nutritiously. Portland, OR, 1986.

possible. As well-described disease entities and processes affect dysphagic patients in differing ways, it is imperative that management of this group of patients should be predicated on individual plans.

EVALUATION

Weight is a critical clinical parameter for monitoring and evaluating the patient during the period of nutritional replenishment (Kamel 1990). Hydration status also must be monitored closely, especially when thin liquids are omitted from the oral dietary regimen. Signs of dehydration include poor skin turgor, dry mucous membranes, lack of axillary sweat, and, in the elderly, mental status changes (Kamel 1990). Laboratory tests that suggest dehydration, such as increased serum osmolality and urine osmolality with an elevated ratio of blood urea nitrogen to creatinine, must be monitored closely (American Dietetic Association 1984). Strict input and output sheets should be kept on all patients who are restricted in free fluid intake. Patients on thickened liquid regimens who complain of dry mouth and thirst require meticulous oral hygiene. The use of lemon glycerine swabs to moisten lips and oral structures and, if tolerated, frozen Popsicles and lemon ice, can bring relief to those who are unable to take additional fluids and to those who complain of an accumulation of stringy, oral mucus associated with the ingestion of milk or other dairy products.

The success of dysphagia therapy and, often, the long-term management strategy for these patients depends largely on the amount of nutrition the patient can safely consume by mouth on a daily basis. Therefore, a convenient and simple method has to be implemented to record how well a patient eats. The use of food intake records or calorie counts is essential during swallowing retraining, especially for patients being tapered from enteral feedings. The nursing staff is generally responsible for documenting food and fluid intake. Dietitians should conduct continuous in-service education on procedures for recording accurate calorie counts, including standard measurements of fluid containers and portion sizes specific to the institution. A small chart with these measurements, attached to calorie-count or input and output sheets, may facilitate more accurate documentation of nutrient intake. Staff also should be aware of the importance of recording all food and fluid taken by the patient by mouth, including calorie-containing condiments (sugar, jelly, margarine), between-meal nourishments and supplements, food or fluid given with medication, and food items brought in by visitors.

If specific dietary modifications and feeding strategies are required after transfer from acute to chronic care facilities, the receiving institution should be alerted to any special feeding or dietary needs to ensure safe oral feeding. In-service education on dysphagia management to staff of chronic care facilities may be necessary.

If it becomes clear that the patient cannot maintain nutritional status when fed any combination of food and fluid consistencies presented orally, supplemental tube feeding may be essential. Gastrostomy tubes may satisfy some quality-of-life issues, since patients may only need to rely on them on sick days when intake is poor or in case a setback is experienced.

SUMMARY

Priorities in managing dysphagic patients include prevention of malnutrition and restoration of optimal nutritional status in those who are compromised. Registered dietitians play primary roles on dysphagia treatment teams and should be instrumental in identifying patients at risk, assessing overall nutritional status, determining the appropriate oral and enteral diet, and monitoring the outcome of the nutritional care plan on an ongoing basis. Providing in-service education to hospital staff at all levels, patients and their caregivers and loved ones, and staff of chronic care facilities presents a challenge to the dietetic professional in ensuring quality patient care in all settings.

REFERENCES

American Dietetic Association. Suggested guidelines for nutrition management of the critically ill patient. Process criteria for nutrition assessment and support of selected conditions. Chicago: American Dietetic Association, 1984.

ASPEN Board of Directors. Guidelines for the use of enteral nutrition in the adult patient. JPEN J Parenter Enteral Nutri 1987;5:435.

Baker JP, Detsky AS, Wesson DE, et al. Nutritional assessment: a comparison of clinical judgment and objective measurements. N Engl J Med 1982;306:969.

Beadle L, Townsend S, Palmer D. The management of dysphagia in stroke. Nurs Stand 1995;9:37.

Bistrian BR, Blackburn GL, Vitale J, et al. Prevalence of malnutrition in general medical patients. JAMA 1976;235:1567.

Blackburn GL. Nutrition in Surgical Patients. In JD Hardy, JS Kukora, HI Pass (eds), Hardy's Textbook of Surgery (2nd ed). Philadelphia: Lippincott, 1988;86.

Blackburn GL, Bistrian BR, Maini BS, et al. Nutritional and metabolic assessment of the hospitalized patient. JPEN J Parenter Enteral Nutri 1977;1:12.

Ciocon JO. Indications for tube feedings in elderly patients. Dysphagia 1990;5:1.

Cluskey MM. The use of texture modified diets among the institutionalized elderly. J Nutr Elderly 1989;9:3.
Cogan R, Weinryb J. Aspiration pneumonia in nursing home patients fed via gastrostomy tubes. Am J Gastroenterol 1989;84:1509.
Detsky AS, Baker JP, Mendelson RA. Evaluating the accuracy of nutritional assessment techniques applied to hospitalized patients: methodology and comparisons. JPEN J Parenter Enteral Nutri 1984;8:153.
Detsky AS, Baker JP, O'Rourke K, et al. Predicting nutrition associated complications for patients undergoing gastrointestinal surgery. JPEN J Parenter Enteral Nutri 1987a;11:440.
Detsky AS, McLaughlin JR, Baker JP, et al. What is subjective global assessment of nutritional status? JPEN 1987b;11:8.
Detsky AS, Smalley PS, Chang J. Is this patient malnourished? JAMA 1994;271:54.
Fleming S, Weaver AW, Brown JM. The patient with cancer affecting the head and neck: problems in nutrition. J Am Diet Assoc 1977;70:391.
Groher ME. Bolus management and aspiration pneumonia in patients with pseudobulbar dysphagia. Dysphagia 1987;1:215.
Heanue P. Enteral Feeding Formulas and Administrative Techniques. In BC Borlase, SJ Bell, GL Blackburn, et al. (eds), Enteral Nutrition. New York: Chapman and Hall, 1994;173.
Hussain A, Cox JCG. Audit of the use of percutaneous endoscopic gastrostomy for enteral nutrition in patients with acute stroke. Gut 1993;34:558.
Hynak-Hankinson MT. Dysphagia evaluation and treatment: the team approach. Nutr Supp Serv 1984;4:33.
Jones PL, Altschuler SL. Dysphagia teams: a specific approach to a nonspecific problem. Dysphagia 1987;1:200.
Kamel PL. Nutritional assessment and requirements. Dysphagia 1990;4:189.
Lang CE, Cashman MD. Nutritional Status. In A Skipper (ed), Dietitian's Handbook of Enteral and Parenteral Nutrition. Rockville, MD: Aspen, 1989;5.
Logemann JA. Factors affecting ability to resume oral nutrition in the oropharyngeal dysphagic individual. Dysphagia 1990;4:202.
Mahan LK, Arlin M. Krause's Food, Nutrition and Diet Therapy (8th ed). Philadelphia: Saunders, 1992.
Mayes C. Puréed diets "come alive" with the right food processor. J Am Health Care Assoc 1985;11:24.
Metheny N, Eisenberg P, McSweeney M. Effect of feeding tube properties and three irrigants on clogging rates. Nurs Res 1988;37:165.
Miller RM. Evaluation of Swallowing Disorders. In ME Groher (ed), Dysphagia: Diagnosis and Management (2nd ed). Boston: Butterworth, 1992;143.
Murray JJ, Healy MD. Drug-mineral interactions: a new responsibility for the hospital dietitian. J Am Diet Assoc 1991;91:66, 73.
Park RHR, Allison MC, Lang J. Randomized comparison of percutaneous endoscopic gastrostomy and nasogastric tube feeding in patients with persisting neurological dysphagia. BMJ 1992;304:1406.
Pasulka P, Crockett C. Selecting Enteral Products. In BC Borlase, SJ Bell, GL Blackburn, et al. (eds), Enteral Nutrition. New York: Chapman and Hall, 1994;115.
Raha SK, Woodhouse KW. Who should have a PEG? Age Ageing 1993;22:313.
Russell A, Hill P. Management of Swallowing and Tube Feeding in Adults: A Team Approach. Boston: Butterworth-Heinemann, 1992.
Schmitz J. Dysphagia. In DJ Gines (ed), Nutrition Management in Rehabilitation. Rockville, MD: Aspen, 1990;141.
Scott A, Austin HE. Nasogastric feeding in the management of severe dysphagia in motor neurone disease. Palliat Med 1994;8:45.
Scott AG, Heughan A. A review of dysphagia in four cases of motor neurone disease. Palliat Med 1993;7(suppl 2):41.

Sitzman JV. Nutritional support of the dysphagic patient: methods, risks, and complications of therapy. JPEN J Parenter Enteral Nutri 1990;14:60.
Smith P, Smith A, Toan B. Nutritional care arts, private pay days. Chicago: Nutrition Care Management Institute, 1989.
Thibault A. Care of Feeding Tubes. In BC Borlase, SJ Bell, GL Blackburn, et al. (eds), Enteral Nutrition. New York: Chapman and Hall, 1994;197.
Thomas S. Gastrointestinal Complications: Diarrhea and High Gastric Residuals. In BC Borlase, SJ Bell, GL Blackburn, et al. (eds), Enteral Nutrition. New York: Chapman and Hall, 1994;188.
Trujillo EB, Queen PM. Transition Feeding. In BC Borlase, SJ Bell, GL Blackburn, et al. (eds), Enteral Nutrition. New York: Chapman and Hall, 1994; 107–114.
Vartan KS. Perspectives on Practice: Understanding Instant Food Thickeners. The Role of Starches and Gums in Hydration. Lancaster, PA: American Institutional Products, 1989.
Vreugde S. Nutritional aspects of dysphagia. Act Otorhinolaryngol Belg 1994;48:229.
Zeman FJ. Clinical Nutrition and Dietetics. Lexington, MA: Heath, 1983;23.

13

Nursing Management of Swallowing Disorders

Barbara A. Griggs

Nurses have the best opportunity to discover a patient who is having difficulty swallowing. A basic knowledge of the anatomy and physiology of normal swallowing helps alert nurses to the potential problems and complications of dysphagia. Initial signs and symptoms include a subtle refusal to eat, coughing, choking, drooling, and pain. Awareness of these signs is important, particularly in older, malnourished, or chronically ill patients with no previous history of a swallowing disorder. Patients who have recently been transferred from special care units also require careful evaluation of swallowing. Prior endotracheal intubation, especially for prolonged periods, can contribute to temporary or permanent vocal cord paralysis, leading to difficulty in swallowing and subsequent aspiration (Shapiro et al. 1975). It is well established that patients with tracheostoma tubes in place have swallowing difficulties and need careful monitoring for aspiration (Cameron et al. 1973; Taylor et al. 1981). Nurses should be conscious of these possibilities as a routine part of daily patient assessment (Loustau and Lee 1985). Patients with documented mechanical or neurogenic swallowing disorders need specialized care plans with specific therapeutic goals. Proper hydration, patent airways, and nutritional support are requisite areas of meticulous and comprehensive nursing care. This chapter addresses each area with emphasis on providing timely and safe nutritional support.

HYDRATION

Thirst is the physiologic mechanism that governs hydration under normal circumstances. It is important to distinguish between thirst that can be sensed by patients who can take nothing by mouth and by intubated or dysphagic patients and that caused by failure to provide sufficient intravenous or oral fluids.

The initial and most common method of hydration in these patients is intravenous (IV) administration of physiologic solutions of water, dextrose, sodium, and potassium chloride. These solutions are administered through a catheter inserted into a peripheral vein. The site of the catheter insertion should be changed every 2–3 days, or more frequently if necessary (Goldmann et al. 1973). Care of the infusion site includes routine inspection for infiltration, pain, inflammation, or infection. Application of a povidone-iodine ointment and change of dry, sterile dressing once a day is generally accepted practice. Solutions are prepared on the patient care unit or under laminar flow hoods in the pharmacy every 24 hours. Administration set tubing, however, may be changed on a 24- to 72-hour basis according to hospital policy (Buxton et al. 1979). The unit nurse hangs the solution and monitors the infusion carefully, recording the rate and volume infused on a flow chart kept at the bedside. Hourly monitoring is necessary to ascertain complete delivery of required solutions and prevent fluid overload. Twenty-four-hour intake and output totals are also recorded as part of the patient's permanent record. Most IV solutions are administered by an infusion-control device.

In addition to basic fluid and electrolyte balance, parenteral solutions may be needed to administer medications. The patient may not be able to swallow the medication or, in the case of certain antibiotics, IV infusion may be the preferred route. Many medications irritate the vein wall, and therefore proper dilution and frequent site monitoring are essential to prevent phlebitis and potentially serious infiltrations.

MAINTAINING CLEAR AIRWAYS

Management of secretions is one of the first concerns encountered by patients who are having difficulty swallowing. This problem may have causes unrelated to dysphagia (e.g., dental work, fractures, oral tumors). It is important to distinguish between oral incompetence (such as drooling) and dysphagia that leads to pooling of secretions in the pharynx. Some patients with obstructive tumors or strictures of the esophagus may respond to surgical or irradiation therapy with relief of the anatomic problem. Swallowing retraining may be possible for those with neurologic disorders (see Chapters 9 and 10). Patients require extra care during the time that they are unable to handle their own secretions. Ambulatory and alert patients take care of their immediate needs when provided with proper receptacles and tissues. Bedridden or partially paralyzed patients require more assistance, including a properly supplied bedside stand that is within reach and an aware nursing staff to respond promptly to their individual needs. Frequent short visits to check on the patient and change receptacles should be routine. The patient should be kept lying on one side and be turned every 2 hours. A protective pad or soft towel arranged over the pillow under the patient's head will collect saliva from drooling. This should be changed as often as necessary and accompanied by routine skin care to prevent unnecessary chapping. A dental suction tip with gentle suction to remove secretions may be helpful for some patients. The tip must be properly supported and repositioned every hour to prevent pressure points and possible skin breakdown. Alert patients can be taught to use this device by themselves.

Patients with tracheostoma tubes in place require special respiratory care. Many hospitals have chest physical therapists working with such patients on a daily basis. Staff nurses, however, must be trained in tracheostoma care, including proper suctioning technique (Fuch 1984; Goodnough 1985; Crow 1986; Hoffman and Moszkiewicz 1987) (Table 13.1).

Table 13.1 How to Suction a Tracheostoma

Procedure	*Rationale*
Prepare equipment. Prepare patient.	Less traumatic for the patient.
Wash hands.	Prevents spread of nosocomial organisms.
Put on sterile gloves.	Apply universal precautions.
Attach catheter to wall outlet.	
Lubricate catheter tip with sterile saline solution.	Aids catheter insertion.
Remove ventilator or humidifier apparatus.	
Hyperoxygenate and hyperinflate the lungs with 100% oxygen.	Prevents hypoxemia.
Insert catheter quickly but evenly into the trachea *without* suction.	Prevents trauma to mucous membranes.
Start to remove catheter before applying suction.	
Gently roll catheter while smoothly withdrawing it.	
Reoxygenate and reinflate the lungs and observe patient.	
Rinse catheter and connecting tubing with saline noting nature of secretions.	Changes of consistency, color, or odor should be documented.
Repeat procedure once if necessary.	Do not suction patient excessively at one time to prevent bronchospasms and hypoxemia.
Suction oropharyngeal cavity.	This is done after tracheal suctioning to prevent contamination (if necessary to do first, a new catheter and glove are required).
Discard catheter, gloves, and saline solution.	Prevents contamination, primarily with *Pseudomonas*.
Reorganize suction materials to be available at all times.	

Adequate ventilation is the first consideration for patients with a tracheostomy tube, whether or not they are using a respirator. Suctioning as necessary prevents mucus build-up, tracheal obstruction, and hypoxemia. Aseptic technique is the second consideration and cannot be overemphasized. Contamination of suction catheters and other related equipment can lead to pneumonia and compromised respiratory function (Shapiro et al. 1975; Egan 1977; Causey 1981). Third is avoiding trauma to the mucous membranes of the trachea by use of proper suctioning (Nielsen 1980). Adequate nutritional support is often overlooked or is initiated too late. Nutritional repletion and maintenance are essential to prevent breakdown of respiratory musculature and progressive inability of the patient to breathe independently (Doekel et al. 1976; Waxman and Shoemaker 1980). Finally, patient education and communication are vital. Patients who are unable to talk or call for help become anxious, which may contribute to a decrease in their ventilatory capacity. Continuous explanations of what is happening and why helps to allay their fears. A clipboard with paper and pencil and a bell or buzzer give them a way to communicate. Patients in special care areas become dependent on the constant presence of nursing staff. Therefore, sufficient preparation must precede the transfer to a regular care unit. A private-duty nurse for several days and particularly at night may ease this transition. For some patients, regular visitations by individual family members may be enough.

A significant complication of tracheostomy is the development of a tracheoesophageal (TE) fistula. This can be caused by an overinflated cuff creating a pressure point with subsequent erosion (Hedden et al. 1969; Cooper and Grillo 1977). Proper inflation and the use of a low-pressure cuff help to minimize this possibility. Coincident use of nasogastric tubes for suction or feeding increases liability to a TE fistula. Large, 16–18 French polyvinylchloride nasogastric tubes should be used only for gastric suctioning; it is no longer necessary or recommended to use them for feeding. The availability of small, soft nasogastric feeding tubes has markedly decreased the risk of TE fistula (Figure 13.1).

The most frequent complication of nasogastric feedings is aspiration of formula or gastric contents. It is important to note that an inflated tracheostoma (or endotracheal) tube cuff is not a guarantee against this. Signs and symptoms of aspiration include increased respiratory rate with labored breathing, pulmonary congestion with decreased breath sounds, cyanosis, and sweating (diaphoresis). These patients may also manifest a persistent low-grade fever. Those who are dependent on a ventilator should not be fed into the stomach because the chances of aspiration are much greater. Nasointestinal or IV feedings are preferred. It is probably best to wait until a patient has been weaned from the respirator before beginning nasogastric or oral feedings. Patients with dysphagia are at high risk for aspiration. Intestinal tube feedings or IV feedings should be continued until there is no evidence of reflux or aspiration through radiographic studies (Sitzmann 1990).

Guidelines for oral feeding of a patient with a tracheostoma are essentially the same as those described for the patient with a swallowing disorder in the following section. Exceptions include:

1. The tracheostoma cuff is moderately inflated before and for 1 hour after the feeding. (Patients may learn to swallow without aspiration and no longer require a cuffed tube.)

2. A test for aspiration consists of adding food coloring to a soft food such as applesauce. The tube is suctioned before the test and the patient is allowed to rest, then fed 2 teaspoons of the colored food. After 15 minutes, the tube is gently suctioned just beyond the end. The returns will be streaked with color if the patient has aspirated; in this circumstance feedings should be discontinued and the patient reevaluated.

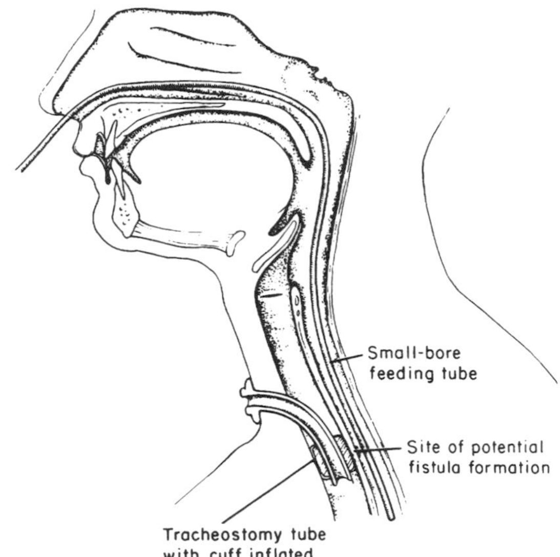

Figure 13.1 Site of potential tracheoesophageal fistula.

NUTRITIONAL SUPPORT

Nosocomial starvation and malnutrition incident to studies and therapy have been reported in up to 50% of hospitalized patients (Bistrian et al. 1974, 1976; Roubenoff et al. 1987). This is especially important to note with the dysphagic patient (Groher and Bukatman 1986; Sitzmann 1990). Caregivers must be aware of the rapid rate of development with which hospital-acquired malnutrition may evolve, and then do something about it by learning the current options that exist and incorporating them into daily patient therapy (Kamel 1990).

All patients should have a nutritional assessment as part of their initial physical work-up. Selected patients who are severely depleted, markedly catabolic, or who exhibit gastrointestinal symptoms require a more extensive evaluation, which is frequently done by a member of a specialized nutritional support service where available (Grant 1980). Anthropometric measurements, nitrogen balance studies, recall antigen skin testing, and oxygen consumption studies are some of the methods of nutritional assessment (Long et al. 1979; Blackburn et al. 1977). The cumulative results are then used to establish an appropriate feeding method and schedule. One must examine the cause and degree of the patient's nutritional deficit, consider the risks and benefits of each modality, and tailor immediate and long-term goals (Sitzmann and Mueller 1988; Ganger and Craig 1990). It is important to note that the evaluation of nutritional status is an ongoing process that requires reassessment as the patient's clinical condition changes.

There are two primary feeding options: enteral, using the gastrointestinal route, and parenteral, using the IV route. The development of parenteral hyperalimentation by Dudrick and colleagues in the late 1960s provided the means of feeding patients with nonfunctioning gastrointestinal tracts (Dudrick et al. 1968). Concurrently, elemental diets of simple protein and calorie sources that require minimal digestive capacity provided an alternate method of using the gastrointestinal tract in selected patients (Winitz et al. 1965). This heralded the beginning of specialized nutritional support as we know it today.

While total parenteral nutrition is an important medical advance, patients with swallowing disorders usually have an intact gastrointestinal tract, and the goal is to use this first. With special training, some patients may be able to return to oral feedings. It is important to remember that nonoral feedings should be gradually decreased, not discontinued, until the patient is able to maintain adequate oral nutrition (Logemann 1990; O'Gara 1990). For those unable to do so, there still remain two means of access to the gastrointestinal tract through noninvasive (nasogastric and nasointestinal feeding tubes) and invasive techniques (percutaneous endoscopic gastrostomy and jejunostomy feeding tubes; and gastrostoma, jejunostoma, and esophagostoma feeding tubes).

FEEDINGS BY MOUTH

The oral route is the ideal way to provide required nutrients. Oral feeding is not always possible in patients with swallowing disorders, although some can be rehabilitated or trained to this method. The patient's nutritional status and the potential risk of aspiration affect the choice of feeding method. Before the availability of total parenteral nutrition, there was an urgency to have patients use the gastrointestinal tract as soon as possible, especially those who were depleted. Total parenteral nutrition may make a significant difference in the early rehabilitation of those with dysphagia, but enteral feeding remains the ultimate goal.

A formal evaluation should always precede the decision to initiate oral feedings. Once approved, the nurse's role includes proper patient preparation and supervision.

Positioning

Correct anatomic alignment helps food pass through pharynx and esophagus with less difficulty in breathing and compromise of swallowing. Patients who can be out of bed are supported in a chair with their head and trunk flexed slightly forward. Those who remain in bed need the head of the bed elevated and a supporting pillow at the lower back. A patient who has difficulty maintaining one position may need additional pillows on either side. A patient who slides may be stabilized by elevating the midsection of the bed or placing a pillow under the knees. A standing position is ideal for patients on circular electric beds. All patients must be relaxed and well supported to eat properly.

Mouth Care

Before the introduction of food, mouth care serves to moisten the mucous membranes of the oral cavity and stimulate salivation to prevent food-sticking and possible choking. It is equally important to assist with mouth care following a meal to be sure that the oral cavity is free of small food particles that could subsequently be aspirated (Silvermann and Elfant 1979).

Suction Equipment

Suction equipment should be kept on standby for patients with a history of swallowing difficulty. It must always be available and functioning properly in case of emergency. It is best, however, to use it only when necessary because suctioning can contribute to gagging with possible regurgitation and aspiration. Patients with permanent tracheostomas requiring frequent suctioning need an organized schedule with sufficient rest time before eating to minimize this possibility.

Choice of Foods

One key to successful feeding is the choice of foods. Water is the easiest to take but the hardest to control. It goes down too fast and has no bulk to stimulate salivation or the action of oral muscles. A semisoft solid is usually better tolerated (Hargrove 1980). (See Chapters 9–12 for the role of food types and their consistency.)

Close Visual Monitoring

The patient should not be left alone at mealtime. A nurse or occupational therapist should be present to assist and observe until the patient can swallow satisfactorily. Later the presence of an aide, a family member, or a volunteer may be sufficient. A formalized program for volunteer training and supervision can increase safety for patients during meals (Lipner et al. 1990). If not in direct attendance, nurses should be alert to potential problems and be prepared to respond quickly if called. Eating takes time and rushing a meal can be hazardous for any patient, especially one with dysphagia, who may also become exhausted by the technical difficulties associated with eating. Smaller, more frequent meals may be better tolerated.

Education

Education of patient and family is a well-established nursing role. Careful explanations of what the nurse is doing and why relieve anxiety and fear and elicit greater cooperation and success. An explanation comes first, but time and patience must follow.

NONINVASIVE TUBE FEEDING METHODS

When a patient is unable to eat by mouth but has a functioning gastrointestinal tract, the best option is tube feeding. Nasogastric feeding tubes and enteral formulas have existed for many years.

Nasogastric or Intestinal Feeding Tube

The decision to use a nasogastric or a nasointestinal feeding tube is, in part, based on the presence or absence of a gag reflex and the risk of aspiration. Patients with some reflex, who are awake and alert, can be fed nasogastrically. For those with absent gag reflexes and a history or incidence of aspiration, the safest method is nasointestinal (Rombeau and Barot 1981). The difference between these tubes is primarily the size of the weighted tip and the length of tube that is inserted. Most nasogastric tubes have small tungsten weights that are as large or slightly larger in diameter as the rest of the tube. Nasointestinal tubes have traditionally had larger bolus weights, also of tungsten, at their tips, which were thought to help with their spontaneous passage through the pylorus into the small intestine. The number of tubes that pass spontaneously within 48 hours varied depending on the patient's position, ambulatory or bedridden status, and the presence of decreased gastric motility. Studies comparing weighted versus nonweighted feeding tubes have shown that the occurrence of spontaneous transpyloric passage has been similar (Levenson et al 1988; Rees et al. 1988). However, the prokinetic agent metoclopramide has been used successfully to aid intestinal passage when given prior to tube insertion (Whatley et al. 1984; Lord et al. 1993). Fluoroscopic (Grant et al. 1983) and endoscopic placement of nasointestinal feeding tubes has become common when immediate nutritional intervention is required. The regular insertion procedure is approximately the same for both. This is outlined step by step in Table 13.2 and Figures 13.2 and 13.3. Modifications for a nasointestinal tube insertion are given in Table 13.3.

Administration

There are two methods of tube feeding—continuous and intermittent. The continuous method is necessary for intestinal feedings or when the patient can tolerate only small volumes of formula at one time. For some patients, continuous feedings are better absorbed, thus increasing the number of calories provided on a daily basis. The term *continuous feeding* implies that it continues 24 hours a day. Some patients, however, can tolerate larger volumes per hour, with feedings running 8–16 continuous hours, either during the day and evening or during the night (Bloch 1987). Intermittent feedings are given hourly or every 3–4 hours. They are generally initiated on an hourly basis and graduated in schedule toward less frequent, larger-volume feedings. This becomes especially important if the patient will be continuing tube feedings after hospital discharge.

Table 13.2 Insertion Procedure for Nasogastric Feeding Tube (with Guide Wire)*

Procedure	*Rationale*
1. Prepare equipment; measure and mark feeding tube.	The tube should be measured for each patient as a guide to ensure proper tip location.
2. Position patient in bed at a 45-degree angle with a pillow behind the shoulders.	Patients seem more secure in bed than in a chair. Bed height can be adjusted to make insertion easier.
3. Have patient blow nose, and check each nostril for the side that allows for greater air passage.	Nose spray may be helpful for some patients.
4. Place protective drape over patient's chest and emesis basin and tissues in patient's lap.	The patient and bed area should be kept clean. Difficulties are not expected but they can arise.
5. Ask patient to hold cup of water with a straw.	
6. Lubricate distal end of feeding tube.	Creates less friction and discomfort in nasal passage.
7. Ask patient to tilt head back slightly.	It is easier to insert tube in this position.
8. Insert tip of tube approximately 2 inches into the nostril.	See Figure 13.2.
9. Ask patient to tilt head down.	Closes trachea and opens esophagus.
10. While advancing tube, ask patient to drink water through the straw.	See Figures 13.3 and 13.4. Swallowing will close epiglottis to allow passage of tube into esophagus rather than trachea.
11. If there is resistance, *stop* and remove feeding tube, then get assistance.	To avoid nasopulmonary intubation.
12. Let the patient rest, then try again, following steps 6 –10.	
13. Continue advancing the tube while the patient swallows water until the mark is reached and the feeding tube is in the body of the stomach.	See Figure 13.5. The tube should go in by gravity, but swallowing makes the procedure easier for the patient. Water seems to work better than ice chips for most patients. Rubbing the throat of an unconscious patient helps to stimulate swallowing.
14. Loop exposed end of feeding tube, hold securely with nondominant hand approximately 3 inches from the nostril, and gently but firmly pull out guide wire with dominant hand.	See Figure 13.6. Patient may feel more comfortable holding tube to keep it from partially pulling out.
15. Check position of feeding tube.	Tube position *must* be checked before feeding begins.
Gently aspirate stomach contents with 60-ml syringe.	An adapter may be needed for a more secure seal. Tubes smaller than 8 French have a tendency to collapse on

Table 13.2 *(continued)*

	Procedure	*Rationale*
		themselves and therefore should be used primarily when aspiration is not a factor or for supplemental feedings (this refers to nasogastric tubes).
	With a stethoscope over the left upper quadrant, instill 10 ml of air into feeding tube with syringe.	The sound of air entering the stomach can be heard. With smaller tubes, 20 ml of air may be necessary.
	Obtain an x-ray either routinely or if there is any question of tube position.	Tubes are radiopaque to enable visualization.
16.	Tape feeding tube in place.	Tube must be secure to prevent accidental slippage.
	Cleanse nose and cheek with alcohol wipe.	To remove perspiration and skin oils.
	Pour tincture of benzoin onto sponge and wipe nose, cheek, and tube. Let air-dry.	To protect skin and aid with adherence of tape.
	Apply small piece of tape, with one split end to nose. Wrap ends in opposite directions around the tube.	Too large a piece can focus patient's attention to tip of his nose. When it is necessary to avoid tape, cotton tracheostomy tape can be tied around tube and then around patient's head. Avoid pressure on nostril to prevent subsequent breakdown.
	Use tape to secure tube to cheek.	See Figure 13.7. Alert, cooperative patients can use only cheek tape to secure feeding tube. Change tape as necessary.

*This is the procedure with a conscious, cooperative patient. An assistant may be necessary if patient is unconscious or uncooperative.

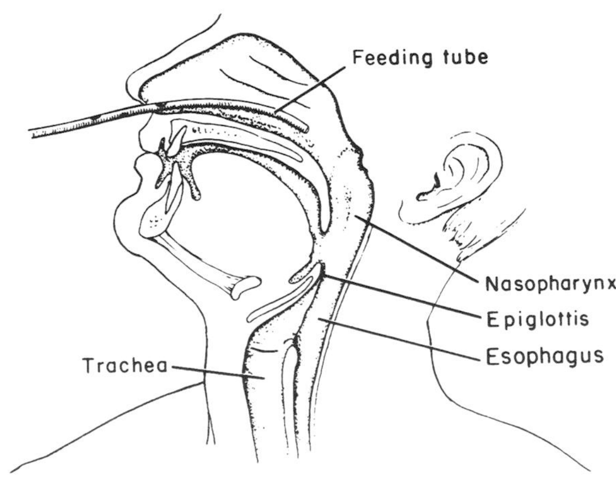

Figure 13.2 Insertion of feeding tube into the nostril.

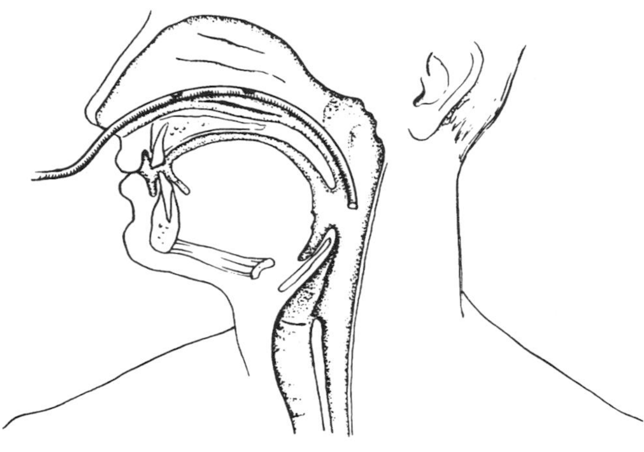

Figure 13.3 The feeding tube is guided into the nasopharynx.

Table 13.3 Modifications for Insertion of Nasointestinal Feeding Tube

Insert an additional 25–35 cm of tubing into stomach.
Wait for tube passage into intestines:
1–2 hrs for ambulatory patients.
24 hrs or more for bedridden patients.
If tube does not pass spontaneously, manual passage by fluoroscopy or endoscopy may be necessary.
Another option may be the use of metaclopramide before insertion.
Document exact position of feeding tube before initiation of tube feeding (Figure 13.8).

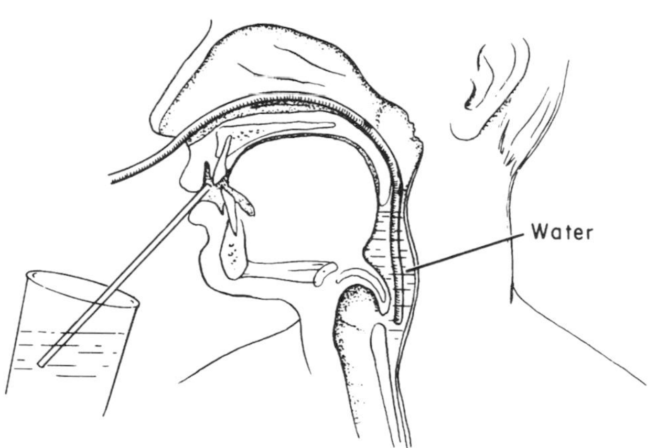

Figure 13.4 Advancement of the feeding tube with the water bolus.

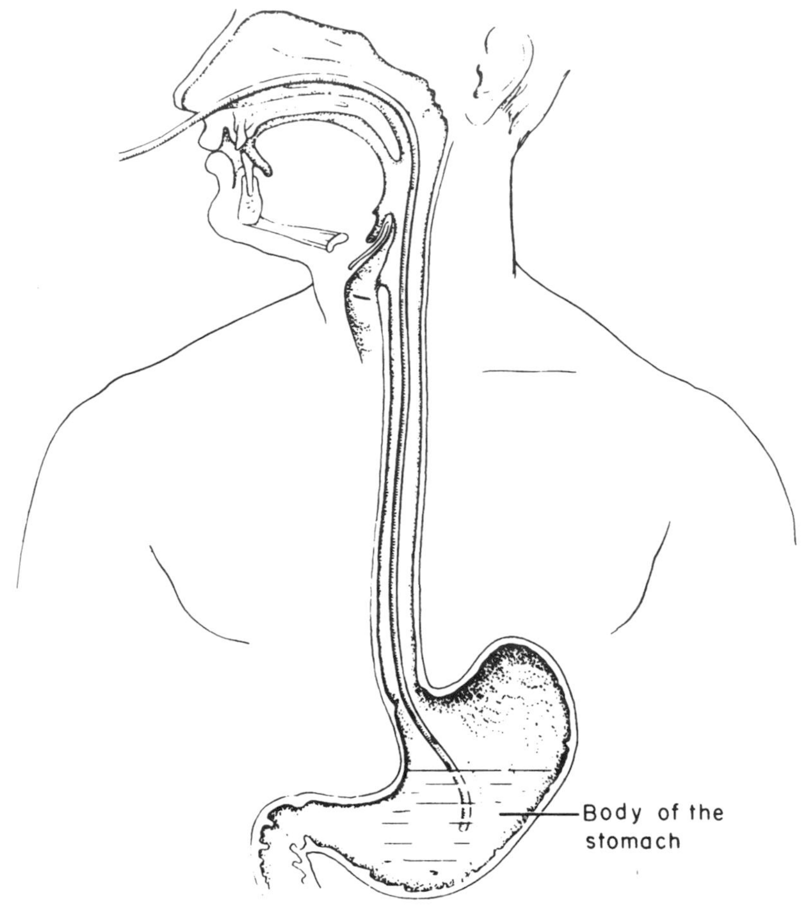

Figure 13.5 Correct positioning of the feeding tube in the stomach.

Tube feedings were once routinely administered by gravity drip, but with the development of enteral hyperalimentation, enteral feeding pumps are predominantly used today for continuous feedings (gravity drip is more common for intermittent feedings). These pumps are less complicated than IV infusion devices. They permit more accurate administration of continuous feedings and save nursing time.

Whether tube feedings are administered continuously or intermittently, by gravity drip or by enteral pump, they all should start slowly with small volumes. Hypertonic formulas should be initially diluted, but it is not necessary to dilute isotonic formulas. The amount is then increased every day, as tolerated, until the patient's caloric requirement has been met. This may take several days, depending on formula osmolality and patient tolerance. When the maintenance rate has

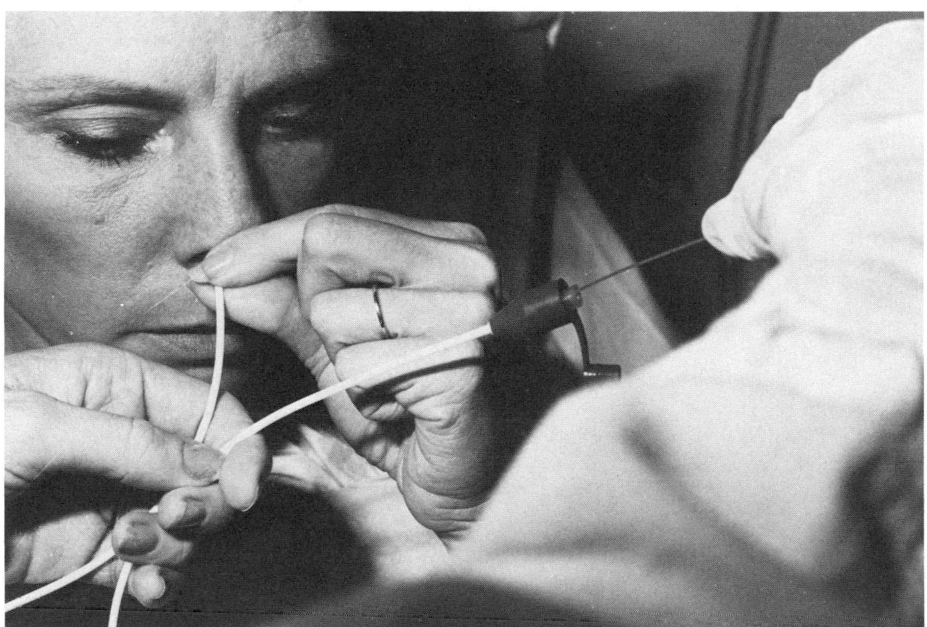

Figure 13.6 Removal of the guidewire from the feeding tube.

been achieved, adjustments can be made in the frequency and total volume of each feeding. The average adult 70-kg male, nonstressed patient needs 30–35 kcal per kg, or a range of 2,100–2,400 calories per day. Surgery and sepsis increase patient requirements to 40–45 kcal per kg (Walters and Freeman 1981).

Complications

The two main complications associated with tube feeding administration are aspiration and diarrhea. Both can be decreased or prevented by adhering to the following guidelines:

1. Elevate the head of the bed at least 30 degrees during continuous feeding and before and 1 hour after intermittent feeding.
2. Aspirate the feeding tube routinely to check for absorption of the formula. Progressively increasing residual volumes, nausea, abdominal distention, and discomfort should alert the nurse to hold the feeding and notify the physician to reevaluate the patient. Residual volumes of more than 100 ml should be questioned.
3. Administer intermittent feedings by slow gravity drip rather than as a bolus.
4. Coordinate with the dietitian the most appropriate formula for the patient.
5. Administer antidiarrheal preparations as necessary.
6. Monitor fluid and electrolyte balance daily.

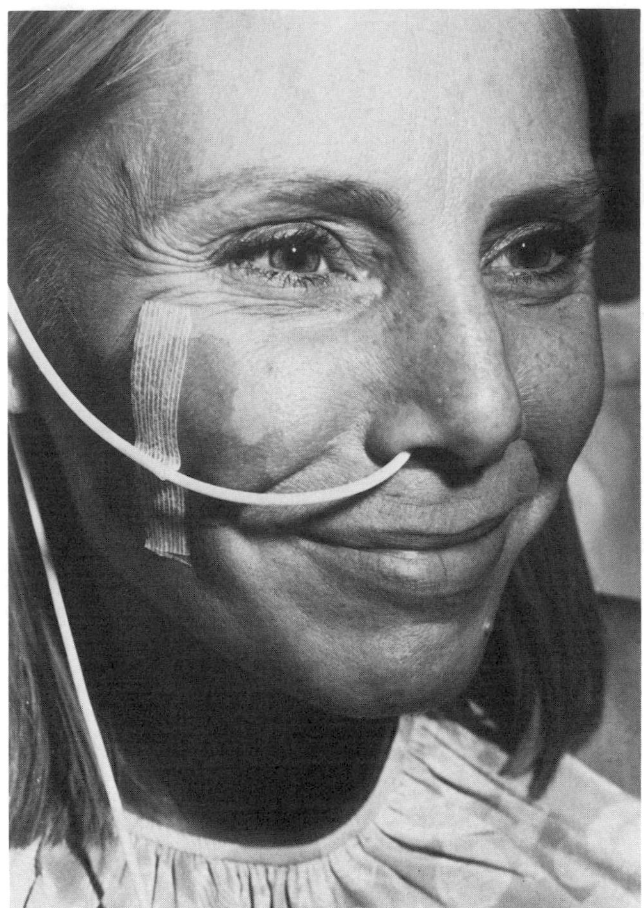

Figure 13.7 Steri-strip taping of the feeding tube.

SURGICAL GASTROSTOMY, JEJUNOSTOMY, AND ESOPHAGOSTOMY

Patients who require tube feedings for prolonged or indefinite periods can be considered candidates for a surgically placed gastrostomy, jejunostomy, or esophagostomy. Surgical insertion of feeding tubes into the stomach, intestine, or esophagus is a sterile procedure that may necessitate general anesthesia. It may be a relatively short, minor procedure or a more extensive, major one depending on the choice of procedure and the patient's condition. Occasionally, procedures are performed under local anesthesia in selected patients when general anesthesia is risky or contraindicated. Development of the needle catheter jejunostomy has increased the use of this access route (Delaney 1973; Delaney et al. 1977). (For a detailed explanation of these surgical procedures see Chapter 14.)

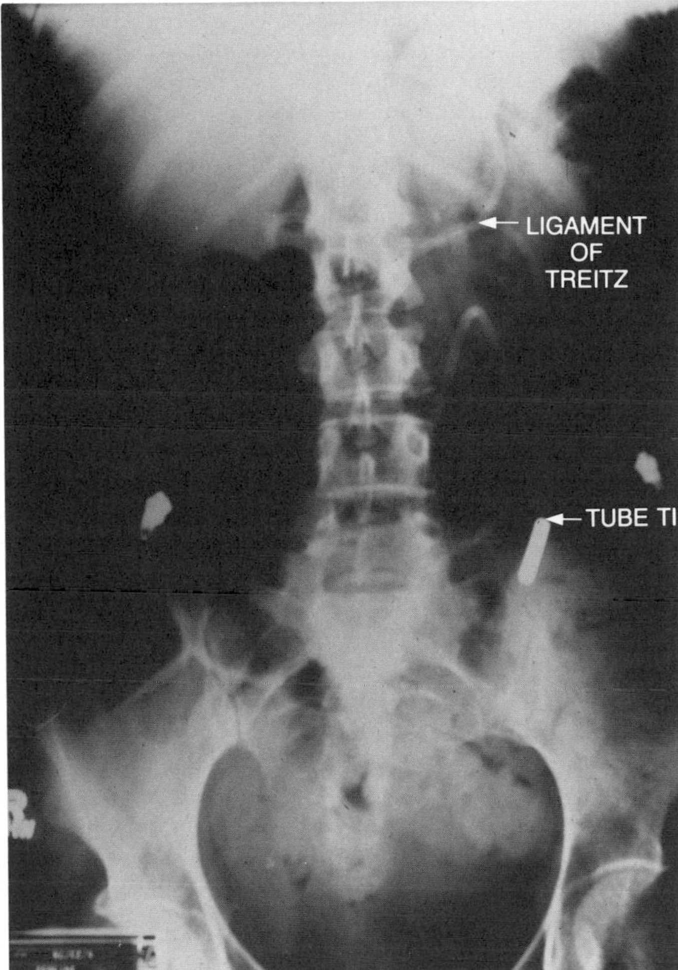

Figure 13.8 Radiographic documentation of the tip of the nasointestinal feeding tube must take place before feedings begin.

The nursing care of a patient with an ostomy tube includes keeping the tube intact and patent, preventing local skin irritation, providing accurate infusions, and monitoring for potential complications.

Procedures for keeping the tube intact and patent depend on the type of tube inserted. All tubes are sutured in place at least initially, but inadvertent tension primarily from the administration tubing and connector can contribute to its dislodgment. Many tubes used for gastrostomies are large—16–18 French—and therefore need to be taped more securely. The tape should be pinched completely around the tube, leaving 1.0–1.5 inches of tape on either side for adherence. Jejunostoma tubes are smaller—5–8 French—but longer. The additional tubing should be coiled and taped securely, with a protective gauze covering, until the site is healed and when not in use. Esophagostoma tubes vary from red rubber catheters to smaller, soft, weighted tubes. The tubes may be sutured until a tract is formed. For some patients, the tube can be removed and reinserted for each feeding. Unlike the noninvasive feeding tubes, gastrostoma-jejunostoma or new esophagostoma feeding tubes require surgical replacement if accidentally pulled out.

Skin cleansing and the application of a skin adherent, such as tincture of benzoin, help to prevent tissue breakdown. Changing the tape as necessary and moving the tube to alternate sides also help maintain skin integrity. The ostomy tube exit site is protected by a dry, sterile dressing. When gastrostoma tubes are used for intermittent feedings, the end of the tube must be clamped and covered with a gauze sponge between feedings to prevent backflow of gastric contents, which are extremely irritating. The area around esophagostoma tubes requires more frequent skin care because of the possibility of saliva draining through the opening.

The administration of ostomy tube feedings is essentially the same as for noninvasive tube feedings, with two exceptions. First, patients with esophagostomies rarely have difficulty tolerating larger volumes of formula (350–500 ml) administered by gravity drip every 3–4 hours. We should always be aware, however, that the patients can aspirate. Second, needle-catheter jejunostomies with a 16-gauge catheter require an elemental diet and an infusion control device to guarantee consistent flow (Freeman et al. 1976).

The complications for ostomy tube feedings include postoperative edema, bleeding, tube dislodgment, and peritonitis as well as aspiration and diarrhea. The surgical procedure is short and nontraumatic for most patients. However, any incision and tissue manipulation can result in edema and bleeding. Small pressure dressings are applied in the operating room and remain in place at least overnight. Proper taping to secure the feeding tube has been previously stressed. Dislodgment could lead to leakage of gastrointestinal secretions into the peritoneal cavity and the possibility of peritonitis (Torosian and Rombeau 1980). Patients with esophagostomas must also be closely monitored for tracheal obstruction in the early postoperative period.

PERCUTANEOUS ENDOSCOPIC GASTROSTOMY AND JEJUNOSTOMY

Another category of invasive feeding tubes includes those that are placed percutaneously. Since first described (Gauderer et al. 1980), the percutaneous endoscopic gastrostomy (PEG) has become a routine procedure in most hospitals. The primary advantage is that the procedure can be performed under local anesthesia in an endoscopy suite. Percutaneously placed gastrostomies require less time to perform and in general have fewer complications compared with surgical procedures.

There are two predominant placement techniques, the Ponsky-Gauderer pull technique (Ponsky et al. 1985) and the Sachs-Vine push technique (Hogan et al. 1986). Choice of technique appears to be based on physician preference. A 20 or 22 French tube is the most common size for adult patients. Less frequently used is the Russell technique (Russell et al. 1984), which uses a 14 French tube. The same formulas are used for nutritional support as with small-bore feeding tubes. PEG tubes have the additional advantage of a larger size, so formulas and medications, when applicable, are easily administered, with a decreased risk of clogging. Formulas may be administered by enteral feeding pump or gravity drip, continuously or intermittently. Feedings are usually initiated the day following the procedure.

The care of the PEG exit site is less involved than that for a surgical gastrostomy. There are fewer complications related to wound dehiscence, gastrointestinal bleeding, and leakage of gastric contents. Povidone-iodine ointment is generally applied at the exit site for 24–48 hours. Frequently no dressing is applied during the postinsertion period nor is one recommended for long-term maintenance. Daily soap and water cleansing, along with exit site inspection, comprises routine care. PEG tubes come with a variety of exit site stabilization devices. Most also require taping the tube to alleviate tension and potential irritation. Exit site complications are managed similarly to surgical gastrostomies.

Initially the complication rate for PEG tubes was low (Ponsky et al. 1983). As this procedure has gained in popularity and higher-risk patients have been selected, the complication rate has increased. It does, however, remain a well-accepted, simple procedure, with a relatively low complication rate (Kirby et al. 1986; Weg and Miskovitz 1987). In general, a patient who requires long-term tube feedings should be considered a candidate for a PEG.

The risk of aspiration in the compromised patient is the same for a PEG tube as for a nasogastric tube. Consequently an 8 or 10 French feeding tube is passed through the PEG tube into the intestines in these patients. When indicated, gastric decompression can be accomplished along with the formula administration. This has been described as a percutaneous endoscopic jejunostomy (PEJ) (Gottsfried and Plumser 1984; Ponsky and Aszodi 1984).

PARENTERAL NUTRITIONAL SUPPORT

The original indication for total parenteral nutrition (TPN) was for the patient with a nonfunctioning gastrointestinal tract. There are additional indications when adequate oral intake is inappropriate or even hazardous. These include patients who are malnourished or severely depleted and those who have obstructions or inflammation of the central nervous system or upper gastrointestinal tract. For example, a patient who has had a recent cerebrovascular accident and has no protective reflexes is at risk of aspiration, as is a patient receiving irradiation therapy to the oral cavity or esophagus who cannot swallow. These patients can benefit from parenteral nutrition support until their conditions stabilize and a long-range nutritional plan is made. There are two methods of providing parenteral nutrition: TPN and peripheral parenteral nutrition (PPN).

Total Parenteral Nutrition

TPN is the administration of a complete metabolic diet through a central venous route. The components are carbohydrates as hypertonic dextrose, protein as synthetic amino acids, plus essential electrolytes, trace minerals, and vitamins (Dudrick et al. 1969; Shils 1972). Fat as either soybean or safflower oil is provided separately (Hansen et al. 1976; Pelham 1981). A typical TPN dextrose–amino acid solution contains approximately 25% dextrose and 50 g amino acids in 1 liter and is equivalent to 1 calorie per ml. The average patient receives 1,800–2,400 ml per day. When used as a caloric source, fat comprises one-third of the daily required calories (Meguid et al. 1982). IV fat emulsion may be administered daily as 3-in-1 solution, combined with the dextrose and amino acids or given twice a week to prevent essential fatty acid deficiency (Riela et al. 1975; Faulkner and Flint 1977).

Hypertonic solution is irritating to peripheral veins and for this reason central venous access is necessary. A subclavian or internal jugular vein is most commonly used as an entry point for the catheter. This is a sterile procedure performed at the bedside for most patients. The catheter is threaded to its correct position in the superior vena cava; its position is documented by x-ray. The solution is ordered by the physician and prepared daily in the pharmacy under a laminar flow hood. The nurse administers the solution by an infusion-control device to ensure accuracy. In addition, the patient is closely monitored through vital signs, weight, intake and output record, urine spot tests, and routine blood tests of electrolytes, glucose, renal and liver function plus selected other values based on the individual's condition.

The complications of TPN therapy can be significant, and awareness and professional skill are required to minimize or prevent them. Pneumothorax is the most common major complication associated with central venous catheterization (Mitchell and Clark 1979). Proper patient preparation and physician training markedly decrease this possibility. The TPN catheter provides direct access to the central bloodstream and the average length of therapy for most acutely ill patients is 4–6 weeks. Therefore meticulous catheter care is essential. Catheter dressings are changed approximately three times a week based on hospital policy and the type of dressing material used. The dressing change is a sterile procedure requiring mask and gloves. A defatting agent may be used initially, then a form of povidone-iodine (solution, ointment, or both) is applied (Figure 13.9). Small gauze dressings are sufficient to protect the catheter exit site because there is no drainage (Figure 13.10). A skin adhesive is recommended and finally the area is occlusively taped by one of the many tapes currently available (Figure 13.11).

The tubing used to administer TPN solution, including pump cassette, is changed every 24 hours (Goldmann and Maki 1973). This can become a routine procedure with the first container of each day. Care in handling the solution and tubing is necessary to prevent contamination and possible infection. Proper taping of the tubing prevents separation at the catheter hub and leakage of solution, blood, or air. A wet dressing increases the chance of infection. Blood back-up can cause the catheter to clot and the solution flow to abruptly cease, leading to a hypoglycemic episode and catheter replacement. Finally, air leakage may mean an air embolism. All three of these potential complications are avoidable through proper attention to details of care.

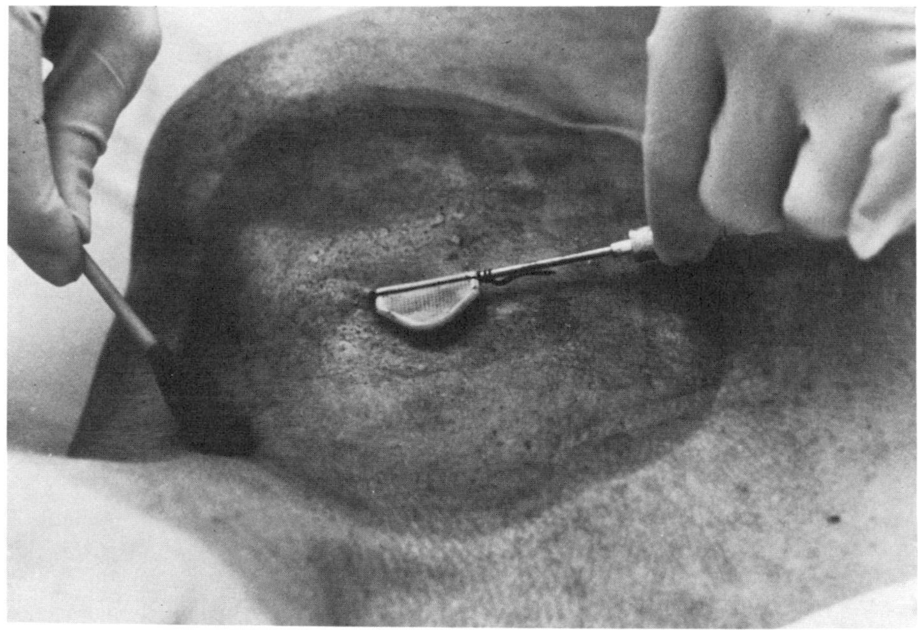

Figure 13.9 Application of povidone-iodine solution.

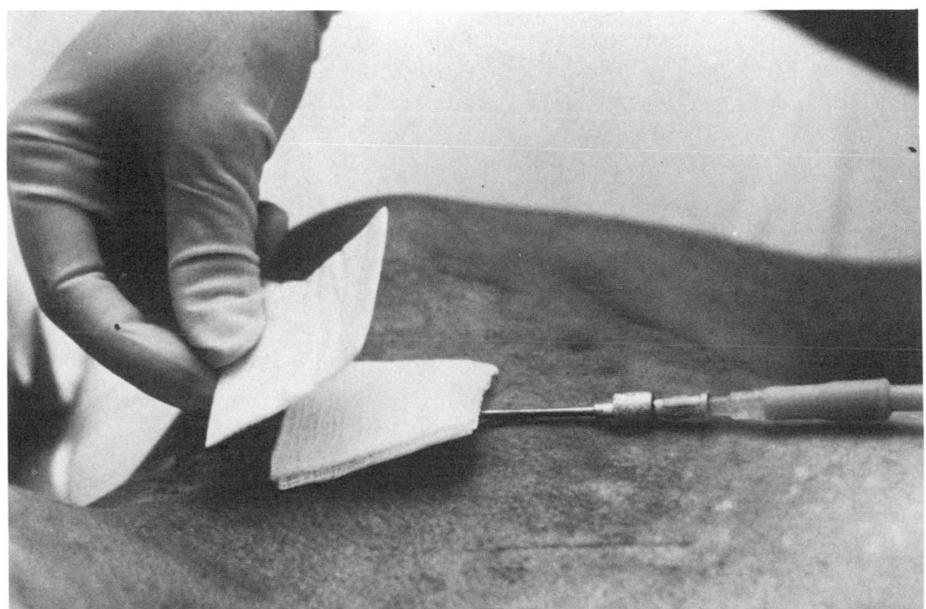

Figure 13.10 Gauze dressings are used to protect the catheter exit site.

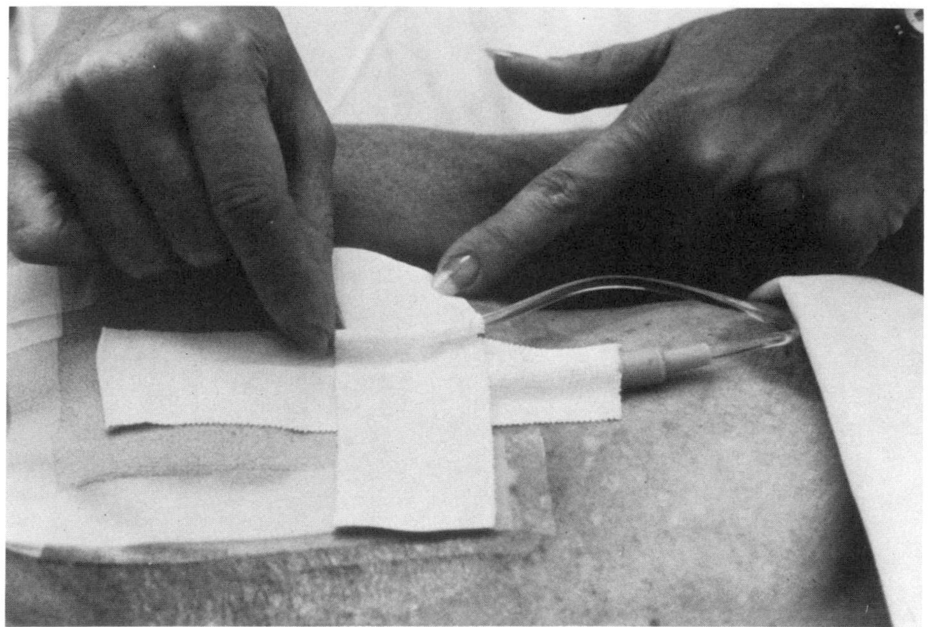

Figure 13.11 The final occlusive dressing.

The most common metabolic complication of TPN is hyperglycemia because of the high concentrations of dextrose that are infused. To prevent this, one should first start at a low infusion rate, about 30–40 ml per hour, and gradually increase the rate over several days while closely monitoring levels of blood and urine sugar. Second, it is important to be aware of patients who are susceptible to glucose intolerance and add regular insulin to the TPN solution as necessary to avoid glucosuria and keep blood glucose levels within normal range (Dudrick et al. 1972). Other metabolic imbalances occur due to the patient's depleted or disease state and can be controlled by additions to or deletions from the TPN solution as determined by regularly scheduled laboratory monitoring. Deficiencies of essential fatty acids and trace minerals were a problem before safe IV fat emulsions and trace mineral preparations became available for routine administration.

Peripheral Parenteral Nutrition

Patients who need only short-term parenteral therapy, for example, 7–10 days, before starting oral or tube feedings may be able to benefit from PPN. It is made up of the same components as TPN, but the dextrose–amino acid solution is less concentrated and comprises only half of the total therapy volume. The other half is administered as fat. Consequently, it takes 1.0–1.5 liters of dextrose–amino acids and 1.0–1.5 liters of 10% fat emulsion to provide approximately 1,400–2,000 calories per day (Deitel and Kaminsky 1974; Freeman 1978). The advantage of PPN solutions is that they can be administered by peripheral vein. Disadvantages are unavailability of peripheral veins and the patient's inability to tolerate the total volume of fluid and fat (Walters and Freeman 1981). Patients with cardiac or renal disorders, severe liver disease, pulmonary disease, or blood coagulation disorders are rarely candidates for this therapy (Silberman et al. 1977). Unless contraindicated, PPN may be used for the dysphagic patient who is undergoing a feeding trial. This provides sufficient calories without interference of a nasogastric or nasointestinal feeding tube.

A peripheral catheter is inserted under sterile conditions and changed every 48–72 hours (Goldmann et al. 1973). The site is inspected hourly for signs of inflammation or infiltration. Solutions are prepared in the pharmacy on a daily basis. They are usually administered by infusion-control devices, with changes of IV tubing every 24 hours. A dry, sterile dressing is changed daily, with similar skin care as with central catheters, although mask and gloves are not worn. Patient monitoring is the same for both TPN and PPN.

Complications of PPN relate mainly to the infusion site. Irritation of the vein wall with painful phlebitis or infiltration is common (Gazitua et al. 1979; Massar et al. 1982). Local infection with bacteremias is rare but does occur. Too-rapid administration may lead to fluid overload and respiratory distress. Each of these complications is preventable with careful and frequent patient observations.

SUMMARY

It is important for all nurses to be familiar with the pathology of swallowing disorders, including the differences between those of neurologic, mechanical, and psychiatric origin. The specific signs and symptoms and the current treatment modalities affect daily and long-term care plans for each patient. The nursing management of dysphagic patients requires knowledge, skill, and patience. Attention to proper hydration and clear airways should be followed by early nutritional intervention. There is no question today that nutritional support should be a consideration for each patient. Enteral and parenteral feeding methods are available and provide options, through one or a combination of therapies, to meet the needs of all of our patients.

REFERENCES

Bistrian B, Blackburn G, Hallowell E, et al. Protein status of general surgical patients. JAMA 1974;230:858.

Bistrian B, Blackburn G, Vitale J, et al. Prevalence of malnutrition in general medical patients. JAMA 1976;235:1567.

Blackburn G, Bistrian B, Maini B, et al. Nutritional and metabolic assessment of the hospitalized patient. JPEN J Parenter Enteral Nutri 1977;1:11.

Bloch A. Nocturnal tube feedings. Dysphagia 1987;2:3.

Buxton A, Highsmith A, Garner J, et al. Contamination of intravenous infusion fluid; effects of changing administration sets. Ann Intern Med 1979;90:764.

Cameron J, Reynolds J, Zuidema G. Aspiration in patients with tracheostomies. Surg Gynecol Obstet 1973;136:68.

Causey W. Infections Complicating Mechanical Ventilation. In C Rattenborg, E Via-Reque (eds), Clinical Use of Mechanical Ventilation. Chicago: Year Book, 1981;280.

Cooper J, Grillo H. Analysis of Problems Related to Cuffs in Intratracheal Tubes. In R Rogers (ed), Respiratory Intensive Care. Springfield, IL: Thomas, 1977;245.

Crow S. Tips for successful respiratory suctioning. RN 1986;31.

Deitel M, Kaminsky V. Total nutrition by peripheral vein—the lipid system. Can Med Assoc J 1974;111:152.

Delaney H, Carnevale N, Garvey J. Jejunostomy by a needle-catheter technique. Surgery 1973;73:786.

Delaney H, Carnevale N, Garvey J, et al. Postoperative nutritional support using needle-catheter-feeding jejunostomy. Ann Surg 1977;186:165.

Doekel R, Zwillich C, Scoggin C, et al. Clinical semi-starvation; depression of hypoxic ventilatory response. N Engl J Med 1976;295:358.

Dudrick S, Macfadyen B, VanBuren C, et al. Parenteral hyperalimentation; metabolic problems and solutions. Ann Surg 1972;176:259.

Dudrick S, Wilmore D, Vars H, et al. Long-term total parenteral nutrition with growth development and positive nitrogen balance. Surgery 1968;64:134.

Dudrick S, Wilmore D, Vars H, et al. Can intravenous feeding as the sole means of nutrition support growth in the child and restore weight loss in an adult? Ann Surg 1969;169:974.

Egan D. Fundamentals of Respiratory Therapy. St. Louis: Mosby, 1977.

Faulkner W, Flint L. Essential fatty acid deficiency associated with total parenteral nutrition. Surg Gynecol Obstet 1977;144:665.

Freeman J. Peripheral parenteral nutrition. Can J Surg 1978;21:489.

Freeman J, Egan M, Millis B. The elemental diet. Surg Gynecol Obstet 1976;142:925.

Fuch P. Streamlining your suctioning techniques, part 3, tracheostomy suctioning. Nursing 1984;39.

Ganger D, Craig R. Swallowing disorders and nutritional support. Dysphagia 1990;4:213.

Gauderer M, Ponsky J, Izant R. Gastrostomy without laparotomy: a percutaneous endoscopic technique. J Pediatr Surg 1980;15:872.

Gazitua R, Wilson K, Bistrian B, et al. Factors determining peripheral vein tolerance to amino acid infusions. Arch Surg 1979;114:897.

Goldmann D, Maki D. Infection control in total parenteral nutrition. JAMA 1973;223:1360.

Goldmann D, Maki D, Rhame F, et al. Guidelines for infection control in intravenous therapy. Ann Intern Med 1973;79:848.

Goodnough S. The effects of oxygen and hyperinflation on arterial oxygen tension after endotracheal suctioning. Heart Lung 1985;14:11.

Gottsfried E, Plumser A. Endoscopic gastrojejunostomy: a technique to establish small bowel feeding without laparotomy. Gastrointest Endosc 1984;30:355.

Grant J. A Team Approach: Handbook of Total Parenteral Nutrition. Philadelphia: Saunders, 1980.

Grant J, Curtas M, Kelvin F. Fluoroscopic placement of nasojejunal feeding tubes with immediate feeding using a nonelemental diet. JPEN J Parenter Enteral Nutri 1983;3:299.

Groher M, Bukatman R. The prevalence of swallowing disorders in two teaching hospitals. Dysphagia 1986;1:3.

Hansen L, Hardie B, Hildalgo J. Fat emulsion for intravenous administration: clinical experience with Intralipid 10%. Ann Surg 1976;184:80.

Hargrove R. Feeding the severely dysphagic patient. J Neurosurg Nurs 1980;12:102.
Hedden M, Ersoz C, Safar P. Tracheoesophageal fistulas following prolonged artificial ventilation via cuffed tracheostomy tubes. Anesthesiology 1969;31:281.
Hoffman L, Moszkiewicz R. Airway management for the critically ill patient. Am J Nurs 1987;39.
Hogan R, DeMarco D, Hamilton J, et al. Percutaneous endoscopic gastrostomy—to push or pull. Gastrointest Endosc 1986;32:253.
Kamel P. Nutritional assessment and requirements. Dysphagia 1990;4:189.
Kirby D, Craig R, Tsang T-K, et al. Percutaneous endoscopic gastrostomies: a prospective evaluation and review of the literature. JPEN J Parenter Enteral Nutri 1986; 10: 155.
Levenson R, Turner W, Dyson A, et al. Do weighted nasoenteric feeding tubes facilitate transpyloric intubation? JPEN J Parenter Enteral Nutri 1988;12:135.
Lipner H, Bosler J, Giles G. Volunteer participation in feeding residents: training and supervision in a long-term care facility. Dysphagia 1990;5:89.
Logemann J. Factors affecting ability to resume oral nutrition in the oropharyngeal dysphagic individual. Dysphagia 1990;4:202.
Long C, Schaffel N, Geiger J, et al. Metabolic response to injury and illness: the establishment of energy and protein needs from indirect calorimetry and nitrogen balance. JPEN J Parenter Enteral Nutri 1979;3:452.
Lord L, Weiser-Maimone A, Pulhamus M, et al. Comparison of weighted vs. nonweighted enteral feeding tubes for efficacy of transpyloric intubation. JPEN J Parenter Enteral Nutri 1993;3:271.
Loustau A, Lee K. Dealing with the dangers of dysphagia. Nursing 1985;47.
Massar E, Daly J, Copeland E, et al. Peripheral vein complications in patients receiving amino acid/dextrose solutions. JPEN J Parenter Enteral Nutri 1982;7:159.
Meguid M, Schimmel E, Johnson W, et al. Reduced metabolic complications in total parenteral nutrition: pilot study using fat to replace one-third of glucose calories. JPEN J Parenter Enteral Nutri 1982;6:304.
Mitchell S, Clark R. Complications of central venous catheterization. Am J Roentgenol 1979;133:467.
Nielsen L. Potential problems of mechanical ventilation. Am J Nurs 1980;80:2206.
O'Gara J. Dietary adjustments and nutritional therapy during treatment for oral-pharyngeal dysphagia. Dysphagia 1990;4:209.
Pelham, L. Rational use of intravenous fat emulsions. Am J Hosp Pharm 1981;38:198.
Ponsky J, Aszodi A. Percutaneous endoscopic jejunostomy. Am J Gastroenterol 1984; 79:113.
Ponsky J, Gauderer M, Stellato T. Percutaneous endoscopic gastrostomy: review of 150 cases. Arch Surg 1983;118:913.
Ponsky J, Gauderer M, Stellato T, et al. Percutaneous approaches to enteral alimentation. Am J Surg 1985;149:102.
Rees R, Payne-James J, Silk D. Spontaneous transpyloric passage and performance of "fine bore" polyurethane feeding tubes: a controlled clinical study. JPEN J Parenter Enteral Nutri 1988;12:135.
Riela M, Broviac J, Wells M, et al. Essential fatty acid deficiency in human adults during total parenteral nutrition. Ann Intern Med 1975;83:786.
Rombeau J, Barot L. Enteral Nutrition Therapy. In J Mullen, L Crosby, J Rombeau (eds), The Surgical Clinics of North America: Symposium on Surgical Nutrition. Philadelphia: Saunders 1981;610.
Roubenoff R, Preto J, Balke C. Malnutrition among hospitalized patients. A problem of physician awareness. Arch Intern Med 1987;147:1462.
Russell T, Brotman M, Norris F. Percutaneous gastrostomy. A new simplified and cost-effective technique. Am J Surg 1984;189:132.

Shapiro S, Harrison R, Trout C. Maintenance of Artificial Airways of Extubation. In S Shapiro, et al. (eds), Clinical Application of Respiratory Care. Chicago: Year Book, 1975;254.

Shils M. Guidelines for total parenteral nutrition. JAMA 1972;220:1921.

Silberman H, Freehauf M, Fong G, et al. Parenteral nutrition with lipids. JAMA 1977;238:1380.

Silverman E, Elfant I. Dysphagia: an evaluation and treatment program for the adult. Am J Occup Ther 1979;33:382.

Sitzmann J. Nutritional support of the dysphagic patient: methods, risks, and complications of therapy. JPEN J Parenter Enteral Nutri 1990;1:60.

Sitzmann J, Mueller B. Enteral and parenteral feeding in the dysphagic patient. Dysphagia 1988;3:38.

Taylor H, Mhoon E, Matz G. Complications Due to Tracheostomy and Endotracheal Tubes. In C Rattenberg, E Via-Reque (eds), Clinical Use of Mechanical Ventilation. Chicago: Year Book, 1981;25:273.

Torosian M, Rombeau J. Feeding by tube enterostomy. Surg Gynecol Obstet 1980;150:918.

Walters J, Freeman J. Parenteral Nutrition by Peripheral Vein. In J Mullen, L Crosby, J Rombeau (eds), Surgical Clinics of North America: Symposium on Surgical Nutrition. Philadelphia: Saunders, 1981;593.

Waxman K, Shoemaker W. Management of Postoperative and Posttraumatic Respiratory Failure in the ICU. In R Bartlett (ed), Surgical Clinics of North America: Symposium on Surgical Nutrition. Philadelphia: Saunders, 1980;1424.

Weg A, Miskovitz P. Percutaneous endoscopic gastrostomy (PEG): a critical appraisal. Dysphagia 1987;1:227.

Whatley K, Turner W, Dey M, et al. When does metoclopramide facilitate transpyloric intubation? JPEN J Parenter Enteral Nutri 1984;6:679.

Winitz M, Graff J, Gallagher N. Evaluation of chemical diets as nutrition for man-in-space. Nature 1965;205:741.

14

Surgical Intervention in Dysphagia

Jonathan R. Workman, Harold C. Pillsbury III, and Gregory Hulka

Surgical intervention in patients with dysphagia is directed toward reestablishing normal physiology or bypassing known lesions and abnormalities of the upper digestive tract. A thorough understanding of the normal anatomy and physiology of this region is therefore necessary to plan surgical therapy for patients with dysphagia. From an evolutionary point of view, the primary function of the larynx is sphincteric protection of the airway, and management of disorders of deglutition must preserve this important function of the upper airway. As a complete discussion of the anatomy and physiology of the upper aerodigestive tract is given elsewhere in this text, only a brief overview is given here. The major sites of surgically treatable dysphagia are discussed, along with methods of intervention.

FUNCTIONAL ANATOMY

The act of swallowing can be broken into three stages (see Chapter 2): oral, pharyngeal, and esophageal. The first stage is voluntary, consisting of mastication, following which the muscles of the mouth and tongue mold the food bolus and push it back toward the posterior wall of the oropharynx. As the bolus moves posteriorly, the pharyngeal stage of swallowing begins as a combination of voluntary and involuntary actions. Contraction of the velopharyngeal muscles of the soft palate and the superior constrictor functions to close off the nasopharynx from the oropharynx. The tongue continues to project the food bolus into the oropharynx, and this dorsal projection bends the epiglottis horizontally to cover the aditus of the larynx. Simultaneous contraction of the stylopharyngeus muscle to elevate the larynx and relaxation of the hypopharynx allows the bolus to descend downward toward the esophageal inlet.

The final stage of swallowing begins with the temporary relaxation of the upper esophageal sphincter (classically described as the cricopharyngeus muscle), located approximately at the level of C6–C7. This allows passage of the bolus into the esophagus, initiating involuntary peristalsis. The upper sphincter then resumes its normal resting tone, the larynx descends, and the epiglottis projects back into its normal upright position.

Oral Stage

Fortunately, dysphagia is least common during this stage of swallowing because surgical treatment is limited. Hypoglossal paralysis, whether following stroke or surgery, is treated with limited success. Some authors describe techniques of cross-innervation for hypoglossal paralysis. Using a midline Z-plasty incision, a portion of the tongue mucosa and underlying muscle from the unaffected side is sewn into the affected side, reintroducing innervation to the paralyzed half of the tongue. This technique is most successful when performed soon after the onset of the paralysis, as the motor end plates have a limited life span following deinnervation.

Patients also may suffer from dysphagia in this stage of deglutition due to mechanical factors. Inflammatory disease, foreign bodies, benign and malignant tumors, and structural abnormalities may all lead toward limitations in the swallowing mechanism. Surgical treatment is aimed at the appropriate management and excision of the endoluminal or extraluminal masses. Treatment of structural abnormalities, including cleft palate and oral webs, is aimed at recreating the normal anatomy of the oral cavity. The variety of techniques for their repair is beyond the scope of this chapter.

Pharyngeal Stage

As in the oral stage, extrinsic and intrinsic compression of the lumen are more amenable to surgical correction than neurogenic lesions. It is also at this level that laryngeal function plays an important role, and it must be considered when treatment plans are determined. Infection and trauma can both result in dysphagia in the pharyngeal stage, with extrinsic compression of the lumen through abscess, hematoma, or traumatic cervical projection into the retropharyngeal or parapharyngeal spaces.

Malignant disease must be seriously considered in any patient presenting with dysphagia in the pharyngeal stage. Although squamous cell carcinoma is the most common type of intrinsic cancer of the oropharynx and hypopharynx, extrinsic compression from parapharyngeal space tumors must also be considered. The Mayo Clinic series of parapharyngeal space tumors revealed the following distribution: mixed tumor, 43%; malignant lymphoma, 25%; schwannoma, 16%; paraganglioma, 12%; hemangiopericytoma, 2%; hemangioendothelioma, 1%; and lipoma, 1%. Sarcomas and glomus tumors also may arise in this space (Heeneman et al. 1980). Any of these parapharyngeal tumors can have dysphagia as a presenting symptom. Surgical management aims at appropriate surgical excision of the tumor.

CERVICAL OSTEOPHYTES

Cervical osteophyte formation occurs in 20–30% of the population and in some individuals results in dysphagia through either mechanical compression of the pharynx or paraesophageal inflammation caused by motion over the osteophytes (Sobol and Ringual 1984; Papadopoulos et al. 1989). Diffuse idiopathic skeletal hyperostosis, characterized by excessive bone growth at the site of attachment of a ligament or tendon to bone, has been reported by several authors (Kibel and Johnson 1987; Fahrer and Markwalder 1988; Shergy et al. 1989) to present with dysphagia. Other conditions, including ankylosing spondylitis, infectious spondylitis, previous surgical fusion of cervical vertebrae, and local trauma (Welsh et al. 1987), all can lead to the development of large osteophytes. While the osteophytes may form throughout the spine, it is typically osteophytes located at C3 through C6 that cause dysphagia.

Treatment of osteophytes is controversial. Nonsteroidal anti-inflammatory agents and oral steroids often are recommended for nonprogressive dysphagia secondary to osteophytes. However, in the case of progressive dysphagia or dysphagia unresponsive to conservative therapy, surgical excision of the osteophytes is recommended.

The surgical approach begins with a transverse incision across the middle of the thyroid cartilage crossing the anterior border of the sternocleidomastoid muscle. The left side of the neck is traditionally chosen because it has a lower incidence of a nonrecurrent laryngeal nerve. The incision is taken down through the platysma, exposing the anterior border of the sternocleidomastoid muscle. Sharp dissection inferiorly along the anterior border of the sternocleidomastoid muscle exposes the carotid sheath and its contents. As these are retracted laterally, the prevertebral fascia can be seen. Structures that may require division to maximize exposure include the superior thyroid artery, the middle thyroid vein, and the omohyoid tendon and muscle. Care must be taken not to divide the external laryngeal nerve. Grasping the midportion of the thyroid ala and rotating it medially exposes the retropharyngeal space. Dissection of this space is carried out from superior to inferior along the midline, care being taken to avoid injury to the recurrent laryngeal nerve. If access below C6 is necessary, the thyroid gland also must be medialized, and the sternocleidomastoid muscle may require division. Identification of the longus coli muscles to each side of midline helps maintain correct midline position. At this point the cervical osteophyte should be apparent. A vertical incision is made through the prevertebral fascia and periosteum, and subperiosteal dissection permits exposure of the osteophytes. A cutting burr is used to remove the bulk of the mass, and a diamond burr is used to smooth and round off all edges. Closure of the periosteum over the bone is the first layer, followed by reapproximation of all divided deep muscles. A deep drain is inserted, the platysma is closed, and the skin is closed. Patients without intraoperative complications are typically permitted peroral intake the evening of surgery.

CRICOPHARYNGEAL DYSFUNCTION

Cricopharyngeal Muscle

A common site for dysfunction resulting in dysphagia is the cricopharyngeal muscle. It has been studied extensively and is generally considered to be the

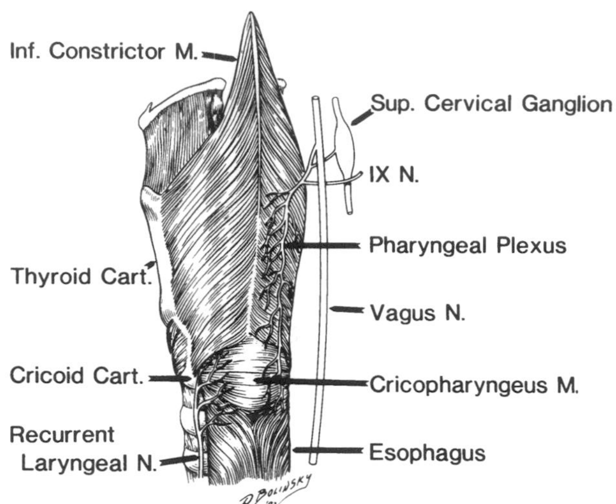

Figure 14.1 Posterior view of the nerve supply to the cricopharyngeal and pharyngeal musculature. (Drawing by David Bolinsky.)

superior esophageal sphincter (Asherson 1950; Kirchner 1958; Lund 1968; Ellis 1971). Inferior to the oblique fibers of the inferior constrictor muscle, the cricopharyngeal muscle forms a sling around the pharyngoesophageal segment from anterolateral attachments to the cricoid cartilage. Inferiorly, the cricopharyngeus is generally continuous with the superior circular fibers of the esophagus (Hollinshead 1968). Manometric measurements reveal a sphincter approximately 3 cm long with a resting pressure of about 40 cm above atmospheric pressure (English 1980). Innervation of the cricopharyngeal muscle (Figure 14.1) in humans remains controversial. In the dog model, Kirchner (1958) demonstrated the motor supply to the cricopharyngeal muscle to be a pharyngeal branch of the vagus nerve. In humans, it is generally considered to be innervated by the pharyngeal nerve plexus, consisting of contributions from the glossopharyngeus, vagus, and superior sympathetic ganglion (Blakley et al. 1968).

Functioning as the superior esophageal sphincter, the relaxation of the cricopharyngeal muscle is considered the terminal event in the pharyngeal stage of deglutition, and abnormal function in this muscle can contribute significantly to dysphagia. The cricopharyngeal muscle has been studied extensively by manometric measurements; in the pathologic state it may be in spasm (Calcaterra et al. 1975; Chodosh 1975), contract prematurely, be delayed in contraction (Ellis et al. 1969), and contribute significantly to the formation of pharyngoesophageal diverticula (Zenker's diverticulum) (Dohlman and Mattson 1960; Lund 1968; Weaver and Fleming 1978). In some diseases involving deglutition, resistance of a normally functioning superior sphincter is too great for weakened pharyngeal constrictor muscles to overcome, resulting in dysphagia (Blakley et al. 1968).

Before surgical intervention for dysphagia, an extensive evaluation of the upper aerodigestive tract must be completed. In addition to identifying a func-

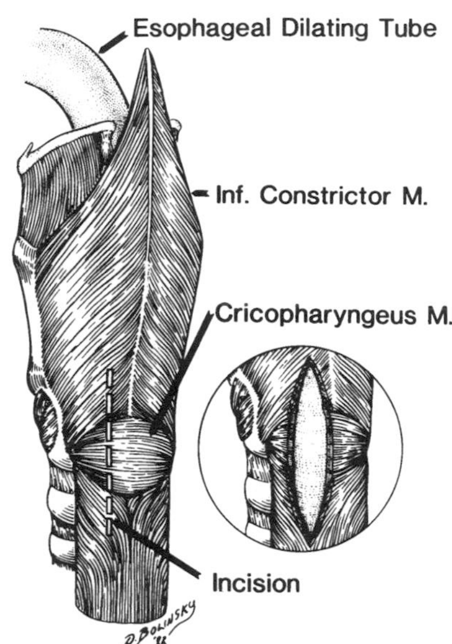

Figure 14.2 Incision for the cricopharyngeal myotomy. The inset shows the mucosa bulging through the excised musculature. (Drawing by David Bolinsky.)

tional disorder, intrinsic or extrinsic masses must be eliminated as possible causes of dysphagia. The most effective preoperative evaluation includes a cine-esophageal barium swallow, esophagoscopy, and manometric measurements (Orringer 1980). The barium swallow often reveals a prominent cricopharyngeal sphincter, a prominent posterior cricopharyngeal "bar" on lateral cervical views, and Zenker's diverticulum.

Cricopharyngeal Myotomy

The most widely practiced surgical management of cricopharyngeal dysfunction has been cricopharyngeal myotomy (Blakley et al. 1968; Chodosh 1975; Mills 1975; Zuckerbraum and Bahma 1979; Ellis 1980; Black 1981; Lindgren and Ekberg 1990) or an extended myotomy (Figure 14.2). Depending on the patient's physical condition, this procedure can be performed under local or general anesthesia (Henderson et al. 1989). Either an oblique incision anterior to the sternocleidomastoid muscle or a horizontal incision at the level of the cricoid cartilage is made. The left side is preferred by most surgeons, because of the decreased likelihood of a nonrecurrent laryngeal nerve. Following sharp dissection through the subcutaneous tissues and the platysma, the larynx is exposed by separating the strap muscles. The larynx is retracted medially, while the carotid sheath and contents are retracted laterally (Calcaterra et al. 1975; Ellis 1980). The middle thyroid vein often must be cut to facilitate exposure. The recurrent laryngeal nerve must be identified and protected. Critical to the success of the myotomy is identification and division of all the cricopharyngeal muscle fibers. To accomplish this, a bougie (weighted rubber tube) can be placed through the mouth into the esophagus, distending the sphincter and allowing all the fibers to be identified and cut, exposing the underlying mucosal membrane (Skolnik et al. 1966). As an additional precaution to prevent recurrent laryngeal nerve injury, the myotomy is performed in the midline on the posterior surface of the esophagus.

Zenker's diverticula are often present in association with cricopharyngeal dysfunction. The base of the diverticulum is located superior to the slinglike band of cricopharyngeus muscle and is inferior to the oblique fibers of the inferior constrictor. Diverticula range from 1–8 cm in length. There is evidence from clinical experience that the size of the diverticulum does not correlate with the degree of dysphagia (Orringer 1980). Subsequently, an adequate myotomy alone may resolve the symptoms of dysphagia when diverticula are present. Many surgeons have demonstrated their disappearance by postoperative esophageal swallow in patients having myotomy alone for small diverticula. For large diverticula, however, surgical resection with two-layer closure in addition to myotomy is indicated (Ellis 1969).

The complications of cricopharyngeal myotomy are few, primarily incomplete division of the cricopharyngeus muscle resulting in persistent dysphagia, damage to the recurrent laryngeal nerve, and fistula formation from unrecognized perforation of the mucous membrane. Because of these complications and the typically poor systemic condition of the patients, some advocate endoscopic resection of the common wall between a diverticulum and the esophagus by coagulating diathermy current (Dohlman and Mattson 1960). This procedure opens the diverticulum and at the same time divides the cricopharyngeus muscle. The procedure has received only modest acceptance because of limited surgical exposure, a high rate of fistulization, and a lower success rate due to the inability to detect when the cricopharyngeus has been completely divided.

Postoperative evaluation of patients having a cricopharyngeal myotomy for dysphagia reveals elimination of dysphagia or only an occasional episode of mild dysphagia in 85% of patients studied (Black 1981). In addition, manometric measurements demonstrate an approximately 50% decrease in the resting pressure of the superior sphincter. Patients who have premature contraction of the sphincter prior to myotomy continue to have it postoperatively (Ellis 1969), although they typically have less dysphagia. Patients with multiple cranial nerve dysfunctions, especially if these include the hypoglossal nerve, or those who have significant ballooning of the pharyngeal constrictor muscles preoperatively, achieve only a modest improvement in dysphagia after cricopharyngeal myotomy (Lebo et al. 1976).

Dilatation of the superior esophageal sphincter using bougie dilators has been advocated as an alternative treatment in patients with idiopathic spasm or achalasia of the superior esophageal sphincter (Calcaterra et al. 1975). This treatment is recommended in systemically debilitated patients who cannot tolerate a more involved surgical procedure. The effectiveness of managing superior esophageal achalasia by dilatation is limited because the procedure must be repeated and relief is of short duration, although a few select patients can be taught self-dilation. Multiple dilatation of the superior esophagus can result in significant risk of esophageal perforation. Because of the necessity for repeated procedures and the significant morbidity and mortality associated with esophageal perforation, superior esophageal sphincter dilatation for dysphagia is only indicated in a select, small group of patients, such as younger persons who are not debilitated but who demonstrate mild to moderate narrowing. Those who do not respond readily to this treatment should not be considered for long-term repeated dilatation.

Laryngeal surgery for carcinoma alters pharyngeal structure and function, and often these patients require weeks to months of practice to relearn the neuromuscular sequence for effective swallowing. By cine-esophageal swallow and manometric pressure measurements, the pharyngeal musculature has been demonstrated to be ineffective in propelling a bolus or secretions through the cricopharyngeal sphincter. Cricopharyngeal myotomy is therefore advocated (Thawley and Ogura 1978) in patients undergoing conservative surgery of the larynx, including hemilaryngectomy and unilateral and bilateral supraglottic laryngectomy. This myotomy is performed by some surgeons at the time of conservative laryngeal surgery (Nicks 1976). Some recommend myotomy in all patients undergoing supraglottic laryngectomy because there is a tendency for the cricopharyngeal muscle to fail to relax properly following the procedure, and aspiration becomes a significant postoperative problem.

ESOPHAGEAL DYSFUNCTION

Dysfunction of the esophageal stage of deglutition must also be considered in patients with dysphagia and aspiration (see Chapter 5). To evaluate esophageal function, the following studies should be considered: cine-esophageal barium swallow, esophageal manometric measurements, pH testing (as subtle acid reflux may not be apparent on manometrics), and endoscopy. Extrinsic or intrinsic structural obstruction of the esophagus must be identified. Neuromuscular dysfunction of the esophagus may result in diffuse esophageal spasm, megaesophagus, lower esophageal achalasia, or hypotensive lower esophageal sphincter with esophageal reflux (Ellis 1980). By precise manometric measurements in patients with spasm of the esophageal body, functional obstruction can be identified at the point of highest resistance. This evaluation can guide the surgical intervention and limit an otherwise overextensive esophageal myotomy.

Typically, surgery is reserved for patients in whom dysphagia is severe and medical treatment has been unsuccessful. The esophagus is approached through a left thoracotomy incision. As in the cricopharyngeus myotomy, the circular fibers of the esophageal musculature are identified and divided longitudinally over the area of dysfunction. Megaesophagus resulting from increased resting tension of the lower esophageal sphincter and lower esophageal achalasia are treated effectively by surgical intervention using the modified Heller procedure (Asherson 1950). A myotomy is performed at the level of the gastroesophageal junction either transthoracically or transabdominally, depending on the necessity for a combined procedure. In cases of megaesophagus in which significant dilatation of the esophagus has been demonstrated preoperatively, partial resection of the esophagus is indicated (Negus 1962; Nicks 1976). Evaluation of patients following myotomy reveals an 18–34% incidence of gastroesophageal reflux (Henderson 1989). Complications from esophageal reflux include esophagitis with stricture formation, profound discomfort, and reflex upper esophageal sphincter achalasia (Ellis 1980; Vantrappen and Hellemans 1980). The mechanism of increased upper esophageal sphincter tension in esophageal reflux is attributed to chronic irritation of the esophagus, followed by a reflex tightening of the sphincter (Henderson and Marryatt 1977). Because of the high incidence of morbidity associated with reflux following a cardiomyotomy, Mansour et al. (1976) advocate a combined procedure, including a reflux-retarding procedure at the time of myotomy. Additionally, patients who have primary esophageal reflux from a hypotensive lower esophageal sphincter may benefit from an antireflux procedure. Several types of antireflux procedures are commonly practiced, including the Belsey Mark IV transthoracic reconstruction of the cardia, the Nissen fundoplication, and the Hill procedure.

In the medically compromised patient with lower esophageal achalasia, dilatation of the cardia may be an effective alternative. A forceful dilation of the sphincter is necessary, using either the Starck dilator, which consists of a balloon of fixed diameter, or the Sippy pneumatic dilator bag (Vantrappen and Hellemans 1980). Following repeated dilatations, patients experience improvement in dysphagia in 75% of cases, with significant reflux occurring only 1% of the time (Vantrappen and Hellemans 1980). The factor limiting the wider use of dilatation techniques is the relatively high incidence (5%) of esophageal perforation. Dilatation of the lower esophageal sphincter is effective and should be performed in patients suffering from severe dysphagia who are not candidates for a major operative procedure.

AORTIC ARCH ANOMALIES

There are multiple anomalies of the aortic arch that lead to dysphagia (Adkins et al. 1986). Bayford (1794) reported compression of the esophagus by an aberrant right subclavian artery originating in the left side of the mediastinum as the most distal branch of the aortic arch and then coursing posterior to the esophagus, leading to dysphagia. Bayford named the syndrome dysphagia "lusoria," or "jest of nature." While this anomaly occurs in 0.5–1.8% of the population, it only occasionally results in dysphagia. The original technique described for the treatment of dysphagia lusoria was simple division of the aberrant artery through a left thoracotomy (Gross 1946; Pome et al. 1987). Bailey et al. (1965) modified the technique to include reimplantation of the artery into the aortic arch to avoid arm ischemia. Thoracotomy has traditionally been the approach used for either simple division (Van Son et al. 1989); however, some authors (Orvald et al. 1972; Valentine et al. 1987) have described extrathoracic approaches to the aberrant arteries because they often course high in the mediastinum. Through a supraclavicular incision, the aberrant artery can be divided and reimplanted into the right carotid artery.

The double aortic arch is the most common vascular ring in infants. If the right and left arches coexist and are of equivalent size, a tight vascular ring will form around the trachea and esophagus, resulting in both breathing and swallowing difficulties. Surgical correction depends on which arch is dominant. In patients with a dominant right posterior arch, division of the left anterior arch between the left common carotid and left subclavian artery is performed (Richardson et al. 1981). When the left anterior arch is dominant, division of the posterior arch as well as the ligamentum arteriosum is performed (Richardson et al. 1981). In these patients, both recurrent laryngeal nerves are long, with the nerves looping around the arch, except on the side of the ligamentum (Nikaido et al. 1972).

Two types of right aortic arch anomalies exist. One type consists of mirror-image branching of the great vessels and is typically associated with a cardiac defect involving the origin of the aorta of the pulmonary artery. In the second type, an aberrant left subclavian artery and left ductus are found. In the child, both airway and esophageal symptoms usually are present, while dysphagia is more often the complaint in the adult (Drucker and Symbas 1980). Most authors agree that for appropriate surgical management, division of the left ligamentum arteriosum and freeing of the esophagus and trachea are imperative. When an aberrant left subclavian artery is present, some authors recommend division of this subclavian artery (Hallman and Cooley 1964; Jung et al. 1978). Disagreement exists as to the importance of reanastamosis of the subclavian artery. Those who choose to reimplant the left subclavian usually implant the artery into the arch or left carotid artery (Wychulis et al. 1971; Jung et al. 1978).

LASER PALLIATION FOR MALIGNANT DYSPHAGIA

Until recently, dysphagia due to unresectable esophageal carcinoma with occlusion of the esophageal lumen has been treated with placement of a feeding gastrostomy. Multiple authors (Ahlquist et al. 1987; Bown et al. 1987; Krasner et al. 1987; Barr et al. 1990) have recently described palliative laser procedures for malignant dysphagia. Following endoscopy under local anesthesia with intravenous sedation, an Nd-YAG laser is used to re-establish an esophageal lumen through excision of tumor. The procedure is not intended to completely excise the lesion, but rather to provide palliative relief to the patient. Symptomatic relief, as measured by subjective improvement in swallowing, was achieved in 80% (Ahlquist et al. 1987) to 85% (Bown et al. 1987) of patients. Endoscopic esophageal intubation following laser therapy did not seem to influence the patient's quality of life (Barr et al. 1990). Mortality due to the procedure is between 0 and 5% (Ahlquist et al. 1987; Krasner et al. 1987, respectively).

Table 14.1 Surgical Routes for Tube Feeding

Procedure	*Advantages*	*Disadvantages*
Esophagostomy	Minimal skin care, tube out between meals, feedings taken upright; reversible as office procedure	Contraindicated in esophageal obstruction, irradiated neck, superior vena cava syndrome
Gastrostomy	Standard procedure; preferable in children	Skin care often troublesome; patient must disrobe for feeding
Jejunostomy	Minimizes gastroesophageal reflux	Increased diarrhea
Pharyngotomy	Local anesthesia, minimal risk	Stoma high in neck, tube changing often difficult

Source: Reprinted with permission from RA Doby. Rehabilitation of swallowing disorders. Am Fam Physician 1978;17:84.

SURGICAL INTERVENTION IN PERSISTENT DYSPHAGIA

When the upper aerodigestive tract fails to perform its role of providing both protected ventilation of the lungs and a passageway for alimentation, separation of these functions by surgical intervention may be required for the patient's survival. A nasogastric tube is an effective temporary means to provide adequate nutrition in the debilitated or unconscious patient who has significant aspiration. Long-term use of the nasogastric tube is limited by discomfort, bleeding, and irritation along the course of the tube, resulting in increased mucous membrane secretions, regurgitation of feedings, and impairment of pharyngeal swallow (Acquarelli et al. 1972). Surgical intervention to provide adequate feedings without associated aspiration include pharyngoesophagostomy, flap esophagostomy, gastrostomy, and jejunostomy (Table 14.1).

Esophagostomy

The pharyngoesophagostomy is an effective means of long-term tube feeding, and in some patients it controls secretions in the pharynx that are difficult to manage (Skolnik et al. 1966; Dobie et al. 1979). A fistula is created from the hypopharynx to the skin anterior to the sternocleidomastoid muscle. A Levin tube or similar feeding tube is placed through the fistula tract into the stomach (Figure 14.3). If secretions in the pharynx create a life-threatening condition because of recurrent aspiration, the fistula tract can be constructed using a skin flap, providing a more permanent fistula and allowing the feeding tube to be removed for short periods of time. Graham and Royster (1967) described a surgical technique that allows placement of a pharyngotomy tube into the piriform sinus. This procedure, performed under local anesthesia at the bedside, is ideal

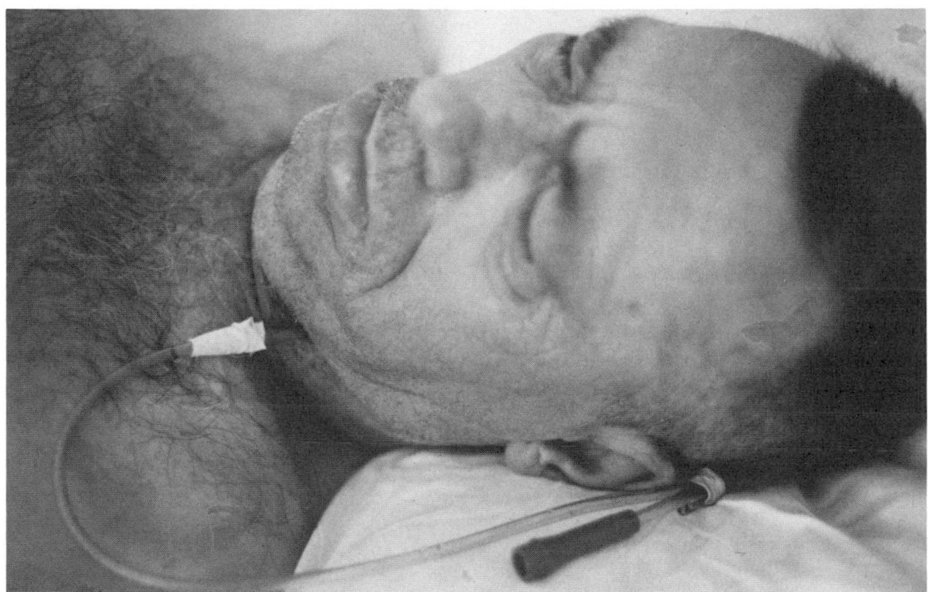

Figure 14.3 Patient with a cervical esophagostoma in place following a brain stem cerebrovascular accident. Note the marked bilateral facial weakness.

for the compromised patient who requires urgent placement of a feeding tube and cannot tolerate general anesthesia or abdominal placement.

Advantages of the esophagostoma over the gastrostoma tube are avoidance of an abdominal procedure, use of local anesthesia, the ability to feed the patient in the sitting rather than the supine position, and the ability to begin feedings immediately following the procedure. Use of an esophagostomy tube poses several disadvantages. In addition to local irritation to skin, it is generally contraindicated in patients with tumor or severe venous congestion in the neck; esophageal obstruction or significant reflux; significant lower respiratory disease, dyspnea, or frequent cough; and frequent emesis or extensive gastroesophageal reflux.

Gastrostomy

The most common surgical approach for placement of a feeding tube is gastrostomy. The popularity of the feeding gastrostomy is best explained by mentioning some of its advantages. The feeding tube is away from the head and neck and therefore can be placed in patients with a head and neck or esophageal tumor. A gastrostomy is technically a straightforward procedure that can be done under local anesthesia. Peristomal irritation is less significant than that in the head and neck region.

In patients with significant esophageal reflux, the gastrostomy, pharyngoesophagostomy, and nasogastric feeding tube should be avoided, as they increase the likelihood of postprandial reflux and aspiration. An exception is the new soft, Silastic pediatric feeding tubes that have proved quite valuable in providing enteral nutrition.

Jejunostomy

When esophageal reflux and associated aspiration are strongly suspected by history or demonstrated by attempted feeding with a nasogastric tube, a feeding jejunostoma tube is indicated. As with gastrostomy, placement of the jejunostoma tube requires an abdominal procedure, but it differs in that a general anesthesia usually is required (Liffman and Randall 1972). The advantage of this type of feeding tube is its placement distal to the duodenum, which minimizes the potential for reflux. Early selection of the appropriate mode of tube placement in the patient with severe dysphagia is a necessity to prevent starvation and aspiration pneumonia associated with attempted feedings.

LARYNGEAL PARALYSIS

In severe dysfunction of the upper aerodigestive tract, a more immediate problem than establishing a mode for feedings is protection of the airway from life-threatening aspiration. The primary function of the larynx is to act as a sphincter for the airway, preventing the aspiration of secretions and food. To provide normal function, the supraglottic mucous membrane, which is innervated by the internal branch of the superior laryngeal nerve, must respond to the presence of foreign material or secretions by initiating glottic closure (this is also accomplished by direct stimulation of the trachea). To complete the sphincter-like action, the intrinsic musculature of the larynx that is innervated by the recurrent laryngeal nerve approximates the vocal cords, thus tightly closing the glottis. Surgical intervention to manage partial or total laryngeal paralysis must be selective, based on the degree and level of paralysis present.

Unilateral low vagal paralysis below the level of the nodose ganglion results initially in paramedian-positioned vocal cords, producing hoarseness and minimal aspiration (Figure 14.4). In the later stages of paralysis the vocal cord moves to the abducted position as the ipsilateral muscles slowly atrophy (Sasaki 1980). In this position the patient may experience mild aspiration and marked hoarseness.

Vocal Cord Injection

Several different materials have been used for vocal cord injection. The three best studied materials are Teflon, absorbable gelatin sponge (Gelfoam), and collagen. By injecting Teflon into a paralyzed cord (Rontal et al. 1976), the glottic space can be partially closed, resulting in improved voice and decreased aspiration. Using the Arnold-Breuning syringe, approximately 0.25 ml of Teflon paste is injected into the paralyzed vocal cord at two points: (1) the middle third of the cord, and (2) immediately above the vocal process of the arytenoid (Figure 14.5). The proce-

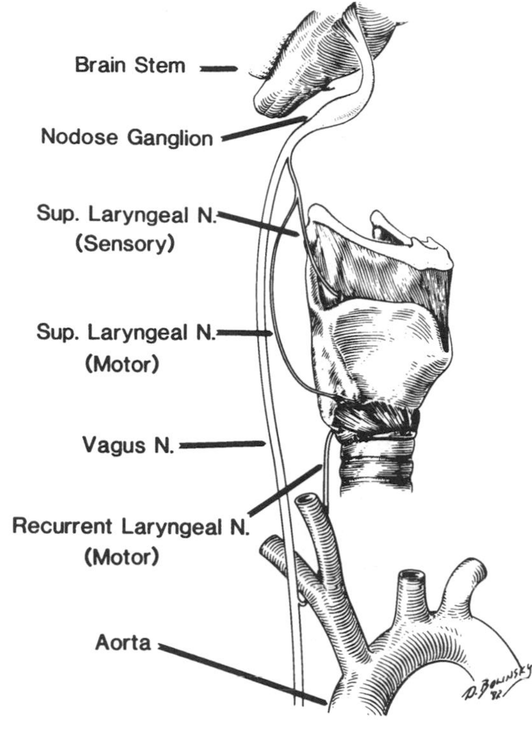

Figure 14.4 Branches of the vagus (superior and recurrent laryngeal nerves) that innervate the sensory and motor aspects of the larynx. Loss of sensory and motor innervation above and below the level of the nodose ganglion produces different pathology. (Drawing by David Bolinsky.)

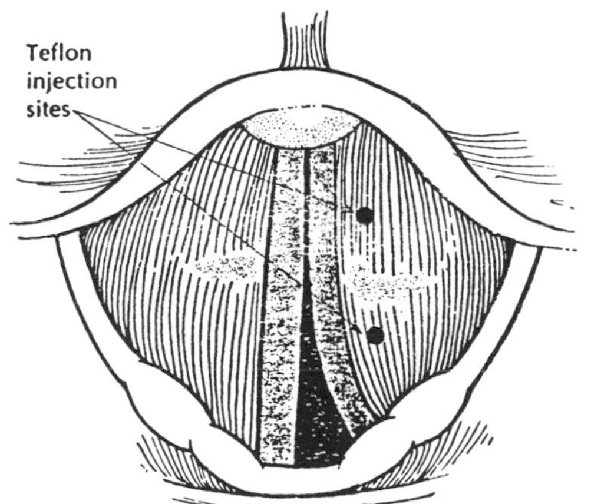

Figure 14.5 Superior view of the vocal cords illustrating the Teflon injection sites on the paralyzed vocal cord. (Reprinted by permission of the publisher, from Doby, American Family Physician, 1978.)

dure is typically performed under local anesthesia, with visualization of the vocal cords by suspension laryngoscopy. By moving the paralyzed cord to the median position, voice quality is markedly improved and aspiration may be decreased.

Before injecting Teflon, the surgeon may elect to inject absorbable gelatin sponge into the paralyzed vocal cord to anticipate the more permanent effects of

Teflon. This material is usually injected with patients who are expected to have return of function or when there is a question as to the efficacy of Teflon. Teflon often is preferred in patients with carcinoma and generalized neurologic deficits because it is a quick, easy procedure, and it may not be prudent to do more than one procedure on patients in this group due to the increased morbidity.

More recently, collagen (Ford and Bless 1986) has been used to inject vocal cords. It is injected in a similar fashion to Teflon, and studies thus far indicate it maintains its volume in the cord without absorption in 3- to 4-year follow-up (Remacle et al. 1989). Thus far this relatively new material has not been used for treatment of aspiration, but it seems like a reasonable alternative.

Arytenoid Adduction

Multiple techniques have been described for arytenoid adduction (Morrison 1948; Montgomery 1966; Isshiki et al. 1978). The basis of these procedures is the surgical repositioning of the paralyzed cord toward the midline. Morrison (1948) describes a "reverse King operation" to displace the arytenoid toward the midline. Using a stainless steel pin, Montgomery (1975) fixes the arytenoid and cricoid cartilages in a new position to medialize the paralyzed cord.

Multiple procedures are attributed to Isshiki et al. (1978). One of the first described was the medialization of the cord by rotating the vocal process of the arytenoid cartilage in a posteromedial fashion and suturing its muscular process through the thyroid cartilage for fixation. This is primarily indicated in the presence of a wide glottic chink and a difference in the height of the two vocal cords. Also described is the placement of a small block of silicone through a window in the thyroid cartilage at the level of the paralyzed vocal cord, thus medially displacing the vocal ligament. One advantage of this procedure is that it is relatively easy to reverse.

While these procedures are not classically indicated for aspiration alone, they should all be considered for patients with dysphagia when medialization of the vocal cord is required.

Nerve-to-Muscle Pedicle

In bilateral low vagal paralysis, deglutition is rarely impaired, and aspiration is often a minimal problem as the vocal cords tend to be in the median position and sensation of the hypopharynx remains intact.

Initial therapy involves providing an adequate airway and protecting against aspiration by the placement of a cuffed tracheostomy tube. Respiration may be improved by fixed lateralization of one of the paralyzed cords; however, permanently widening the glottic space for increased respiration increases aspiration, which may pose a difficult management problem. An alternative surgical approach that has achieved some popularity is the use of a nerve-to-muscle pedicle transferred from the omohyoid muscle to the paralyzed posterior cricoarytenoid (Tucker 1976). Inspiratory activity of the omohyoideus mediated by the ansa hypoglossi results in phasic vocal cord abduction, which may be adequate to allow increased ventilation and at the same time protect the airway against aspiration.

Tympanic Neurectomy

High unilateral vagus paralysis above the nodose ganglion results in vocal cord and pharyngeal paralysis that produces significant dysphagia and aspiration of stagnated material retained in the hypopharynx (see Figure 14.5). Surgical intervention in these cases requires a combination of procedures to facilitate deglutition and protect the airway from aspiration. Initially, a cuffed tracheostomy tube is placed, followed by the insertion of a feeding tube, Teflon injection of the paralyzed vocal cord, and cricopharyngeal myotomy (Glenn et al. 1980). If persistent aspiration of secretions in the pharynx continues, bilateral chorda tympani and tympanic nerve sections may be performed by a transtympanic approach under local anesthesia (Townsend et al. 1973; Mills 1975). Sectioning the chorda tympani and tympanic nerve interrupts the parasympathetic innervation of the submandibular and parotid glands, markedly decreasing the oral secretions (Figure 14.6). These nerve sections are often effective in controlling secretions, but approximately 30% of patients have a recurrence of symptoms within the first 6 months following the operation.

Laryngeal Closure

In high bilateral vagal nerve paralysis, immediate airway control is required to maintain life. As soon as practical, a cuffed tracheostomy tube and a feeding tube (usually gastrostoma) are placed. In the past, this condition and cases in which the ninth, tenth, eleventh, and twelfth cranial nerves are involved required laryngectomy to prevent recurrent aspiration, pneumonia, and death. There are now alternative procedures, including diversion of the larynx (Lindeman 1975), an epiglottic flap (sewing the epiglottis over the false cords and into the arytenoids) (Habal and Murray 1972), and laryngeal closure (Sasaki et al. 1980). The most practical and effective approach is the laryngeal closure described by Montgomery (1975) and modified by Sasaki (1980). Both procedures close the larynx and are reversible if there is significant neurologic improvement.

Following placement of a permanent tracheostoma, a horizontal skin incision over the cricoid is made to approach the larynx. The larynx is entered by a vertical midline thyrotomy. Mucous membrane between the free edges of the vocal and vestibular folds is resected. The glottis is then closed, beginning superiorly by approximating the denuded edges of the vestibular folds. A superior-based sternohyoid muscle pedicle is then passed through the thyroid notch and sutured to the interarytenoideus muscle at the posterior commissure. The vocal

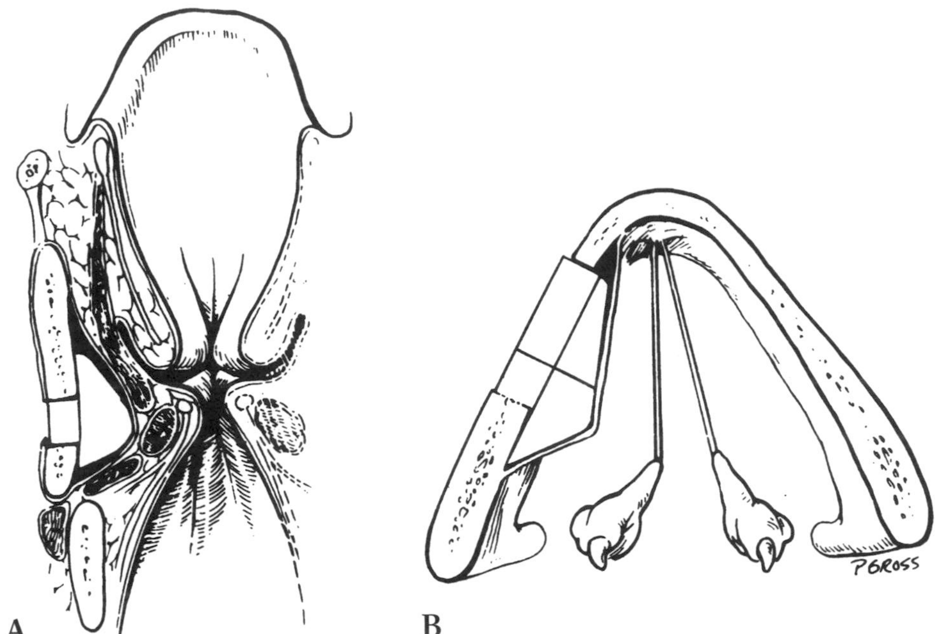

Figure 14.6 A. Coronal view of the larynx with the implant in position demonstrating medialization of the vocal fold. B. Axial view showing the posterior extension of the implant (which can be adjusted) that medializes the vocal process of the arytenoid cartilage. (Reprinted by permission of the publisher, from MS Benniger, et al. Evaluation and treatment of the unilateral paralyzed vocal fold. Otolaryngol Head and Neck Surg 1994;111;497.)

folds are then approximated, followed by closure of the thyrotomy and the skin incision. Placement of the sternohyoid muscle pedicle eliminates the dead space between the vocal and vestibular folds, and the larynx is closed in three layers. The major advantage of laryngeal closure is the protection of the respiratory tract from aspiration while allowing the upper aerodigestive tract to be used for alimentation.

SUMMARY

The goals of surgical intervention in patients with dysphagia should be to re-establish normal physiology or bypass known lesions and abnormalities of the upper digestive tract. It is crucial to separate the airway from the passage of secretions and feedings. Appropriate surgical management requires an extensive knowledge of the normal anatomy and physiology of the upper aerodigestive tract in addition to an understanding of the methods of evaluating dysphagia.

REFERENCES

Acquarelli MJ, Fenno G, Ward PH. Cervical esophagostomy (an improved technique for alimentation of the debilitated patient). Arch Otolaryngol 1972;96:453.

Adkins RB, Maples MD, Graham BS, et al. Dysphagia associated with aortic arch anomaly in adults. Am Surg 1986;52:238.

Ahlquist DA, Gostout CJ, Viggiano TR, et al. Endoscopic laser palliation of malignant dysphagia: a prospective study. Mayo Clin Proc 1987;62:867.

Asherson N. Achalasia of the cricopharyngeal sphincter: record of cases, with profile pharyngograms. J Laryngol Otol 1950;64:747.

Bailey CP, Hirose T, Alba J. Re-establishment of the continuity of the anomalous right subclavian artery after operation for dysphagia lusoria. Angiology 1965;16:509.

Barr H, Krasner N, Raouf A, et al. Prospective randomized trial of laser therapy only and laser therapy followed by endoscopic intubation for the palliation of malignant dysphagia. Gut 1990;31:252.

Bayford D. An account of a singular case of obstructed deglutition. Mem Med Soc Lond 1794;2:275.

Black RJ. Cricopharyngeal myotomy. J Otolaryngol 1981;10:145.

Blakley WR, Garety EJ, Smith DE. Section of the cricopharyngeus muscle for dysphagia. Arch Surg 1968;96:745.

Bown SG, Hawes R, Matthewson K, et al. Endoscopic laser palliation for advanced malignant dysphagia. Gut 1987;28:799.

Calcaterra JC, Kadell BM, Ward PH. Dysphagia secondary to cricopharyngeal muscle dysfunction. Arch Otolaryngol 1975;101:726.

Chodosh PL. Cricopharyngeal myotomy in the treatment of dysphagia. Laryngoscope 1975;85:1862.

Delisa JA, Mikulic MA, Miller RM, et al. Amyotrophic lateral sclerosis: comprehensive management. Am Fam Physician 1979;19:137.

Dobie RA, Cox KW, Larsen GL. Skin flap esophagostomy: a new procedure. Arch Otolaryngol 1979;105:200.

Dohlman G, Mattson O. The endoscopic operation of hypopharyngeal diverticula: a roentgenocinematographic study. Arch Otolaryngol 1960;71:744.

Drucker MH, Symbas PN. Right aortic arch with aberrant left subclavian artery: symptomatic in adulthood. Am J Surg 1980;139:432.

Ellis FH. Upper esophageal sphincter in health and disease. Surg Clin North Am 1971;51:553.

Ellis FH. Surgical management of esophageal motility disturbances. Am J Surg 1980;139:752.

Ellis FH Jr, Schlegel JF, Lynch VP, et al. Cricopharyngeal myotomy for pharyngo-esophageal diverticulum. Ann Surg 1969;170:340.

English GM. Otolaryngology. New York: Harper & Row, 1980.

Fahrer H, Markwalder T. Dysphagia caused by diffuse idiopathic skeletal hyperostosis. Clin Rheumatol 1988;7:117.

Ford CN, Bless DM. Clinical experience with injectable collagen for vocal cord augmentation. Laryngoscope 1986;96:863.

Glenn WWL, Hoak B, Sasaki C, et al. Characteristics and surgical management of respiratory complications accompanying pathologic lesions of the brainstem. Ann Surg 1980;191:655.

Graham W, Royster HP. Simplified cervical esophagostomy for long-term extraoral feeding. Surg Gynecol Obstet 1967;125:127.

Gross RE. Surgical treatment for dysphagia lusoria. Ann Surg 1946;124:532.

Habal MB, Murray JE. Surgical treatment of life endangering chronic aspiration pneumonia. Plast Reconstr Surg 1972;49:305.

Hallman GL, Cooley DA. Congenital aortic vascular ring. Surgical considerations. Arch Surg (Chicago) 1964;88:666.
Heeneman H, Gilbert JJ, Rood SR. Paralaryngeal Space: Anatomy and Pathologic Conditions with Emphasis on Neurogenous Tumors—A Self Instructional Package. Rochester, NY: American Academy of Otolaryngology, 1980.
Henderson RD, Hanna WM, Henderson RF, et al. Myotomy for reflux-induced cricopharyngeal dysphagia. Five-year review. J Thorac Cardiovasc Surg 1989;98:428.
Henderson RD, Marryatt G. Cricopharyngeal myotomy as a method of treating cricopharyngeal dysphagia secondary to gastroesophageal reflux. J Thorac Cardiovasc Surg 1977;74:721.
Hollinshead WH. Anatomy for Surgeons. New York: Harper & Row, 1968.
Isshiki N, Tanabe M, Sawada M. Arytenoid adduction for unilateral vocal cord paralysis. Arch Otolaryngol 1978;104:555.
Jung JY, Almond CH, Saab SB, et al. Surgical repair of right aortic arch and aberrant left subclavian artery and left ligamentum arteriosum. J Thorac Cardiovasc Surg 1978; 75:237.
Kibel SM, Johnson PM. Surgery for osteophyte-induced dysphagia. J Laryngol Otol 1987;101:1291.
Kirchner JA. The motor activity of the cricopharyngeus muscle. Laryngoscope 1958;68:1119.
Krasner N, Barr H, Skidmore C, et al. Palliative laser therapy for malignant dysphagia. Gut 1987;28:792.
Lebo CP, Kwei SU, Norris PH. Cricopharyngeal myotomy in amyotrophic lateral sclerosis. Laryngoscope 1976;86:862.
Liffmann KE, Randall HT. A modified technique for creating a jejunostomy. Surg Gynecol Obstet 1972;134:663.
Lindeman RC. Overting the paralyzed larynx: a reversible procedure for intractable aspiration. Laryngoscope 1975;85:157.
Lindgren S, Ekberg O. Cricopharyngeal myotomy in the treatment of dysphagia. Clin Otolaryngol 1990;15:221.
Lund WS. The cricopharyngeal sphincter: its relationship to the relief of pharyngeal paralysis and the surgical treatment of early pharyngeal pouch. J Laryngol 1968; 82:353.
Mansour KA, Symbas P, Ellis J, et al. A combined surgical approach in the management of achalasia of the esophagus. Ann Surg 1976;42:192.
Mills CP. Cricopharyngeal sphincterotomy and bilateral division of the chorda tympani in bulbar palsy. Proc R Soc Med 1975;68:644.
Montgomery WW. Cricoarytenoid arthrodesis. Ann Otol Rhinol Laryngol 1966;75:380.
Montgomery WW. Surgery to prevent aspiration. Arch Otolaryngol 1975;101:679.
Morrison L. The "reverse King operation." Ann Otol Rhinol Laryngol 1948;57:945.
Negus VE. Comparative Anatomy and Physiology of the Larynx. New York: Hafner, 1962.
Nicks GR. Webs, dysrhythmias and diverticulae of the esophagus. N Z Med J 1976;84:179.
Nikaido H, Riker WL, Idriss FS. Surgical management of "vascular rings." Arch Surg 1972;105:327.
Orringer MB. Extended cervical esophagomyotomy for cricopharyngeal dysfunction. J Thorac Cardiovasc Surg 1980;30:669.
Orvald TO, Scheerer R, Jude JR. A single cervical approach to aberrant right subclavian artery. Surgery 1972;71:227.
Papadopoulos SM, Chen JC, Feldenzer JA, et al. Anterior cervical osteophytes as a cause of progressive dysphagia. Acta Neurochir 1989;101:63.
Pome G, Vitali E, Mantovani A, et al. Surgical treatment of the aberrant retroesophageal right subclavian artery in adults (dysphagia lusoria). Report of two new cases and review of the literature. J Cardiovasc Surg (Torino) 1987;28:405.

Remacle M, Marbaix E, Hamoir M, et al. Initial long-term results of collagen injection for vocal and laryngeal rehabilitation. Arch Otorhinolaryngol 1989;246:403.
Richardson JV, Doby DB, Rossi NP, et al. Operation for aortic arch anomalies. Ann Thorac Surg 1981;31:426.
Rontal E, Rontal M, Morse G, et al. Vocal cord injection in the treatment of acute and chronic aspiration. Laryngoscope 1976;86:625.
Sasaki CT. Paralysis of the larynx and pharynx. Surg Clin North Am 1980;60:1079.
Sasaki CT, Milmoe G, Yanagisawa E, et al. Surgical closure of the larynx for intractable aspiration. Arch Otolaryngol 1980;106:422.
Shergy WJ, Nunley JA, Caldwell DS. Dysphagia due to diffuse idiopathic skeletal hyperostosis. Am Fam Physician 1989;39:149.
Skolnik EM, Tenta LT, Massair FS. Pharyngo-esophagostomy. Arch Otolaryngol 1966;84:534.
Sobol SM, Rigual NR. Anterolateral extrapharyngeal approach for cervical osteophyte-induced dysphagia. Ann Otol Rhinol Laryngol 1984;93:498.
Thawley SE, Ogura JH. Cricopharyngeal myotomy. Laryngoscope 1978;88:872.
Townsend G, Morimoto AM, Kralemann H. Management of sialorrhea by transtympanic neurectomy. Mayo Clin Proc 1973;48:776.
Tucker HM. Human laryngeal reinnervation. Laryngoscope 1976;86:769.
Valentine RJ, Carter DJ, Clagett GP. A modified extrathoracic approach to the treatment of dysphagia lusoria. J Vasc Surg 1987;5:498.
Van Son JA, Vincent JG, van Oort A, et al. Translocation of aberrant right subclavian artery in dysphagia lusoria in children through a right thoracotomy. Thorac Cardiovasc Surg 1989;37:52.
Vantrappen G, Hellemans J. Treatment of achalasia and related motor disorders. Gastroenterology 1980;79:144.
Weaver AW, Fleming SM. Partial laryngectomy: analysis of associated swallowing disorders. Am J Surg 1978;136:486.
Welsh LW, Welsh JJ, Chinnici JC. Dysphagia due to cervical spine surgery. Ann Otol Rhinol Laryngol 1987;96:112.
Wychulis AG, Kincard OW, Weidman WH, et al. Congenital vascular ring: surgical considerations and results of operation. Mayo Clin Proc 1971;46:182.
Zuckerbraum L, Bahma MS. Cricopharyngeus myotomy as the only treatment for Zenker's diverticulum. Ann Otol 1979;88:798.

15

Establishing a Swallowing Program

Michael E. Groher

It may seem somewhat ironic that this book ends with a discussion devoted to beginning a swallowing program. The preceding chapters help provide the clinician with the basic theoretical and technical knowledge needed to evaluate and treat swallowing disorders. A thorough, working understanding of the issues and topics discussed is the first step in developing a program. It is necessary to become familiar with the literature and professional staff involved and with the evaluation and treatment procedures recommended. All can serve as important resources when problems and questions arise.

Putting this knowledge into place in a clinical setting may be the greatest challenge of all. This chapter focuses directly on organizing and developing a dysphagia program. Clinicians who have had direct experience in managing swallowing disorders on a regular basis would agree that certain key organizational steps must be taken. By accepting that good dysphagia programs do not evolve overnight one can adjust to the potential psychological disappointments that may be frequent in the initial stages. Most programs take 3 full years before becoming a viable and recognized part of the hospital's life. Others take longer.

ESTABLISHING GOALS

Many kinds of programs can be established. Each of the contributors to this book has had a different experience, whether in a hospital-wide, multidisciplinary dysphagia clinic or as a single therapist incorporating the techniques into a personal schedule of rehabilitation treatment. The size and type of patient population, the attitudes of the staff toward rehabilitation, the available personnel, the real opportunity for program development, and most important, the individual interest in dysphagia are essential considerations in defining a program suitable to a particular setting. Some settings will not have the laboratory (videoradiography, scintigraphy) or consultive (gastroenterology, neurology) support that may be necessary in diagnosis. In this circumstance, treatment will be more conservative, emphasizing correct feeding postures during enteral and oral intake and monitoring intake in an effort to avoid medical complications secondary to malnutrition. Jones and Altshuler (1987) found that an absence of videoradiographic studies would not impede a functional approach to treatment if the clinicians were skilled in recognizing physical signs and symptoms that predispose one to aspiration (see Chapter 7).

The type of program ultimately established depends on the goals defined. Three goals should be universal to all dysphagia programs: (1) identification of the patient who may be at risk for aspiration, (2) prevention of aspiration, and (3) prevention of malnutrition. The minimal requirement of the staff to achieve these goals is careful evaluation and re-evaluation of the patient to determine the extent to which he or she tolerates oral foods. It can be argued that the additional goal of improving swallowing behavior should be included whenever possible.

Ideally, the patient should achieve a nutritionally complete oral diet. If this is not possible, nonoral supplements or total feedings should be recommended. The rudiments of a successful dysphagia program can be established based on evaluation and careful monitoring to achieve the first three goals. Following the diagnostic evaluation described earlier, it is preferable to attempt the active intervention described in the treatment chapters where potential for improvement has not been ruled out.

Depending on the capabilities of the staff and the extent to which the dysphagia program is incorporated into general rehabilitation, other goals may be expressed, such as increasing the patient's independence in eating (or in self-administration of tube feedings) and helping the family care for the patient's special nutritional needs at home. Some centers have established outpatient clinics or a system of outpatient follow-up to provide continuing care to their dysphagic patients. How long and how often patients should be followed has not been established, although some evidence suggests that in patients with head and neck cancer, functional swallow may change at different rates up to 1 year following their first postsurgical evaluation (Rademaker et al. 1993).

ASSEMBLING A TEAM

The contributors to this book represent diverse fields of health care management, all of whom share a common interest in swallowing disorders. Those in other disciplines, such as psychiatry, dentistry, social services, general surgery, respiratory therapy, and physical therapy, also have an interest. Dysphagia management is best if each participates, either directly and on a daily basis or by periodic consultations. An organizational chart of the potential participants in both clinical and research contributions is presented in Figure 15.1. If possible, one or more persons with a particular interest in dysphagia can be identified from each service and serve as direct resource persons for consultations or in-service training. For a section head or supervisor to give tacit approval for the department as a whole to participate is not as useful as specifically designating an individual to be an active representative.

The continuity of care and specialization of knowledge needed to manage dysphagic patients are facilitated if one individual assumes direct responsibility and it is clear to the rest of the team who that individual is. This individual should be familiar with each participating discipline's potential for interaction with the dysphagic patient. He or she will be the most visible member and therefore the one to whom consultations will be directed. The team leader probably

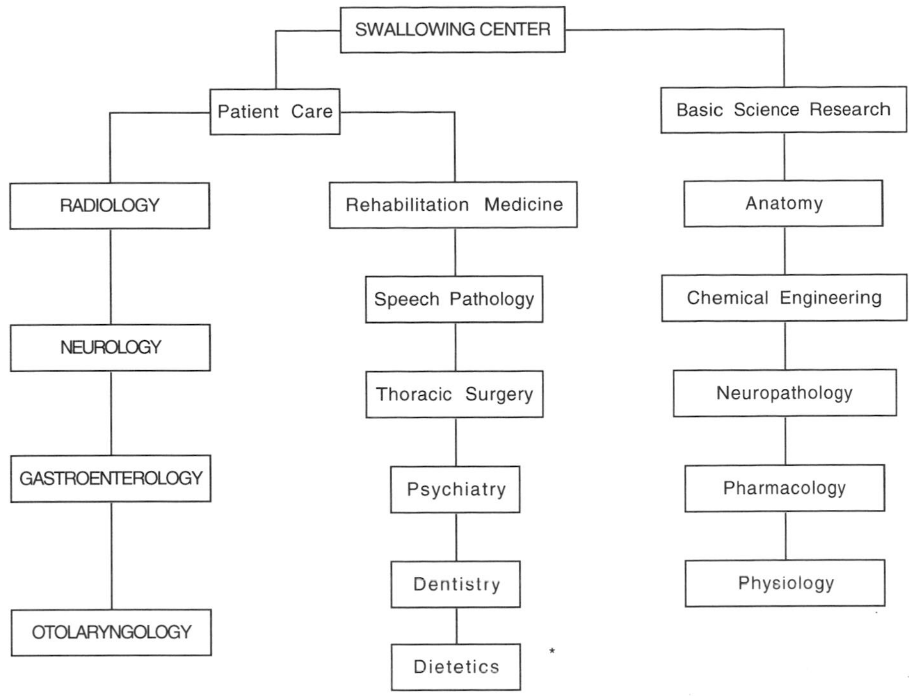

Figure 15.1 Proposed interdisciplinary organization of a swallowing center. (Reprinted with permission of Springer-Verlag from WJ Ravich, MW Donner, H Kashima, et al. The swallowing center: concepts and procedures. Gastrointest Radiol 1985;10:255.)

will be the prime participator in dysphagia management on a daily basis. In increasing numbers, this role has been assumed by the speech pathologist. Responsibilities usually include accepting consultations, completing the evaluation with appropriate recommendations, coordinating the necessary rehabilitation or further diagnostic tests, and providing some direct feeding training. A team leader employed in a hospital or rehabilitation center setting eventually has to devote 35–45% of total working hours to dysphagia management. In medical centers where dysphagia management is a priority, the team leader's time is devoted solely to this function.

Hutchins and Giancarlo (1991) describe an eight-step process for assembling, implementing, and sustaining a program focused on managing dysphagic patients. The steps are (1) providing clinical education, (2) collecting and analyzing data, (3) gaining administrative support, (4) identifying team members, (5) developing a referral and treatment structure, (6) providing in-service training, (7) facilitating the program, and (8) demonstrating the program's efficacy.

The role played by each member of the dysphagia management team may differ from clinic to clinic, but most contributions are established as part of traditional roles. A specialized interest or demonstrated expertise in dysphagia management may lead to some overlapping of responsibilities. This should not be viewed by other team members as encroachment, but as a way to complement and verify information to improve care. One entire journal issue has been devoted to providing details about the team roles of the speech pathologist, radiologist, gastroenterologist, pediatrician, dentist, neurologist, and occupational therapist (Bosma 1990). Mody and Nagai (1990) present a model for patient allocation when similar competencies and roles for care overlap. Some dysphagia rehabilitation programs have failed to sustain themselves because of the failure of team members to define and accept their roles. The following may serve as useful guidelines.

Nursing Staff

The nurses, through physician orders, have the direct responsibility of monitoring the patient's medical and nutritional status. In many institutions, they coordinate dysphagia consultations and as such serve as dysphagia team leaders. Overall responsibilities usually include administration and care of nonoral feeding including hyperalimentation and tube feedings, recording oral and nonoral intake (particularly of fluids), care and suctioning of tracheostoma tubes, maintaining good oral hygiene, and assigning nursing staff or volunteers to assist with feeding at mealtimes. Nurses should be responsible, in part, for reporting successes and failures during oral feedings. These impressions are recorded in the progress notes. The patient's intake and output usually are recorded on a separate sheet at the bedside.

Occupational Therapist

Concern for manual feeding skills has been a traditional part of an occupational therapist's involvement in improving the patient's daily living skills. Experience in training patients with motor weakness or loss of function to adapt to new feeding techniques has often led the occupational therapist to coordinate dysphagic rehabilitation (Weiss et al. 1992). These therapists are specialists in suggesting which types of adaptive equipment would be best suited for the patient's needs and in providing specific technical assistance at mealtimes; they are also well trained in general physical rehabilitation techniques (see Chapter 10). In conjunction with the physical therapist, the occupational therapist may provide preliminary therapy to reduce muscle spasticity, improve muscle strength and coordination, and prevent primitive reflex patterns from interfering with swallowing.

Dietitian

The dietitian monitors the patient's overall nutritional status, ensuring that the patient's intake of fluids and nutrients meets the requirements as appropriate to the medical condition (see Chapter 12). The dietitian coordinates special diet orders with the kitchen, helps obtain a dysphagia evaluation tray, takes a dietary history when possible, and makes specific recommendations relating to food textures and nutritional values (Curran and Groher 1990). If the patient is receiving tube feedings, the dietitian can make recommendations about the type, adequacy, and regulation of the feedings. The dietitian also is a consultant on the visual presentation of food items, including the environment in which food is served (Hotaling 1990).

The dietitian is the most important resource when treatment involves providing specialized nutrition and food technology. An example might be to combine foods that provide high-caloric or low-salt content with gelatin to facilitate swallowing, together with some special spices to appeal to the patient's taste. This person, who serves as the liaison between the team and the kitchen, may find it useful to develop a specialized dysphagia diet that facilitates swallowing while maintaining nutritional integrity (Clusky 1989; Curran and Groher 1990).

Speech Pathologist

Many patients with swallowing difficulty also have accompanying disorders of speech production (Martin and Corlew 1990). It follows that the speech pathologist would become directly involved with both the diagnosis and management of dysphagic patients. Many times the patient's swallowing disorder must be managed before speech rehabilitation can begin. The speech pathologist is expert in muscle re-education of the oral and laryngeal structures. In many institutions the speech pathologist is the team leader. In 100 dysphagia treatment programs in the Department of Veterans Affairs, the speech pathologist is the team leader in 92% (Mills 1991). The knowledge and skills necessary for the speech pathologist to assume this role have been documented (Erlichman 1989; ASHA 1990). Speech pathologists have taken an active role in both clinical and basic research in establishing diagnostic and treatment protocols for patients with swallowing impairments (Groher 1990b).

Neurologist

The neurologist is one of the primary diagnosticians on the swallowing management team (Chapters 2 and 3). It is this person's responsibility to help differentiate neurologic from mechanical and psychogenic swallowing disorders. The neurologist combines the results of physical examination with those of radiography, electromyography, electroneurography, and muscle and nerve biopsy to arrive at an etiologic diagnosis. Recommendations for special techniques may be combined with prescriptions for medications that assist in swallowing management by modifying the neurologic disease.

Otolaryngologist–Head and Neck Surgeon

The otolaryngologist–head and neck surgeon has a special interest in the differential diagnosis of mechanical swallowing disorders. Usually he or she is the team member most familiar with the sensory and motor abnormalities of the pharynx and larynx, including surgical management of the majority of head and neck cancers and postsurgical swallowing disorders and subsequent nutritional status. The otolaryngologist may perform specialized surgical procedures such as cricopharyngeal myotomy or esophagostomy to manage persistent dysphagia (see Chapter 14). Fiberoptic endoscopy is a valuable tool in evaluating the patient's ability to protect the airway during swallow (Langmore et al. 1988).

Gastroenterologist

The gastroenterologist serves as a diagnostician and surgical consultant for patients with suspected dysphagia related to the esophagus or gastrointestinal tract (see Chapter 5). While usually not directly involved in daily dysphagia behavioral treatment, an interested gastroenterologist can be an important member of the swallowing management team. The gastroenterologist provides direct visualization of the esophagus and stomach, recommending surgical evaluation and providing medical management, which may include dilatation or drug therapy regimens. The gastroenterologist is consulted for percutaneous endoscopic placement of gastrostoma tubes (Weg and Miscovitz 1987).

Pulmonologist–Respiratory Therapist

The pulmonologist–respiratory therapist is not usually directly involved on the dysphagia team but does provide valuable information relating to patients with respiratory disorders and tracheostoma tubes. This includes monitoring pulmonary toilet and helping the physician by making recommendations for removal of the tracheostoma tube. Often this therapist provides expert consultation on the choice of tracheostoma tube and how it should be used during feedings. Some are important resources in developing strategies for feeding patients who need ventilator support and can provide valuable insights into the consequences of aspiration (Elpern et al. 1987; Terry and Fuller 1989).

Attending Physician

Although each patient's attending or primary physician is not necessarily an active member of the dysphagia team, all communications must include this person. As coordinator of the patient's total medical and surgical management, the physician must order the original consultation to the dysphagia team or medical specialist. It is imperative that orders be written clearly. The dysphagia evaluation should be prescribed specifically. If the patient is a candidate for oral intake, the orders should reflect the physician's concurrence because of the potential risks of aspiration and subsequent illness. Any changes in dietary management should also be accompanied by written orders. Sometimes these orders are privileged to the dysphagia team leader to facilitate care. The question of liability is often the first issue to be raised when a dysphagia program is introduced in a new setting. The primary care physician must agree with each step in the patient's dysphagia management, since he or she ultimately carries the responsibility for that patient's care.

Team Coordination

Some dysphagia teams find it necessary to have regular meetings. Such meetings might focus on patient management, quality assurance issues, or research strategies. The frequency of these meetings varies depending on the scope and design of the dysphagia management program. Some groups meet weekly, others quarterly. Of the 100 dysphagia management programs in the Department of Veterans Affairs, about one-third had no meetings, one-third met once per week, and one-third met monthly (Mills 1991). The dysphagia team at the Tampa VA Medical Center initially had a regular monthly meeting, but it was canceled because of poor attendance. The team now is linked by an electronic mail system that allows members to consult one another on a daily basis at any time during the day. In acute care settings, communication among team members most often is by chart notes alone; formal meetings are more frequent in rehabilitation settings (Mirro and Patcy 1991). An excellent example of how multidisciplinary teams can meet and discuss difficult diagnostic and treatment issues is presented by Jones and Ravich (1989).

Time Assessment

The amount of time needed to serve as team leader may appear excessive, especially for an individual who is already fully involved in specialized patient care. The team leader should first try to free this amount of time through direct reassignment of responsibilities within the hospital or clinic. Attaining this goal is facilitated by presenting rationales for the position, by offering data on the incidence of dysphagia, by comparing successful programs in similar settings, and by obtaining support from other team members.

The major activity in a dysphagia rehabilitation program is feeding patients at mealtimes. Although this should be overseen by the team leader, feeding training sessions may be carried out by assigned (trained) nursing or therapy personnel. Volunteers and, when possible, family members should be so assigned only after a patient has demonstrated repeated success at swallowing and requires no more than standby assistance. The time expended by staff who are involved in training volunteers or directly involved in feeding at mealtimes may be exorbitant, especially in the initial stages of program development. However, the net result of this initial time expenditure is to reduce the time needed to manage dysphagic patients. Weekends and holidays are the most difficult times for program coordination and implementation. Therefore, the need arises to develop a dependable corps of trained volunteers or family members who can be instructed to follow a prescribed feeding program without direct assistance. Lipner et al. (1990) have described the use of volunteers to meet this need.

Team members also must make some personal commitments to changes in their work schedules. Working between 8 or 9 and 4 or 5 with an hour off for lunch is incompatible with caring for dysphagia patients. Most in-patient settings serve meals at 7 AM, noon, and 5 PM. Therefore, if one is to assist in feeding, consideration must be given to rearranging working hours.

IDENTIFYING THE POPULATION

A dysphagia team may wish to limit the scope of its initial efforts to a small segment or service of the hospital population—for example, rehabilitation, neurology, and otolaryngology and head and neck service. The team might decide to run a demonstration diagnostic and treatment dysphagia program on one of these services to evaluate the efficacy of beginning such a program and to eliminate some of the problems that can arise as it is established before offering the service to the entire hospital.

As the program develops, the need for diagnostic and swallowing treatment services becomes apparent. One new consultation a week quickly turns into five and perhaps ten as word of the program spreads. Dysphagia programs in the initial stages usually treat 12–15 patients per week. The number of dysphagic patients in a given institution may vary depending on the setting and patient population (see Chapter 1).

Growth of the program depends on available staff time and efficient coordination of team effort. Team members who can spend only a limited time per day with dysphagic patients normally limit their efforts to those who can benefit the most. The same principle holds for very active programs that attempt to provide services to more patients than their resources can support.

Some centers have found it necessary to provide outpatient clinics for patients who continue to have episodes of dysphagia following hospital discharge and for those who do not need hospitalization but who complain specifically of swallowing difficulty. Such clinics require additional space and staff time, both of which must be carefully budgeted. Clinics are usually formed only after the dysphagia program has become well recognized both in the hospital and in the immediate community.

OUTLINING THE PROGRAM AND PROCEDURES

At this point it should be possible to outline the structure of the dysphagia program in terms of who will participate, how much they will participate, where they will participate, and finally, the rationale for beginning such an effort. This information is usually passed through the hospital's chain of command for final approval. A statement of procedures is a useful attachment to the program outline. The following are questions to consider:

1. How will dysphagic patients be identified?

2. To whom will consultations and follow-up orders be directed?
3. What is the process for constructing and ordering a swallowing evaluation diet?
4. Will the need to have dysphagic patients eat smaller portions more times per day require procedural changes between the dietary service and the kitchen?
5. Who will be responsible for monitoring the results of dysphagia rehabilitation?
6. How are the results to be documented?
7. What medical precautions must be taken when dysphagia therapy is initiated?

Following administrative approval, a policy memorandum or directive authorizing the team's activities may need to be developed. A sample policy memorandum is presented in the appendix to this chapter. Question number 7 above requires some elaboration. As pointed out in Chapter 8, one can minimize risks of aspiration after introducing food orally by completing a thorough evaluation of the patient's neuromuscular and cortical potentials before beginning. Patients can and do aspirate during trial periods of swallowing rehabilitation, and the dysphagia team must delineate the types of precautions to be taken. This includes knowing suctioning and emergency medical procedures, and of course, getting clearance from the attending physician. Some centers begin by having the attending physician or registered nurse present during all first-time attempts at oral feeding; as the feeder becomes more experienced, this support may not be as necessary. The therapist who provides feeding training should receive special clinical privileges from the hospital's chief of staff before independent first-time feedings begin.

Finally, a pilot study might be initiated at this stage with permission from the appropriate medical or research committee. When the program has been outlined and the dysphagia team has become familiar with the procedures, such a study may facilitate final acceptance of the program. A small sample of patients should be drawn from those identified as being most in need of the team's services. Physicians who support the program may be enlisted to refer candidates from among their patients. For example, a neurologist may refer a patient who has recently had a cerebrovascular accident. By carefully documenting evaluation and treatment results, the team can make a preliminary assessment of the success of the program. Before the formal recognition of their dysphagic team, Martens et al. (1990) sought to gather appropriate incidence data and conduct a prospective study to ascertain the effects of the team on caloric intake, body weight, instances of aspiration pneumonia, and feeding independence.

INITIATING THE PROGRAM

After final approval has been given, announcements should be sent to each service director and ward physician briefly describing the program's intent and consultation procedures.

At this point, training should begin, focusing on the types of services the team will offer and their importance to the patient's medical recovery. Training should be offered first to staff physicians and nurses. It is best accomplished if the physician and nursing members of the dysphagia team teach their peers; however, to enhance collaboration and improve the visibility of the program, the team leader should be included in all educational sessions. Members from the allied health sector (dietetics, speech pathology, rehabilitation) can provide training to their own peers and can help train volunteers to serve as feeders. Publicity should be ongoing to alert nonrelated hospital staff and consumers that such a specialized program exists. This may be especially important in active medical centers with constant changes of house staff assignments. Grand rounds presentations and hospital newsletter articles can communicate achievements and help gain wider acceptance of the program.

Volunteer training should focus on the basics of the swallowing act and the importance of strictly adhering to the prescription for feeding designed by the rehabilitation team. Such prescriptions should be clearly posted at bedside with a copy in the nursing files to facilitate communication among day, evening, and night shifts. Each prescription should be clearly signed and provide an appropriate telephone or call number of a person to contact for additional assistance. An example of such a prescription follows.

1. Make sure the patient is sitting upright during and one-half hour after eating.
2. Pull curtains around the bed to minimize distractions.
3. Let the patient feed himself, making sure he takes one bite and swallows before taking another. He will require reminders to do so.
4. Do not talk with the patient while he is eating as this distracts him and interferes with swallowing. For more information call: R.Y., Ext. 212. Beeper: 303.

In some centers these instructions cannot be posted at the bedside because it violates the patient's privacy, but recommendations should be available in another well-defined place. When appropriate, the prescription should also include the types of foods and liquids that are and are not permitted. This helps to eliminate confusion that may result from a patient receiving the wrong food tray. These prescriptions greatly facilitate the passing of information from shift to shift and from volunteer to volunteer, as most volunteers do not come each day, nor do they always feed the same patients.

The team leader should monitor any changes needed in diets and procedures for feeding. Ideally, one member from the dysphagia team makes rounds with the ward physicians to report progress in dysphagia rehabilitation and to keep informed of changes in the patient's medical status that may preclude oral feeding or dictate different nutritional requirements. The importance of passing clear and relevant information from the team leader to the nursing staff and volunteers cannot be overestimated. Dysphagia rehabilitation efforts can change from day to day, and unless requests and orders are easily translated and implemented, they can be hampered and lead to undue frustration.

MAINTAINING RECORDS

Daily notes are generally kept by physicians and therapists, while nurses record progress notes for each shift. The team leader should ensure that progress is addressed at least once a day or as often as each meal. An immediate notation should be made of any occurrence or suspicion of significant aspiration, including which staff member was notified and the action taken. Immediate notation should also be made after diet changes, either to add a newly tolerated food or to delete an item that is not well tolerated. A change in the patient's alertness, physical appearance, metabolism, or mental status, as well as new evaluative findings such as the return or absence of swallowing reflexes, should be reported as soon as they are observed.

Routine daily notes should review the gains and losses that occur during dysphagia rehabilitation. They should indicate both the training techniques used and the success or failure of the prescribed diet. The nursing staff and dietitian are usually responsible for recording fluid intake and output. In addition, a daily record of food intake can be charted, identifying the exact quantity of each item actually consumed as closely as can be estimated. Allowance should be made for spillage or drooling, because this may significantly alter estimates made from leftovers on the tray.

Close examination of these charts often shows patterns of food intake that might otherwise have gone unnoticed. For instance, it may become clear that a patient seems to swallow best when macaroni rather than ground meat is on the menu. Another patient may swallow better at the noon meal, which may be related to the level of alertness at that time, or to the diet or therapist. This specific information can prove useful for supporting changes in diet or modifications of training techniques.

Charting food consumption gives a good picture of the patient's progress in eating and of daily nutritional intake in the absence of a calorie count. In the event a calorie count is ordered, the dietitian keeps a careful record of the daily calorie intake, usually over a period of several days (see Chapter 12).

MEASURING RESULTS

If a pilot study is completed before the program begins, a follow-up study should be done to measure the effectiveness of the program in progress. An excellent example of a prospective pilot dysphagia program with recommendations for change following the program's implementation is presented by Young and Durant-Jones (1990). It is essential to determine the program's success in achieving its objectives, such as reducing the incidence of aspiration pneumonias, reducing dependence on tube feedings (measured by days of use or incidence), shortening total dysphagia recovery time, and promoting a normal oral diet (measured by the diet achieved at the conclusion of the program or at discharge). The efficacy of instituting a dysphagia team on a 26-bed neurology-neurosurgery unit was studied prospectively by Martens and her colleagues (1990). They divided their patients into those who received a team evaluation and those who were managed without a team approach. Those who had team management had a significant improvement in weight gain and caloric intake. Presumably this would have positively affected the patient's nutritional status, although this was not measured due to administrative restrictions. Using the reduction in the occurrence of aspiration pneumonia as an outcome measure, Kasprisin and her colleagues (1989) found that their team approach produced a significant reduction in the incidence of aspiration pneumonia even for patients with moderate to severe dysphagia. In a retrospective review of their dysphagia teams, Jones and Altschuler (1987) discussed findings after comparing the records of patients before and after an interdisciplinary management approach. They included (1) increased and earlier use of feeding tubes (to prevent malnutrition), (2) a decrease in pulmonary aspiration, (3) increased intradepartmental cooperation, (4) earlier documentation of the problem, and (5) improved oral intake.

The dysphagia team must keep careful records on each patient referred for evaluation. Maintaining separate files can facilitate data collection for future use. Data should be organized so that they specifically describe the patient population, including age, cause of dysphagia, and significant contributing medical history. Evaluation techniques and results should be coded for each patient. These basic data eventually can be compared with the goals originally set. They can also serve as a program evaluation tool, as the basis for scientific investigation, or as a part of a quality-assurance program. The use of a quality-assurance audit to establish the need for services and the demonstration of intervention with dysphagia patients in a chronic care setting is described by Musson and her colleagues (1990).

The study might seek to evaluate treatment techniques, such as the effects of manipulation of diet versus cognitive training without diet manipulation. Unfortunately, some experimental designs of this nature involve depriving a control group of selected intervention. One way to avoid this ethical dilemma is to use the chart audit procedure now routinely performed in many institutions. By establishing outcome criteria for the chart review, a sample can be selected and charts collected from a specific, predetermined time period. A matched group of charts then can be drawn for comparison from a previous time period (prior to initiation of the program, but recent enough to ensure similar medical management). This step is not essential to the chart audit, as the first sample is intended to be measured only against its own criteria. Even if chart audit fails, it provides a valuable tool for identifying and correcting problems that surface during the review. A subsequent reaudit should succeed if the program is, in fact, effective.

Finally, administrators and colleagues must be informed of both the positive and negative results of the studies, as they can be important for keeping the program visible and viable.

ETHICAL CONSIDERATIONS

As the dysphagia management team develops, its members often become involved in issues relating to the ethics of providing or withholding nutrition.

For this reason it is important that the dysphagia team hold discussions with their medical center's ethics committee. Each medical center should develop policy that directs the medical personnel in situations in which the patient refuses to be fed, when the family wishes that the patient not be fed, or when the risks of providing nutrition outweigh the benefits (Quill 1989; Groher 1990b). Having the patient or family execute an advance directive stating preferences for long-term alimentation can help manage the nutritional needs of the dysphagic patient (Silverman et al. 1992; Ouslander et al. 1993).

SUMMARY

The diagnosis and management of dysphagic patients has become a subspecialty for many professions. It is generally agreed that a multidisciplinary approach provides the care necessary to justify the use of the resources. The number of centers developing teams that interact on behalf of the dysphagic patient has grown steadily. In the Department of Veterans Affairs in 1986, 17 of 172 medical centers had established teams. By 1990 the number had grown to 97. A growing scientific basis for understanding the mechanisms of swallow has given the dysphagia team improved rationales for treatment. The efficacy of team treatment approaches in controlled studies remains to be established.

REFERENCES

ASHA. Skills needed by speech-language pathologists providing services to dysphagic patients/clients. ASHA 1990;32(suppl 2):7.

Bosma JF. Recent advances in the evaluation and care of neurologic feeding impairments. J Neurol Rehab 1990;4:57.

Clusky MM. The use of pureed diets among the elderly. Diet Curr 1989;16:17.

Curran J, Groher ME. Development and dissemination of an aspiration risk reduction diet. Dysphagia 1990;5:6.

Elpern EH, Jacobs ER, Bone RC. Incidence of aspiration in tracheally intubated adults. Heart Lung 1987;16:527.

Erlichman M. The Role of Speech Pathologists in the Management of Dysphagia. National Center for Health Services, Research and Health Care Technology Assessment, U.S. Department of Health and Human Services, 1989;1:1.

Groher ME. Ethical dilemmas in providing nutrition. Dysphagia 1990a;5:102.

Groher ME. The role of the speech-language pathologist in the evaluation and care of oral and pharyngeal dysphagia. J Neurol Rehab 1990b;4:5.

Hotaling DL. Adapting the mealtime environment: setting the stage for eating. Dysphagia 1990;5:77.

Hutchins BF, Giancarlo JL. Developing a comprehensive dysphagia program. Semin Speech Lang 1991;12:209.

Jones PL, Altschuler SL. Dysphagia teams: a specific approach to a nonspecific problem. Dysphagia 1987;1:200.

Jones B, Ravich W. Multidisciplinary case discussion panel. Dysphagia 1989;3:209.

Kasprisin AT, Clumeck H, Nino-Murcia M. The efficacy of rehabilitation management of dysphagia. Dysphagia 1989;4:48.

Langmore SE, Schatz K, Olsen N. Fiberoptic endoscopic examination of swallowing safety: a new procedure. Dysphagia 1988;2:216.

Lipner HS, Bosler J, Giles G. Volunteer participation in feeding residents: training and supervision in a long-term care facility. Dysphagia 1990;5:89.

Martens L, Cameron T, Simonsen M. Effects of a multidisciplinary management program on neurologically impaired patients with dysphagia. Dysphagia 1990;5:147.

Martin BJ, Corlew MM. The incidence of communication disorders in dysphagic patients. J Speech Hear Disord 1990;55:28.

Mills RH. Survey of Dysphagia Services in the Veterans Affairs Health Care System 1988–1991. Murfreesboro, TN: Department of Veterans Affairs Medical Center, 1991.

Mirro JF, Patey C. Developing a dysphagia dietary program. Semin Speech Lang 1991;12:218.

Mody M, Nagai J. A multidisciplinary approach to the development of competency standards and appropriate allocation for patients with dysphagia. Am J Occup Ther 1990;44:369.

Musson ND, Kinkaid J, Ryan P, et al. Nature, nurture, nutrition: interdisciplinary programs to address the prevention of malnutrition and dehydration. Dysphagia 1990;5:96.

Ouslander JG, Tymchuck AJ, Krynski MD. Decisions about enteral tube feeding among the elderly. J Am Geriatr Soc 1993;41:70.

Quill TE. Nasogastric feeding tubes in a group of chronically ill elderly patients in a community hospital. Arch Intern Med 1989;149:1937.

Rademaker AW, Logemann JA, Pauloski BR, et al. Recovery of postoperative swallowing in patients undergoing partial laryngectomy. Head Neck 1993;15:325.

Silverman HJ, Vinicky JK, Gasner RM. Advance directives: implications for critical care. Crit Care Med 1992;20:1027.

Terry PB, Fuller SD. Pulmonary consequences of aspiration. Dysphagia 1989;3:179.

Weiss DR, Conyers KH, Epstein CF. A systems approach to eating skills programming in long-term care. Occup Ther Prac 1992;3:65.

Weg AL, Miskovitz PF. Percutaneous endoscopic gastrostomy (PEG): a critical appraisal. Dysphagia 1987;1:227.

Young EC, Durant-Jones L. Developing a dysphagia program in an acute care hospital: a needs assessment. Dysphagia 1990;5:159.

Appendix: Sample Policy for a Dysphagia Team

I. **Purpose.** To define the organization and functions of an interdisciplinary dysphagia team for the management of patients with swallowing disorders. The intent of this dysphagia team is to implement protocol and procedures for the identification, assessment, and treatment of patients with dysphagia in order to optimize nutrition, promote feeding independence of the patients, minimize the need for feeding tubes, and reduce the incidence of complications of dysphagia (e.g., aspiration pneumonia, dehydration, and/or malnutrition).

II. **Policy.** To provide diagnostic and rehabilitative services to all eligible inpatients and outpatients with dysphagia (swallowing problems). It is necessary that these patients be identified and treated in a coordinated manner by the appropriate clinical services.

III. **Definition.** Dysphagia is difficulty in one or more stages of deglutition from placement of food in the mouth, oral motor manipulation and control of the bolus, and triggering of the swallowing action and pharyngeal peristalsis, through relaxation of the cricopharyngeal sphincter, which allows the bolus to pass into the esophagus. Etiologies of such disturbances include varied neuropathologies and head and neck disease, in addition to other medical and psychological problems that may affect oral nutritional intake.

IV. **Responsibilities**

A. Team membership shall include representation from the following services/sections:

1. Speech-language pathology
2. Physician
3. Dietetics
4. Nursing

Other specialists may participate on an as-needed basis (e.g., gastroenterology, digestive diseases and nutrition section, radiology, surgery, social work, hospital-based home care, oncology, pulmonary, etc.).

B. Team responsibilities

1. Facilitate identification of patients with swallowing problems.
2. Recommend, implement, and modify dysphagia management plans in cooperation with the primary care physician.
3. Hold regularly scheduled patient care staff meetings for purposes of reviewing patients referred and developing, recommend-

ing, and monitoring the interdisciplinary patient care plans for further evaluation and/or treatment.

4. Request consultation with other services as needed.
5. Document clinical activities.
   a. Response to consultation request
   b. Flowsheet data on each team referral
   c. Progress notes by individual team members
6. Educate medical center personnel about the dysphagia team's purpose and increase their awareness of dysphagia as a patient problem.
7. Promote continuing education of team members.
8. Propose and generate research where issues of dysphagia are unclear.

C. **Specific responsibilities of team members**

1. **Speech-language pathologist.** Serves as coordinator of the dysphagia team. The speech-language pathologist obtains a history and description of the problem and performs the initial screening of the patient to determine his or her candidacy for further evaluation of the dysphagia problem by the team. The initial screening and further evaluation of the dysphagia patient by the speech-language pathologist may include evaluation of oral motor function and integrity of the components of the swallowing process (as observed on physical examination as well as via video-fluoroscopic study in conjunction with the radiologist). Treatment activities of the speech-language pathologist may include direct activities such as oromuscular strengthening, thermal stimulation to improve the swallowing mechanism, and exercises to increase adduction of the vocal folds. Direct treatment activities may include recommendations regarding compensatory adjustments (e.g., posture, protective swallow techniques, and prostheses) as well as participation in the determination of appropriate food consistencies for the dysphagic patient.
2. **Physician.** Participates in patient examination with the speech pathologist to relate findings to the patient's general medical condition and to act as a liaison with the patient's attending physician.
3. **Dietitian.** Coordinates the nutritional assessment, recommendations, and documentation of plans with the ward dietitian to accomplish nutritional goals. Serves as a liaison between the team, patient, and food service personnel to ensure the order and the food served are consistent with the patient's nutritional needs. Participates in the determination and provision of texture/consistency needs to optimize oral intake and monitors nutrient intake as needed to ensure adequacy and/or tolerance of texture. Recommends enteral/parenteral feeding modalities

as appropriate. Provides education to the patient and/or caregiver on diet modification, weight gain or loss, and so forth before discharge. Arranges follow-up visit with the outpatient dietitian if needed.

4. **Nurse.** Integrates the dysphagia program into the total patient needs. Participates during the evaluation process by providing nursing assessments of the patient in the following areas: cognitive, functional, sensory, communicative, learning ability, and social support. The nurse member will communicate the recommendations of the team to the nursing staff caring for the patient. Will also be available for consultation for the nursing staff caring for the patient and/or the patient's caregiver.

D. **Procedures**

1. Authorized medical staff will send a Consultation Request (SF 513) to: Dysphagia Team Speech Pathology, Mail Code 126.
2. The speech-language pathologist will contact the dysphagia team members after the initial review of the problem.
3. Dysphagia team members will perform their respective assessments and document the same on progress notes, as delineated in the responsibilities section.
4. The findings of the dysphagia team and recommendations for management will be discussed at the next scheduled patient care meeting. The patient's primary physician and charge nurse will be informed of the recommendations. Recommendations for management may include:
   a. Oral vs. nonoral feeding; oral feeding with assistance
   b. Head, neck, and body posture and positioning
   c. Food textures and consistencies
   d. Food placement
   e. Adaptive equipment
   f. Oral-motor facilitation techniques
   g. Reflex sensitization techniques

Index

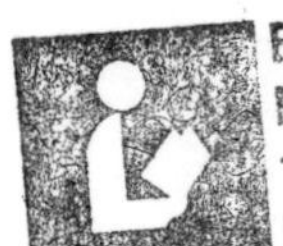